Promoting Adherence to Medical Treatment in Chronic Childhood Illness: Concepts, Methods, and Interventions

Promoting Adherence to Medical Treatment in Chronic Childhood Illness: Concepts, Methods, and Interventions

Edited by

Dennis Drotar
Case Western Reserve University
School of Medicine

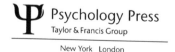
Psychology Press
Taylor & Francis Group

New York   London

First published by

Lawrence Erlbaum Associates, Inc., Publishers
10 Industrial Avenue
Mahwah, New Jersey 07430

This edition published 2013 by Psychology Press

Psychology Press   Psychology Press
Taylor & Francis Group   Taylor & Francis Group
711 Third Avenue   27 Church Road, Hove
New York, NY 10017   East Sussex, BN3 2FA

First issued in paperback 2014

Psychology Press is an imprint of the Taylor & Francis Group, an informa business

Library of Congress Cataloging-in-Publication Data

Promoting adherence to medical treatment in chronic childhood illness : concepts,
methods, and interventions / edited by Dennis Drotar.
    p.   cm.
Based on a conference held at Case Western Reserve University, on Oct. 30–31, 1998.
Includes bibliographical references and index.
ISBN 0-8058-3348-X
1. Chronic diseases in adolescence—Congresses.   2. Chronic diseases in
children—Congresses.   3. Patient compliance—Congresses.   I. Drotar, Dennis.
[DNLM: 1. Chronic Disease—Adolescence—Congresses.   2. Chronic
Disease—Child—Congresses.   3. Patient Compliance—Congresses. WS 200 P9645 2000]
RJ380 .P76 2000
618.92—dc21
                                                                99-089283

ISBN 13: 978-0-8058-3348-5 (hbk)
ISBN 13: 978-1-138-01264-6 (pbk)

Dedication

This book is dedicated to my parents,
Helen and Donald Drotar, and my sister, Patty,
who are deceased but not forgotten.

Contents

Preface

The need for this volume arose from several sources. Large numbers of children and adolescents are affected by chronic physical illnesses (Newacheck & Halfon, 1998; Newacheck & Taylor, 1992). Optimal management of such conditions and reduction of associated morbidity require children and families to adhere to demanding treatment regimens. At the same time, there is widespread recognition that patient and family noncompliance with treatment regimens for pediatric chronic illness is an important clinical problem that can lead to unnecessary hospitalizations, increased risk for illness-related complications, and increased medical care costs.

Moreover, recent trends in medical care have increased the significance of patient compliance as a clinical problem. Although advances in medical technology have resulted in potentially more effective treatments for some chronic conditions, some have increased the necessity for more intensive medical management and hence problems in compliance. For example, technologies such as blood glucose monitoring are now available to help children with diabetes to conduct intensive treatment, which has been shown to decrease the rate of complications in this condition (Diabetes Control and Complications Trial Research Group, 1993). However, intensive treatment regimens are much more demanding on children and families and more difficult to follow than traditional approaches. Moreover, shorter duration of hospital stays and limitations on the amount of time practitioners can spend with their patients have shifted increasing burdens for management of chronic illness treatment to children and families. However, not all families are prepared or able to assume such increased treatment-related responsibilities effectively without additional support from their providers or health care team.

All of these developments heighten the need for scientific data to inform pediatric practitioners' abilities to enhance their patients' adherence to medical regimens and for data to document interventions that are effective in reaching this difficult goal. Unfortunately, scientific advances regarding the efficacy of interventions to enhance adherence in pediatric chronic illness have been limited by several problems. These include (a) limited conceptual models of adherence to treatment, (b) limitations in measurement of adherence to treatment, (c) lack of data concerning the impact of treatment adherence on children's health status and quality of life, and (d) relatively limited information concerning the effectiveness of interventions to promote treatment adherence in pediatric chronic illness (La Greca & Schuman, 1995).

Recent progress in measuring treatment adherence in pediatric chronic illness, identifying family influences on treatment adherence, and developing new interventions to promote adherence with treatment regimens for children and adolescents heightens the need to summarize and synthesize the current state-of-the-art research in this area. For example, progress has been made in identifying the factors that predict adequate versus problematic compliance to medical treatment regimens among children and adolescents with chronic conditions (La Greca & Schuman, 1995). Moreover, promising new interventions have been designed to promote successful adherence and reduce noncompliance to treatment among children and adolescents with chronic health conditions.

PURPOSE OF THE VOLUME

To address the previous needs for summary and synthesis, a conference was sponsored by the Genentech Foundation for Growth and Development. It was held on the campus of Case Western Reserve University from October 30 to 31, 1998. This conference brought together experts on treatment adherence in pediatric chronic illness from the fields of anthropology, pediatrics, psychology, and sociology. These experts presented new data and conceptual models of treatment adherence in childhood chronic illness and discussed the implications of their work for next directions of the field. Developed from the work of the conference participants, this volume is a synthesis of new concepts of treatment adherence, recent research concerning the measurement of treatment adherence in pediatric chronic illness and intervention approaches, and methodological issues in assessing adherence.

Designed to address critical gaps in scientific understanding of adherence/compliance to treatment regimens in chronic health conditions for children and adolescents, the work presented in this volume includes the following areas: (a) conceptual models that have been used to define treatment adherence and conduct research and clinical care on this topic, (b) influences on treatment adherence to chronic illness in children, (c) impact of treatment adherence on children's health and psychological development, (d) new strategies of interventions to promote adherence and reduce rates of noncompliance among children and adolescents with chronic health conditions, (e) methodological and measurement problems in the assessment of treatment adherence, and (f) recommendations to advance scientific knowledge concerning the measurement of adherence, interventions to promote treatment adherence in pediatric chronic illness, and training providers to promote adherence.

ORGANIZATION OF THE VOLUME

This book is divided into eight parts: (a) overview and introduction, (b) historical foundations of the concept of adherence compliance, (c) conceptual models of adherence to chronic illness treatment, (d) measurement issues, (e) influences on treatment adherence, (f) impact of treatment adherence on children's health and psychological outcomes and research, (g) results of interventions to promote treatment adherence in specific chronic illnesses, and (h) summary of implications for the development of research methods, clinical interventions to promote treatment adherence, and training of providers.

REFERENCES

Diabetes Control and Complications Trial Research Group. (1993). The effect of intensive treatment of diabetes on the development and progression of long-term complications in insulin-dependent diabetes mellitus. *New England Journal of Medicine, 329*, 977–986.

La Greca, A. M., & Schuman, W. B. (1995). Adherence to prescribed treatment regimens. In M. C. Roberts (Ed.), *Handbook of pediatric psychology* (2nd ed., pp. 55–83). New York: Guilford.

Newacheck, P. W., & Halfon, N. (1998). Prevalence and impact of disabling and chronic conditions in childhood. *American Journal of Public Health, 88*, 610–617.

Newacheck, P. W., & Taylor, W. R. (1992). Childhood chronic illness: Prevalence, severity, and impact. *American Journal of Public Health, 82*, 364–371.

Acknowledgments

I acknowledge the support of the Genentech Foundation for Growth and Development without whose sponsorship the conference and this book could not have been completed. The Board of Directors of the Genentech Foundation including the Foundation leadership of Robert Blizzard, Foundation president and director, and members including Ann E. Johanson, Kim Amer, Raymond Hintz, Richard Fine, Thaddeus Kelly, John Curd, and James Strain facilitated the planning and conduct of the conference. Special thanks are owed to Juanita Bishop, assistant treasurer and office manager of the Genentech Foundation, who provided her usual excellent administrative support for this project.

The conference and this book were clearly facilitated by students in the graduate training program in pediatric psychology at Case Western Reserve University. Special thanks to Kristin Riekert, who took a leadership role in planning and conducting this project from beginning to end. In addition, Natalie Walders, Erika Burgess, Astrida Seja Kaugars, Chantelle Nobile, and Rachel Levi all provided important assistance in making the conference a success. Preparation of this volume was also supported in part by NIH HL 47604 Trial of Family Intervention in Cystic Fibrosis. The efforts of Elisabeth Rogers, who worked hard to process and organize the information in this book, are gratefully acknowledged. Finally, a debt is owed to the conference participants and chapter authors who have given the field much food for thought in this volume. This work is theirs.

Contributors

Dana E. Alliger, Children's Hospital of Buffalo, 219 Bryant Street, Buffalo, NY 14222-2006

Barbara J. Anderson, Joslin Diabetes Center, Mental Health Unit, 1 Joslin Place, Boston, MA 02215

Laurie J. Bauman, Preventive Intervention Research Center for Child Health, Albert Einstein College of Medicine/Montifore Medical Center, NR 7 South 15, 1300 Morris Park Avenue, Bronx, NY 10461

Bruce G. Bender, National Jewish Medical Research Center, 1400 Jackson Street, Denver, CO 80206

Julienne Brackett, Joslin Diabetes Center, Mental Health Unit, 1 Joslin Place, Boston, MA 02215

John Buchlis, Children's Hospital of Buffalo, 219 Bryant Street, Buffalo, NY 14222-2006

Erika Burgess, Department of Psychology, Case Western Reserve University, 10900 Euclid Avenue, Cleveland, OH 44106-7123

Thomas L. Creer, 144 East, 4620 North, Provo, UT 84604

Alan M. Delamater, Department of Pediatrics, Mailman Center for Child Development, D-820, P.O. Box 016820, Miami, FL 33101

M. Robin DiMatteo, Department of Psychology, University of California, Riverside, CA 92521

Dennis Drotar, Department of Pediatrics, Rainbow Babies and Children's Hospital, 11100 Euclid Avenue, Cleveland, OH 44106-6038

Peggy Greco, Nemours Children's Clinic, 807 Nira Street, Jacksonville, FL 32207

Michael A. Harris, Department of Pediatrics, Washington University School of Medicine, One Children's Place, Box 8116, Room 1002, St. Louis, MO 63110

Rebecca A. Hazen, Children's Hospital of Buffalo, 219 Bryant Street, Buffalo, NY 14222-2006

Joyce Ho, Joslin Diabetes Center, Mental Health Unit, 1 Joslin Place, Boston, MA 02215

Carolyn E. Ievers-Landis, Department of Pediatrics, Rainbow Babies and Children's Hospital, 11100 Euclid Avenue, Cleveland, OH 44106-6038

Jenifer R. Jacobs, Center for Child Health Outcomes, Children's Hospital and Health Center, 3020 Children's Way, MC 5053, San Diego, CA 92123

Jessica Jacobsen, Riley Children's Hospital, 702 Barnhill Drive, Indianapolis, IN 44602-5128

Suzanne Bennett Johnson, Center for Pediatric Psychology, University of Florida, Box 100195, Gainesville, FL 32610-0195

Barbara M. Korsch, Department of Pediatrics, Children's Hospital of Los Angeles, 4650 Sunset Boulevard, Los Angeles, CA 90027

Lori M. B. Laffel, Joslin Diabetes Center, 1 Joslin Place, Boston, MA 02215

Rachel Levi, Department of Psychology, Case Western Reserve University, 10900 Euclid Avenue, Cleveland, OH 44106-7123

Margaret H. MacGillivray, Children's Hospital of Buffalo, 219 Bryant Street, Buffalo, NY 14222-2006

Stephanie N. Marcy, Department of Pediatrics, Children's Hospital of Los Angeles, 4650 Sunset Boulevard, Los Angeles, CA 90027

Doreen M. Matsui, Children's Hospital of Western Ontario, 800 Commissioners Road East, London, Ontario, Canada N6C 2V5

Tom A. Mazur, Children's Hospital of Buffalo, 219 Bryant Street, Buffalo, NY 14222-2006

Henry Milgrom, National Jewish Medical Research Center, 1400 Jackson Street, Denver, CO 80206

Chantelle Nobile, Department of Psychology, Case Western Reserve University, 10900 Euclid Avenue, Cleveland, OH 44106-7123

Alexandra L. Quittner, Department of Clinical and Health Psychology, University of Florida, Health Sciences Center, P.O. Box 100165-HSC, Gainesville, FL 32610-0165

Cynthia Rand, Department of Medicine, Pulmonary Critical Care, JHACC, 5501 Bayview Circle, Baltimore, MD 21224

Michael A. Rapoff, Department of Pediatrics, University of Kansas Medical Center, 3901 Rainbow Boulevard, Kansas City, KS 66160-7330

Kristin A. Riekert, Department of Medicine, JHACC, 5501 Bayview Circle, Baltimore, MD 21224

David E. Sandberg, Children's Hospital of Buffalo, 219 Bryant Avenue, Buffalo, NY 14222

Michael Seid, Center for Child Outcomes, Children's Hospital and Health Center, 3020 Children's Way, MC 5053, San Diego, CA 92123

Dawn Seidner, Department of Educational and Counseling Psychology, Indiana University, Bloomington, IN 47405

Astrida Seja Kaugars, Department of Psychology, Case Western Reserve University, 10900 Euclid Avenue, Cleveland, OH 44106-7123

Nancy Slocum, Department of Pediatrics, Rainbow Babies and Children's Hospital, 11100 Euclid Avenue, Cleveland, OH 44106-6038

Lori J. Stark, Children's Hospital Medical Center, Psychology Service OSB-4, 3333 Burnet Avenue, Cincinnati, OH 45229

James A. Trostle, Anthropology Program, Trinity College, 300 Summit Street, Hartford, CT 06106

James W. Varni, Center for Child Health Outcomes, Children's Hospital and Health Center, 3020 Children's Way, MC 5053, San Diego, CA 92123

Natalie Walders, Department of Psychology, Case Western Reserve University, 10900 Euclid Avenue, Cleveland, OH 44106-7123

Frederick Wamboldt, National Jewish Medical Research Center, 1400 Jackson Street, Denver, CO 80206

Neil H. White, Department of Pediatrics, Washington University School of Medicine, One Children's Place, Box 8116, St. Louis, MO 63110

Tim Wysocki, Nemours Children's Clinic, 807 Nira Street, Jacksonville, FL 32207

PART I

OVERVIEW AND INTRODUCTION

Adherence to Medical Treatment in Pediatric Chronic Illness: Critical Issues and Answered Questions

Kristin A. Riekert
Dennis Drotar
Case Western Reserve University and Rainbow Babies and Children's Hospital, Cleveland, OH

Large numbers of children and adolescents have chronic physical conditions requiring treatment regimens that are complex, are time-consuming, and need to be managed over the course of a lifelong illness (Newacheck & Taylor, 1992). Increasing numbers of children and adolescents with life-threatening chronic conditions now survive into adolescence and early adulthood. The quality of life for these children/adolescents and their families may be influenced by their abilities to successfully manage their treatments. Child and family nonadherence with treatment regimens for pediatric chronic illness has also been recognized as an important clinical problem that can lead to unnecessary hospitalizations, increased risk for illness-related complications, and more costly medical care costs (La Greca & Schuman, 1995). Recent trends in health care have also increased the importance of treatment adherence to ensure optimal medical outcomes. For example, advances in illness management such as intensive therapy for conditions such as diabetes have been shown to decrease the rate of diabetes-related complications (Diabetes Control and Complications Trail Research Group, 1993). Moreover, new anti-retroviral treatments that are now available to treat HIV infection (Vernazza et al., 1997) offer new hope to affected children, adolescents, and adults. However, such intensive treatments are quite demanding and often difficult for children, adolescents, and their families to manage.

Other recent developments in health care, such as shorter duration of hospital stays and limitations in reimbursement, place significant constraints on the amount of time practitioners can spend with their patients and have shifted increasing responsibility for treatment management to children and their families (Kuhthau et al., 1998). For example, parents now administer at home some medications that were formerly given in hospitals and clinics for conditions such as childhood cancer (Tebbi, Richards, Cummings, Zevon, & Mallon, 1988). However, not all families are prepared or able to assume such treatment-related responsibilities. Moreover, cost-containment in health care makes it difficult to support a coordinated, interdisciplinary approach to management that provides maximal support to children and families to maintain adherence to chronic illness treatment (Klerman, 1985).

THE SCOPE OF TREATMENT NONADHERENCE
FOR CHILDHOOD CHRONIC ILLNESS

Rates of nonadherence vary as a function of the specific health condition, regimen requirements, measures of adherence, and criteria for classifying adherence and related behaviors (Rapoff, 1999). Nevertheless, available evidence concerning medication use across various chronic conditions suggests that, although nonadherence rates vary considerably, they are substantial (e.g., 40%; Alessandro, Vincenzo, Marco, Marcello, & Enrica, 1994; 25%, Conley & Salvatierra, 1996; 52%, Ettenger et al., 1991; 48%–52%, Festa, Tamaroff, Chasalow, & Lanzkowsky, 1992; 21%, Meyers, Thomson, & Weiland, 1996; 52%, Schoni, Horak, & Nikolaizik, 1995; 25%, Weisberg-Benchell et al., 1995). Typically between 50% and 60% of children and adolescents with adherence problems underuse their medication and less than 10% overuse medication (Chmelik & Doughty, 1994; Coutts, Gibson, & Patton, 1992).

Although there are much less data on rates of adherence-related behaviors other than medication use, researchers have typically found that adherence to more complex and intrusive treatments, such as dietary modifications, glucose monitoring, and physical therapy, is even lower than adherence to medication treatment (Rapoff, 1999). For example, Passero, Remor, and Salomon (1981) found that 93% of their sample of children with cystic fibrosis (CF) followed the prescribed antibiotic treatments, but only 40% adhered to chest physiotherapy and even fewer (20%) to dietary recommendations. Similarly, Hentinen and Kyngas (1992) found that, compared with 3% of their sample of adolescents with diabetes who were rated as nonadherent with insulin injections, 34% and 38% had poor adherence to dietary restrictions and glucose monitoring, respectively. Furthermore, 43% of parents of children with juvenile rheumatoid arthritis reported that it was difficult to get their children to take their medication, and 60% noted difficulty getting their children to perform prescribed exercises (Rapoff, Lindsley, & Christophersen, 1985).

IMPACT OF TREATMENT NONADHERENCE ON THE CLINICAL OUTCOMES OF CHILDHOOD CHRONIC ILLNESS

The health consequences of treatment nonadherence to chronic physical illness are not well documented in pediatric populations (Johnson, 1994). Nevertheless, there is suggestive evidence that problematic adherence can lead to serious medical complications and increase the risk for chronic illness-related morbidity and mortality (see Walders, Nobile, & Drotar, chap. 9, this volume). Consequently, practitioners in medical settings struggle to manage children and adolescents whose treatment adherence is so problematic that it can compromise their medical care. Serious nonadherence can contribute to such problems as recurrent ketoacidosis in juvenile diabetes (Golden, Herold, & Orr, 1985; Liss et al., 1998) as well as recurrent symptoms (Weinstein & Faust, 1997), compromised functional status (Taylor & Newacheck, 1992), and mortality (Sly, 1988) in pediatric asthma. Problematic adherence in CF may relate to compromised pulmonary functioning (Patterson, Budd, Goetz, & Warwick, 1993).

In some instances, problematic treatment adherence may also account for some of the unexplained relapses seen in children and adolescents with certain chronic health conditions, such as losses of pediatric cadaver renal transplants (Conley & Salvatierra, 1996; Ettenger et al., 1991). Children with renal transplants who have poor adherence to treatment have been found to have a shorter length of graft survival, need more grafts, and be at greater risk for graft rejection and death (Meyers, Weiland, & Thomson, 1995). Moreover, Dolgin, Katz, Doctors, and Siegel (1986) judged the level of nonadherence with treatment as a significant threat to the health of many teenagers with cancer.

Not surprisingly, in light of the prior findings, significant numbers of referrals are made to mental health providers who work in pediatric hospital settings to evaluate and manage problematic adherence to medical treatment for chronic illness (Olson et al., 1989). Nevertheless, in our experience, many children and adolescents with adherence-related problems are not referred for intervention until their problems have become serious and potentially intractable. Such compelling clinical needs heighten the importance of developing empirically validated interventions that can prevent as well as treat adherence problems.

Financial Impact

Although there has been little research on the financial implications of non-adherence to treatment in pediatric chronic illness, noncompliance with treatment of chronic medical conditions in adults has been linked with increased medical costs due to hospital admissions, length of stay, and health care expenditures (Sclar et al., 1991; Swanson, Hull, Bartus, & Schweizer, 1992). The annual cost of nonadherence to medical treatment in the United States (including adult and pediatric patients) has been estimated to be $100 billion (Berg, Dischler, Wagner, Raia, & Palmer-Shevlin, 1993).

Impact of Nonadherence to Chronic Illness Treatment on the Quality of Scientific Data

Although the impact of nonadherence on the clinical management of pediatric chronic illness appears to be substantial, the impact of nonadherence on the quality of data obtained from scientific studies, especially from clinical trials of medical treatment efficacy, is less well recognized but may be significant (see Johnson, chap. 13, this volume; Rand, in press). For example, less than optimal adherence to treatment during clinical trials can obscure data concerning the efficacy of medical treatments for chronic health conditions (Tebbi, 1993). The erroneous conclusions that are drawn from such problematic data may have serious consequences (e.g., leading to a potentially effective medication being declared as ineffective or to setting recommended dosages of medications at unnecessarily high levels; Lasagna & Hutt, 1991; see Johnson, chap. 13, this volume, for a comprehensive discussion of this problem). Undetected nonadherence in clinical trials can lead to distortion of outcome data and overestimation of required dosage of a medication; it also can obscure the true rate of adverse reactions to medications (Matsui, 1997).

Nonadherence to treatment is also reflected in patients who terminate early from trials (see Johnson, chap. 13, this volume). When dropout rates disproportionately occur within a certain group (i.e., more severely in all patients) and when nonadherence is the cause of termination, generalizability of the findings is problematic. Moreover, validity of data obtained before termination can also be questionable.

DEFINITIONS: COMPLIANCE, ADHERENCE, AND ALTERNATIVES

Although the prevalence and impact of treatment nonadherence for pediatric chronic illness are formidable, there is much less agreement on how best to define and study this problem. Because definitions of compliance and adherence are important insofar as they influence the conduct of research and guide clinical management, they are considered briefly here. The dictionary definition of *compliance* includes the following: a complying, or giving in to a request, wish, or demand, acquiescence, and a tendency to give in readily to others (Newfeldt & Guralnik, 1988). Several scholars have expressed concern that the use of the term compliance to treatment overemphasizes the patient's subservient role as well as the power of the physician relative to the patient, but underestimates the importance of patients' and families' contributions to illness management (see Bauman, chap. 4, this volume; Creer, chap. 5, this volume).

The dictionary definition of *adherence* includes the following: the act of adhering, attachment to a person, cause, etc., devotion and support (Newfeldt & Guralnik, 1988). Some, but not all, researchers and practitioners find the term adherence preferable to compliance because it implies less emphasis on the patient and family's obedience in conforming to physicians' recommendations and underscores patients' and families' more active roles in making treatment-related decisions.

Problems that are inherent in the operational definitions of adherence and/or compliance should be recognized. One fundamental problem with each of these definitions is that the specific criteria against which a child's adherence to or compliance with treatment is evaluated are not usually well defined. Most studies do not carefully compare the child's or family's behaviors concerning the treatment regimen with the specific treatments that are actually prescribed by physicians partially because it is difficult to ascertain specific prescriptions for chronic illness treatment from clinical records (La Greca, 1990a). Consequently, the similarities and differences between a child's performance of treatment-related tasks and the treatment regimen that has been prescribed by the physician cannot be objectively defined. For this reason, La Greca (1990a) suggested that terms such as *self-care* and *disease management* may provide more accurate and functional descriptions of treatment-related behaviors than either compliance or adherence (see Bauman, chap. 4, this volume; Creer, chap. 5, this volume).

The terms adherence and compliance also define implicit models of relationships among the child, family, and physician that do not adequately characterize the potential for their partnership in the management of a chronic illness. For example, neither definition emphasizes the active role children and parents can play in helping determine their treatment goals and define how best to fit the treatment of a chronic illness into their lives. Moreover, neither term encompasses activities such as negotiation, mutual decision making, or communication among children, patients, physicians, and families, which may be important in determining what treatment is prescribed and how the chronic illnesses are managed (see

Bauman, chap. 4, this volume; Creer, chap. 5, this volume, for more extensive discussion). Finally, the terms adherence and compliance reflect ideologies that overemphasize patients' response to treatment and the broader context of illness management (see Trostle, chap. 2, this volume).

For ease of understanding, the terms adherence and compliance are used interchangeably throughout this book. However, readers may wish to keep these caveats in mind as they consider the work in this volume.

WHY IS A CONCEPTUAL MODEL OF COMPLIANCE/ADHERENCE TO CHRONIC ILLNESS TREATMENT NEEDED?

Clinical Implications

One of the important but neglected needs in research and practice on treatment adherence is the development of conceptual models that inform and guide these activities (La Greca & Schuman, 1995). What is the clinical utility of a conceptual model? In clinical care, practitioners' working models of adherence can guide the goals of clinical interactions, set expectations for patients, and help understand reasons for nonadherence, including barriers. Consider the potential clinical implications of alternative models of adherence or compliance. For example, a narrow definition or model of compliance might emphasize the physician's role in prescribing a treatment and the patient's role in carrying out the prescription. This model neglects potentially important factors such as the physician's contribution to parent or child misunderstanding of prescribed or problematic adherence. In contrast, a more comprehensive model of adherence to treatment emphasizes the contribution of the patient–physician relationship in promoting adherence (see DiMatteo, chap. 10, this volume; Feldman, Ploof, & Cohen, 1999).

Conceptual models of treatment adherence can also be used to help guide and inform communications among children, parents, and practitioners concerning illness management. For example, physicians who define their roles in chronic illness treatment as providing technical support, advocacy, or coaching in accord with a *driving instructor* model (see Creer, chap. 5, this volume) operate differently from those who believe that they are *experts* who need to impart their wisdom concerning illness management to children and their families.

Conceptual models of treatment adherence can also help researchers and practitioners set priorities concerning the information they need to obtain to evaluate potential barriers to treatment and specific adherence-related behaviors in an informed manner. For example, a broad conceptual model of adherence that emphasizes the contextual determinants of medical treatment (Quittner, DiGirolamo, Michel, & Eigen, 1992) would suggest targeting parent, family, and peer influences on adherence behaviors for routine assessment. In contrast, a child-centered model would logically focus on assessing the child's or adolescent's specific adherence behaviors and individual strategies of chronic illness management.

Finally, practitioners' models of adherence can inform clinical care by helping set specific targets for clinical interventions. For example, to the extent that practitioners believe that children's behaviors and attitudes toward treatment are critical for adherence promotion, they focus their efforts on changing these factors rather than on modifying other potential influences on treatment adherence (e.g., family members' behaviors or the treatment team's approach to chronic illness management).

Research Implications

Conceptual models can also facilitate research on adherence to treatment for pediatric chronic health conditions by guiding the following key tasks: (a) identification of variables that influence adherence to treatment, (b) documentation of the key influences on adherence to treatment, (c) formulation of testable hypotheses concerning the factors that predict adherence to treatment, and (d) development and evaluation of interventions that promote adherence to treatment. Unfortunately, most research concerning treatment adherence among children and adolescents with chronic health conditions has lacked a clear and cogent theoretical justification for the selection of intervention models and has not led to clear hypotheses concerning specific variables that should be manipulated in interventions (Dunbar-Jacob, Dunning, & Dwyer, 1993).

The complexity of chronic illness management undoubtedly contributes to this relative lack of theoretical guidance. Consider the key ingredients of an effective conceptual model or framework of adherence to pediatric chronic illness treatment. Ideally, a model should accomplish the following: (a) specify the key independent variables (e.g., what influences treatment adherence?), (b) define the relevant dependent variables (e.g., what are the components of treatment adherence?), (c) specify the important interrelationships between independent and dependent variables (e.g., what is the direction of influences on a child or family's response to treatment?), and (d) specify the interventions that are necessary to enhance adherence to treatment (e.g., what variables need to be manipulated to improve adherence to chronic illness treatment?).

To be most useful for research and practice, a conceptual model of adherence needs to account for a complex, multidimensional set of variables and specify their interrelationships. The many possible influences on treatment adherence for childhood chronic illness, coupled with the multiple domains of adherence to treatment (e.g. medication, diet, etc.), makes such model building a formidable task (see Varni et al., chap. 12, this volume).

ALTERNATIVE CONCEPTUAL MODELS
OF TREATMENT ADHERENCE

Various models have been used to conceptualize treatment adherence in childhood chronic illness. These include social-cognitive theories, stages of change models, and integrated models.

Social-Cognitive Theories

Four social-cognitive theories have led to useful predictions of medical adherence behaviors for adults with chronic illnesses. These include: (a) Health Belief Model, (b) Protection Motivation Theory, (c) Theory of Planned Behavior and Reasoned Action, and (d) Self-Efficacy Theory (Bandura, 1997; Boer & Seydel, 1996; Janz & Becker, 1984; Maddux & DuCharme, 1997; Rogers & Prentice-Dunn, 1997). Unfortunately, with the exception of the Health Belief Model, these models have not been tested in research on treatment adherence for pediatric chronic illness.

All of the social-cognitive models consider the perceived threat of the chronic health condition and/or expectancies regarding the consequences of performing adherence behaviors to be important in predicting adherence but use different names and definitions of these constructs (Norman & Conner, 1996). For example, outcome expectancies are defined as perceived benefits and barriers in the Health Belief Model, as response efficacy and self-efficacy in the Protection Motivation Theory, and as attitudes, subjective norms, and perceived behavioral control in the Theory of Planned Behavior and Reasoned Action.

For the most part, research—including studies with pediatric populations—have generated empirical support for social-cognitive theories. For example, greater maternal- or child-perceived severity, defined as the perception of the seriousness of the child's chronic health condition if left untreated, has been shown to relate to treatment adherence (Brownlee-Duffeck et al.,1987; Charron-Prochownik et al., 1993; Jamison, Lewis, & Burish, 1986; Palardy, Greening, Holderby, & Atchison, 1998; Radius et al., 1978; Shope, 1988; Smith, Ley, Seale, & Shaw, 1987). Similarly, maternal-perceived susceptibility (e.g., the perception of risks related to health problems or complications that arise if the treatment regimen is not followed) has been shown to correlate positively with treatment adherence (Radius et al., 1978; Shope, 1988; Smith et al., 1987). However, adolescents with cancer and diabetes with higher perceived susceptibility to risk have poorer adherence to treatment (Bond, Aiken, & Somerville, 1992; Brownlee-Duffeck et al., 1987; Tamaroff, Festa, Adesman, & Walco, 1992).

Outcome expectancies are a second key set of variables in social-cognitive models of treatment adherence. Outcome expectancies include perceived benefits, defined as one's judgment of the benefits of following the recommended treatment regimen, and perceived barriers or costs of following a treatment regimen. Greater maternal- and child-perceived benefits and fewer perceived barriers have been found to relate to better treatment adherence in children with a range of chronic illnesses (Bobrow, AvRuskin, & Siller, 1985; Bond et al., 1992; Brownlee-Duffeck et al., 1987; Charron-Prochownik et al., 1993; Flynn, Lyman, & Prentice-Dunn, 1995; Glasgow, McCaul, & Schafer, 1986; Palardy et al., 1998; Radius et al., 1978; Schafer, Glasgow, McCaul, & Dreher, 1983; Smith et al., 1987; Tamaroff et al., 1992; Wood, Casey, Kolski, & McCormick, 1985).

Several studies have found that adolescents who demonstrate higher self-efficacy for completing a treatment regimen (i.e., they believe they are capable of completing their treatment) are more adherent with such treatments (Clark et al., 1988; Czajkowski & Koocher 1987; Littlefield et al., 1992). Such relationships may also hold for parental self-efficacy. In the only study we identified that examined the relationship between parental level of self-efficacy and treatment adherence, Flynn et al. (1995) found that, with regard to children with muscular dystrophy, parents' ratings of their self-efficacy were positively correlated with adherence to a physical therapy regimen.

Despite the promising results described earlier, differences in concepts and measures have limited the development of standardized measures and replication of tests of social-cognitive models of adherence to treatment for childhood chronic illness (Corcoran, 1995; Janz & Becker, 1984; Strecher, Champion, & Rosenstock, 1997). Moreover, the independent variables (e.g., attitudes or beliefs) that are measured in studies of social-cognitive models typically account for only a small proportion of variance in adherence behaviors (Rapoff, 1999; Stroebe & Stroebe, 1995). Finally, models of treatment adherence have been tested primarily in descriptive studies of the relationships among a range of independent variables and treatment adherence. To our knowledge, no one has demonstrated that clinical interventions designed to modify child or family members' perceptions of key constructs of social-cognitive models have improved child or family adherence behaviors (La Greca & Schuman, 1995; Rapoff, 1999).

Personal Meanings of Treatment Adherence

The personal meaning of treatment adherence to children with chronic illness and their families is related to but much broader than the variables typically tested in social-cognitive theories. Conrad (1985) noted that a wide range of personal meanings of treatment adherence may contribute to individual differences in the quality of adherence. Such relevant personal meanings include testing, control or dependence, and/or stigmatization. In some situations, adolescents and young adults may decide to stop taking their medications as an experiment to determine whether these medications make a difference for their health and well-being (Conrad, 1985). Yet because many treatments do not result in obvious short-term changes in physical symptoms or health, some children and adolescents may incorrectly conclude that their treatments are not effective or necessary. Treatment regimens may also be perceived as a sign of unwanted dependence on family and doctors, especially by adolescents. Moreover, to reduce their perceptions of dependence, some children, adolescents, and adults with chronic conditions may decide to limit or even abandon their treatments (Stein, 1999).

Another salient personal meaning of adherence that may influence treatment-related behaviors among children and adolescents, which has not received much empirical scrutiny, concerns feelings of stigma. Many chronic illnesses, especially those that are visible to peers, engender powerful social stigma. Even chronic illnesses that are not obvious to peers and others may be experienced as potentially stigmatizing by affected children and adolescents. For this reason, taking medications and conducting treatment can be perceived as acknowledging one's difference from others. Some individuals with chronic illnesses may try to reduce the stigma of their conditions by avoiding taking their medication in front of others or sometimes eliminating treatments entirely (Conrad, 1985; see also La Greca, 1990b, for a discussion of the role of peer support in managing a chronic illness such as diabetes).

Although nonadherence with medical treatment is generally perceived as problematic by practitioners, in some instances, nonadherence may have a positive personal meaning to patients and their families and, in some cases, reflect a well-reasoned decision concerning treatment (Donovan & Blake, 1992). In support of this idea, Deaton (1985) described adaptive parental nonadherence with the management of pediatric asthma and found that the level of adaptiveness of parental decision making with asthma treatment was actually associated with better medical outcomes in children. Similarly, Koocher, McGrath, and Gudas (1990) defined educated nonadherence among children and adolescents with CF as an informed choice for medical management that is based on a full understanding of the treatment regimen and the implications of not following the prescribed treatment (e.g., a patient whose illness has progressed to the point where treatment does not make a difference). Such observations underscore the need to develop a more informed scientific understanding of children's and adolescents' personal models of their chronic illnesses and how they influence the management of their chronic illnesses.

Stages of Change Models

The models of treatment adherence most appropriate to understand how children and adolescents with chronic health conditions manage their illness should include longitudinal and developmental perspectives (La Greca, 1990a; La Greca & Schuman, 1995). A developmental perspective is needed because expectations for treatment adherence vary as a function of the stage of the children's adaptations to their illness as well as their developmental levels. For example, a child who is newly diagnosed with a chronic illness such as diabetes cannot be expected to perfectly adhere to a treatment regimen that involves an unfamiliar and personally demanding set of skills. By the same token, children's attainment of an acceptable level of adherence to treatment of a chronic illness at one point in time does not guarantee that they will sustain comparable levels of adherence over the course of their condition.

To our knowledge, conceptual models of treatment adherence that focus explicitly on the stages of acquisition and change of adherence behaviors have not been developed or tested for children and adolescents with chronic health conditions. Nevertheless, the Transtheoretical Model, which postulates stages of change in the acquisition of health-enhancing behaviors (e.g., smoking cessation) and has received empirical support (Prochaska, DiClemente, & Norcross, 1992; Prochaska et al., 1994; Ruggiero & Prochaska, 1993), is applicable to research on treatment adherence in pediatric chronic illness. The five stages of change in this model include: (a) precontemplation (i.e., not thinking about making changes in treatment), (b) contemplation (i.e., considering a change in treatment regimen in the future), (c) preparation (i.e., considering change in the treatment regimen in the immediate future), (d) action (i.e., changing behavior concerning adherence to treatment in a chronic illness), and (e) maintenance (i.e., continued change over time).

In this model, progression through these stages of change is not always linear. Individuals may relapse back through various stages. Moreover, individuals and families may be at different stages of change for the various specific components of adherence-related tasks (e.g., medication vs. diet; La Greca & Schuman, 1995). Other interesting and potentially important key variables in the Transtheoretical Model include decisional balance (e.g., the process of weighing the benefits vs. the costs of desired behaviors) and self-efficacy, defined as the personal confidence in the patient's ability to make the desired behavior change.

Despite its conceptual appeal, the Transtheoretical Model of behavioral change is limited by the absence of empirical data to support its validity or clinical utility in populations of children with chronic health conditions. Moreover, the stages of change/concept may oversimplify the behavior of children and families especially because it may be difficult to categorize children and adolescents into one stage of change (Bandura, 1997; Rapoff, 1999). Finally, the definition of stages of change are circular in that they are defined in terms of the behaviors they are meant to explain (Rapoff, 1999).

Integrated Models

Some researchers have developed integrated models of adherence to chronic illness treatment that incorporate a wide range of factors (see Varni et al., chap. 12, this volume). One of these is Hanson's (1992) model of psychosocial factors of health outcomes, adherence, and metabolic control in youths with insulin-dependent diabetes mellitus (IDDM). In this model, family factors such as cohesion, parental support of treatment, and quality of family relationships have been identified as salient influences on children's coping strategies and level of psychological stress, which, in turn, are hypothesized to influence treatment adherence and blood sugar control. Other potentially influential factors in this model include knowledge and family attitudes toward the health care system, peer pressure to engage in normal activities, and salient developmental variables (e.g., the child's age). Hanson, Henggeler, and Burghen (1987) found that older adolescents had less positive family relations, which in turn were associated with poorer adherence to treatment. As adolescents became older and more independent, the decisions that they made regarding their behaviors were less likely to be based on health reasons and more on personal and social factors (Hanson et al., 1987; see also Hampson, Glasgow, & Toohert, 1992, for similar findings with adults).

NEGLECTED FACTORS IN MODELS
OF TREATMENT ADHERENCE

One salient limitation of current research is that the available conceptual models of adherence behavior have not been used to develop interventions to promote adherence to chronic illness treatment and/or to test them. Nevertheless, each of these models suggests important variables that need to be assessed to document the nature of adherence problems and that should be included in the design of relevant interventions. For example, interventions can be designed to match the type of intervention that is delivered with the specific adherence problems and barriers to adherence that are identified.

Several additional factors have been largely neglected in available conceptual models of treatment adherence in childhood chronic illness, but are important to mention and are described briefly. These are illness-related factors, the role of the physician and treatment setting, cultural factors, and developmental issues.

Illness-Related Factors

Children with chronic health conditions and their families are required to learn a complex set of specific treatment-related behaviors and skills. Because the demands of treatment adherence vary as a function of disease severity and illness stage or duration, condition-specific factors are important in the development of conceptual models of influence on treatment adherence. One example is the *honeymoon* period that follows the diagnosis of diabetes: The specific task demands on children and families to maintain a reasonable level of blood sugar control through their adherence behaviors are much less following the initial diagnosis of diabetes because the pancreas continues to produce some insulin, which helps naturally maintain blood sugar control.

Role of the Physician and Treatment Setting

Despite the importance of physician behavior in managing adherence to treatment (see DiMatteo, chap. 10, this volume, for a more extensive discussion), the quality of physician–family interactions have been neglected in models of treatment adherence in chronic illness in children and adolescents. Moreover, the specific setting in which treatment is received as well as the nature and level of comprehensive care provided to the child and family may be highly relevant to adherence to chronic illness treatment but has not been considered in conceptual models.

Cultural Factors

Cultural factors have also been largely neglected in developing conceptual models of research and practice in treatment adherence in childhood chronic illness. In this regard, one of the key distinctions that should be made in models of treatment adherence is between *disease*, which is defined as the measurable deviation of an organic system or malfunction of biologic structure, and *illness*, which is defined as the human experience of suffering or distress (Dressler & Oths, 1997). A child or family's explanatory model of illness and relevant treatment can be influenced by available cultural knowledge and support and is not a direct reflection of the physicians' diagnosis (Kleinman, 1980). Although largely unexplored in childhood chronic illness, culturally based norms and meaning may be important in defining sickness and sick role, seeking and accepting advice about health and illness, choosing a treatment for an illness, and communicating with physicians and health care professionals concerning diagnosis and treatment (Dressler & Oths, 1997).

Developmental Issues

Despite that developmental issues are important in the clinical management of treatment adherence in childhood chronic illness, they have been neglected in most conceptual models of adherence (see Hanson, 1992, for an exception). Key developmental issues relevant to treatment adherence in childhood chronic illness include age-related changes in developmental competencies, differences in treatment-related expectations for children's adherence behavior, and changes in allocation of treatment-related responsibilities among the child and other family members.

Individual practitioners' expectations vary widely for how much independence in treatment-related responsibilities children with chronic conditions such as diabetes should assume at a particular age (Wysocki et al., 1992). However, relatively little is known about the age-related allocation of responsibilities among parents and children and increases in children's self-management skills for many chronic illnesses (for exceptions, see Anderson, Auslander, Jung, Miller, & Santiago, 1990; Wade, Islam, Holden, Kruszon-Moran, & Mitchell, 1999). In the absence of such data, it may be difficult for physicians and nurses to set realistic expectations for family allocation of responsibilities for treatment of various chronic illnesses or to implement adequate developmental updates of treatment-related responsibilities (Koocher et al., 1990).

MEASUREMENT OF ADHERENCE
TO PEDIATRIC CHRONIC ILLNESS TREATMENT

The measurement of adherence to treatment in childhood chronic illness is extremely challenging and raises many difficult methodological problems (Rand, 2000). For example, it is widely recognized that, in the absence of a gold standard of adherence measurement in pediatric populations (La Greca & Schuman, 1995), a range of different methods need to be employed. These are: (a) direct versus indirect measures, (b) single versus multiple adherence behavior measures, and (c) categorical versus continuous measures. Relevant methodological issues for each of these dimensions are discussed briefly. For a more complete discussion of the costs versus benefits of various measurement techniques, readers are referred to Bender et al. (chap. 7, this volume), Rand (2000), and Rapoff (1999).

Direct Versus Indirect Measures

Direct measures of adherence include drug assays, such as body fluid levels of the prescribed drug or of a systemic marker. Although direct methods provide the most objective and quantifiable method for assessing treatment adherence, practical problems such as cost often prohibit their systematic use in research and clinical practice. Moreover, other problems limit the use of objective measures. First, results obtained from objective measures are affected by individual differences in metabolism, drug absorption rates, and food interactions (Epstein & Cluss, 1982; Pedersen & Moller-Petersen, 1984). Second, drug assays may be difficult to implement and interpret when tracking multiple medication regimens due to drug interactions (Hazzard, Hutchinson, & Krawiecki, 1990). Finally, drug assays become less useful when an investigator wants to examine medication adherence in individuals with different conditions and/or who are taking different medications.

Other direct measures include pill counts and electronic/computer monitoring devices. Pill counts are inexpensive and easy to accomplish, but rely on patients to return their unused medications. Furthermore, direct measures cannot measure patients' consumption of medications, which can be quite problematic if patients *dump* their unused medication prior to their appointment. Electronic/computer monitoring devices, which have the advantage of monitoring when and how often the pill container is open, facilitate the identification of dumping of used medication, but still cannot address whether pills have actually been consumed. Moreover, electronic/computer monitoring devices are costly, can malfunction, and, to our knowledge, cannot be used with liquid medication.

Indirect measures include self-report (i.e., interview) and physician ratings. Reports of adherence obtained from adolescents and their parents are most frequently employed in research because they are relatively easy to obtain and are cost-effective (La Greca & Schuman, 1995). However, questions have been raised about their validity. For example, self-report measures are highly sensitive to demand or social desirability effects (Rapoff, 1999). Adolescent and parent reports have been found to be biased in the direction of overreporting adherence (Epstein & Cluss, 1982; Mathews & Christophersen, 1988). Nevertheless, those patients who admit to being nonadherent are typically also identified through other more direct methods (Epstein & Cluss, 1982; Liptak, 1996; Tebbi et al., 1986).

The quality of adherence assessment using self-report methods has been improved by the use of the 24-hour recall interview (Johnson, Silverstein, Rosenbloom, Carter, & Cunningham, 1986), which, as its name implies, asks adolescents and their parents to report on adherence behaviors for a short time period. The 24-hour recall interview may give more accurate results because its questions are highly specific, time limited, and less likely to be judgmental. However, the typical 24-hour recall protocol, which involves interviewing the child and/or parent on three different occasions over a 2-week period, is time-consuming and costly.

Validity for the 24-hour recall interview among children and adolescents with diabetes has been demonstrated by comparisons of behavioral observations with the 24-hour recall interview data, exploratory and confirmatory factor analyses, and studies that have linked the interview data with indexes of diabetes control (Johnson, Freund, Silverstein, Hansen, & Malone, 1990; Johnson et al., 1986; Johnson, Tomer, Cunningham, & Henretta, 1990; Reynolds, Johnson, & Silverstein, 1990). For example, Freund, Johnson, Silverstein, and Thomas (1991) found statistically significant parent–child agreement for 13 different adherence behaviors reported using the 24-hour recall interview. Moreover, adherence behaviors assessed in the recall interview remained relatively stable over 3 months (Freund et al., 1991).

Physician reports have been found to be inaccurate at predicting their patients' levels of adherence, particularly when compared with more direct measures of adherence such as drug assays (Riekert, Wiener, Drotar, & Sprunk, 1999; Rudd, 1993). For example, in a study of pediatricians in private practice, ratings of adherence were no better than chance and adherence tended to be overestimated (Charney et al., 1967). More recently, Finney, Hook, Friman, Rapoff, and Christophersen (1993) found that provider predictions of adherence were highly specific (i.e., providers were able to accurately predict who would be adherent, but were not very sensitive—that is, they did not accurately identify those patients who were nonadherent). The overall accuracy of provider predictions was only 65%.

Multiple Adherence Behaviors and Outcomes

Another significant challenge in measuring adherence to treatment in chronic pediatric health conditions is that these treatment regimens often require children, adolescents, and their families to manage several different behaviors at once, such as taking medicine, altering diet, and/or participating in physical therapy or exercise programs. Depending on the specific chronic illness and its severity, individual treatment regimen components may have variable therapeutic significance and impact on the children's health status. Other difficult measurement problems are raised by varying levels of adherence for various components of treatment. Furthermore, individual children and adolescents with a chronic condition such as diabetes may adhere fully to some aspects of treatment (e.g., taking insulin injections) while being partially or even completely noncompliant with other aspects of the regimen (e.g., exercise or dietary restrictions; Kaplan & Simon, 1990; Kasi, 1983; Orme & Binik, 1989). For these reasons, global adherence measures that summarize a wide range of required treatment behaviors may obscure potentially important profiles of strengths and weaknesses in individual domains of adherence. Consequently, separate scores for each adherence behavior give a more complete and accurate picture of the individual's pattern of adherence than does a summary score of overall adherence.

Categorical Versus Continuous Measurement

One frequently used research strategy has been to categorize individuals into groups of *compliant* or *noncompliant* patients. A significant limitation of this approach is that the cut point to identify a compliant versus noncompliant patient can be arbitrary and is not based on valid criteria concerning the level of adherence necessary to achieve a clinically meaningful impact on health status. One of the problems in ascertaining such levels is that the normative or expected levels of treatment adherence for children and adolescents of various ages have not been established empirically for many chronic health conditions.

An alternative to this approach is to assess adherence to chronic illness treatment behaviors on a continuum. A clear advantage of this approach is that it avoids the use of arbitrary cutoff scores and allows a comparison of adherence rates to treatment across different behaviors, studies, and pediatric conditions (La Greca & Schuman, 1995). However, the clinical significance of treatment adherence data that are measured on a continuum is not always possible to determine.

INTERVENTIONS TO PROMOTE TREATMENT ADHERENCE
FOR CHRONIC HEALTH CONDITIONS
IN CHILDREN AND ADOLESCENTS

One of the most important areas of research on treatment adherence in pediatric chronic illness concerns the evaluation of the efficacy and effectiveness of interventions to enhance adherence. An extensive review of intervention studies is beyond the scope of this chapter. Interested readers are referred to Kibby, Tyc, and Mulhern (1998), La Greca and Schuman (1995), Rapoff (1999), and Roter et al. (1998) for reviews of adherence-related interventions for children with chronic health conditions. This section describes promising directions for interventions to enhance treatment adherence for childhood chronic illness and relevant methodological issues.

La Greca and Schuman (1995) divided interventions to promote adherence to chronic illness treatment into five categories that reflect the primary focus of the approach. These include: (a) interventions that emphasize learning new skills and behaviors such as educational approaches and modeling and behavioral rehearsal programs (Sergis-Davenport & Varni, 1982, 1983), (b) approaches that emphasize close medical monitoring of adherence (Delamater et al., 1990) and reminders and/or self-monitoring (Lowe & Lutzker, 1979), (c) programs that emphasize incentives for adherence behaviors (Greenan-Fowler, Powell, & Varni, 1987), (d) interventions that emphasize family support and/or problem solving (e.g., social support and involvement from family and peers; Satin, La Greca, Zigo, & Skyler, 1989) or reducing family barriers to adherence (Schafer, Glasgow, & McCaul, 1992), and (e) multicomponent approaches (e.g., Anderson, Wolf, Burkhart, Cornell, & Bacon's [1989] intervention with adolescents in peer groups as well as parents).

Examples of Interventions to Improve Treatment Adherence

In the research and clinical literature, most interventions to promote adherence to medical treatment of pediatric chronic health conditions have focused on improving the child and/or family's knowledge about the illness and treatment or implement behavior modification techniques (e.g., shaping, positive reinforcement). In contrast, recent innovative interventions have noted a positive impact on adherence behaviors and health outcomes. For example, two studies of adolescents with diabetes have investigated peer-group interventions designed to improve illness-management problem solving (Anderson, Wolf, Burkhart, Cornell, & Bacon, 1989) and social skills related to peer influences on illness management (Kaplan, Chadwick, & Schimmel, 1985). Both of these studies found that adolescents in the experimental group demonstrated better metabolic control postintervention than adolescents who received standard diabetes education. Similarly, the results of family-based group interventions that have focused on improving the families' problem-solving skills related to diabetes management have demonstrated significant improvements in metabolic control and adherence behaviors when compared with families that received standard care (Delamater et al., 1990; Satin et al., 1989).

Other innovative studies have used computer and telecommunication technology as a method to improve adherence. Horan, Yarborough, Besigel, and Carlson (1990) demonstrated that a computer-based self-management program for adolescents with diabetes resulted in more frequent blood glucose testing as compared with standard printed educational and problem-solving materials. Brown et al. (1997) demonstrated that an educational video game designed to promote diabetes self-care behaviors resulted in significantly more self-care behaviors 6 months later relative to a control group that received a nonhealth-related video game.

Erickson, Ascione, Kirking, and Johnson (1998) provided individuals with asthma message-based pagers that were programmed for multiple daily reminders to take the medication as well as specific directions about which medicines to take and subdirectories with administration steps or techniques (e.g., proper inhaler technique, what to do if having an asthma attack). Preliminary data for this intervention suggest that this can be a viable and cost-effective means to improve adherence behaviors.

Some investigators have evaluated the efficacy of interesting behavioral self-management programs on medical outcomes. For example, Colland (1993) compared the effectiveness of comprehensive self-management training in a group of children with asthma using games and learning materials designed for school-age participants to controls who either received no program or information only. Children in the experimental group had a reduction in the number of medical visits and less frequent occurrence of symptoms than controls. This study is noteworthy because children were selected to participate on the basis of inadequate self-management abilities that were objectively assessed.

Another example of an innovative intervention, again with pediatric asthma, is Greinder, Loane, and Parks' (1995) study of the effectiveness of an individualized outreach treatment program that included instruction in asthma management medications, triggers, and use of inhalers and peak flow meters. Personal telephone contact was maintained with families to enhance compliance. The intervention was associated with significant reductions in rates of emergency room visits and hospital admissions in a group of predominantly African-American children and adolescents drawn from an inner-city population.

Methodological Problems of Intervention Studies

Although a number of intervention studies have shown positive effects on adherence to treatment for pediatric chronic illness, the findings are not consistent. Moreover, conclusions that can be drawn from these data have been limited by the small number of large, randomized, controlled trials of intervention. Moreover, interventions to promote treatment adherence have rarely been studied in some chronic conditions, such as sickle cell anemia.

Moreover, owing to short follow-up periods employed in available studies, data demonstrating the long-term impact of interventions on treatment adherence in childhood chronic illness have been largely nonexistent. Consequently, we do not know whether interventions designed to impact adherence also affect children's long-term health-related outcomes, including illness-related morbidity or other relevant outcomes such as family adaptation.

Another problem with research on adherence-promotion interventions is that, although most adherence interventions have a primary focus (e.g., education or support), they often include several components (e.g., reinforcement and problem solving) and may involve different participants (e.g., parents and children). Consequently, when such interventions are found to be successful, it is difficult to identify the specific components that accounted for the success.

A significant methodological problem is that the impact of interventions designed to enhance treatment adherence in pediatric chronic illness has not been described and summarized in a systematic manner. We were able to locate only one meta-analysis that specifically focused on interventions to improve patient adherence (Roter et al., 1998). However, only 22 of the 153 published studies from 1977 to 1994 that were included in this review involved children. Nevertheless, the main conclusions of this meta-analysis were interesting and potentially applicable to children and families. For example, although no single strategy of intervention showed clear advantage over another, comprehensive interventions combining educational, behavioral, and affective components were more effective than a single-focus approach (Roter et al., 1998). These findings coincide with those of the Kibby et al. (1998) meta-analysis, which included a range of interventions, including disease management, for children with chronic health conditions. Although the effect sizes for interventions that were focused on disease management reported in the analysis were large (1.28), it was not clear which of the studies in this review focused explicitly on treatment adherence in pediatric chronic illness.

To address the need for empirical studies of interventions, some of the work in this volume describes the results of new intervention models designed to enhance child, adolescent, and family treatment adherence. These include: behavioral family systems therapy for adolescents with diabetes (Wysocki, Greco, Harris, & White, chap. 16, this volume), intervention with parents to promote adherence with nutritional requirements of young children with CF (Stark, chap. 18, this volume), family-centered problem solving and education with adolescents with CF and their families (Quittner et al., chap. 17, this volume), office-based interventions with children and adolescents with diabetes (Anderson, Brackett, Ho, & Laffel, chap. 15, this volume), comprehensive approaches to improve treatment adherence for juvenile rheumatoid arthritis (Rapoff, chap. 14, this volume), and ways to promote adherence to treatment for growth hormone therapy (Sandberg et al., chap. 19, this volume). Readers are referred to these chapters for descriptions of design issues and results of these ongoing studies.

UNANSWERED QUESTIONS AND RECOMMENDATIONS FOR FUTURE RESEARCH CONCERNING TREATMENT ADHERENCE

Despite the large number of studies that have focused on adherence/compliance (Trostle, chap. 2, this volume), in many ways the development of generalizable scientific knowledge concerning treatment adherence in pediatric chronic illness is still in its infancy. Some of the more significant unanswered questions are addressed by the contributions to this volume. Others remain unanswered. Several potential priorities for future research are described in this chapter, whereas others are noted in the summary of the conference participants' discussions and recommendations. Interested readers are referred to this chapter.

Develop Integrated, Clinically Relevant Models of Treatment Adherence

Integrated models of treatment adherence based on empirical data potentially need to be developed (see Hanson et al., 1987). Moreover, these models should be used to develop interventions that target specific situational barriers and enhance the support that influences day-to-day management of pediatric chronic illness, including treatment adherence. Potential targets of interventions include situations that children and families regard as difficult or interfering with their chronic illness treatment (e.g., see Quittner et al., chap. 17, this volume) or management and allocation of treatment-related responsibilities among children and family members (see Anderson et al., chap. 15, this volume).

Use Prospective Research Designs to Evaluate Treatment Adherence

Despite that treatment adherence in pediatric chronic illness is a lifelong endeavor, most empirical research on this topic has not involved prospective research (La Greca & Schuman, 1995). The work of Hauser, Jacobson, and colleagues, who have conducted long-term studies of relationship of

family factors to adherence and psychosocial outcomes in juvenile diabetes, is an important exception (Hauser et al., 1990; Jacobson et al.,
1990). Both short- and long-term prospective studies are needed to
extend this work: Short-term prospective studies are necessary to assess
the development of adherence behaviors in response to the diagnosis of
a chronic condition and/or in response to exacerbations in symptoms,
complications, or specific critical changes in treatment (e.g., maintenance
of organ transplants). Long-term studies are needed to understand how
treatment adherence can be maintained over time and to evaluate the
long-term impact of adherence-promoting interventions on health behaviors and outcomes to assess the influence of developmental change on
adherence behaviors.

Define the Behavior of Practitioners
and the Treatment Team Concerning
Illness Management

One of the most important needs for future research is to describe and
define the behaviors of professional caregivers in managing pediatric
chronic illness treatment and their relationship to treatment adherence.
Research on adherence needs to define whether and how practitioners
provide support for adherence management; how such care is typically
delivered in terms of continuity, frequency of contact, and accessibility to
families; and the relationship of patient and family adherence to treatment. Researchers also need to address the following questions concerning clinical management of adherence to pediatric chronic illness treatment: What information and expectations are transmitted to the child and
family in critical areas (e.g., skills, knowledge of illness, and treatment
plan)? How is such information transmitted to children and families (e.g.,
is it repeated and reinforced?)? How are treatment plans for chronic illness and adherence monitored over time? What modifications are made
in response to developmental changes in the child or changes in health
status?

Assess the Impact of Treatment Adherence
on Medical Outcomes and Families

Empirical studies that document the impact of excellent versus problematic adherence to treatment on medical and psychological outcomes are
very much needed. From the standpoint of children and families, the
strenuous demands for adherence to chronic illness treatment stand in
stark contrast to the lack of direct evidence for the impact of treatment
adherence on children's long-term health outcomes (Johnson, 1994).

Moreover, another key area of future study is to assess the burden of treatment adherence in a range of chronic conditions on children and families relative to the benefits of treatment on the quality of life for children and families.

Develop Studies of the Measurement of Treatment Adherence in Childhood Chronic Illness

Despite significant advances in the measurement of treatment adherence in pediatric chronic illness (Johnson, Tomer, et al., 1990), much of the most important work in this area of research remains to be done. In particular, there is a need to develop reliable and valid approaches to adherence measurement within and across different chronic conditions, especially approaches that combine self-report and objective measures.

A large gap exists between how adherence behaviors are measured in research versus clinical practice and it needs to be closed. Researchers tend to use costly and/or time-consuming methods, such as electronic monitoring devices or 24-hour recall interview procedures, to assess adherence to treatment; these often are not feasible to use as part of standard care within clinical settings. Consequently, there is a need for valid, yet feasible cost-effective methods of measuring adherence behaviors that can be used in clinical practice and research.

Evaluate the Effectiveness of Interventions to Promote Adherence

Little is known about the impact of adherence-related interventions on children's long-term health and psychological outcomes. Consequently, there is a need for controlled clinical trials to establish the empirical validity of adherence-promotion interventions as well as the impact of these interventions on the long-term health and psychological development of children and adolescent with chronic illness Moreover, there is a need for well-described and documented case studies and series that assess the effectiveness of clinical interventions for serious, potentially intractable compliance problems that compromise the effectiveness of medical treatment and clinical care.

Integrate Research and Practice Concerning Treatment Adherence in Pediatric Chronic Illness Treatment

The limitations of research on adherence to pediatric chronic illness treatment are similar to those encountered in research on psychological interventions with children with emotional disorders (i.e., most research has been conducted on populations of children that are different than those seen in practice; for an exception, see Anderson et al., chap. 15, this volume). Consequently, integration of research and practice is a clear priority for future work concerning treatment adherence in pediatric chronic illness. To date, most controlled trials of interventions to improve adherence behaviors have focused on prevention of adherence problems. That is, participants in such intervention studies were not selected because of significant adherence difficulties (for an exception, see Rapoff, chap. 14, this volume). Children who participate in the majority of studies on treatment adherence in pediatric chronic illness are different than those who have serious and clinically significant adherence problems. In addition, adherence-promotion interventions that have been tested in highly controlled clinical trials with children have not been evaluated in *trials by fire*, which can only occur in clinical practice situations. Consequently, there is the need to develop a research agenda that applies available research findings concerning assessment and intervention concerning adherence to pediatric chronic illness treatment to practice situations.

CONTRIBUTION OF THIS VOLUME

The work presented in this volume represents a step in the direction of addressing the considerable research and clinical needs concerning treatment adherence in pediatric chronic illness. Many of the important scientific and clinical questions concerning treatment adherence in childhood chronic illness have yet to be addressed. This is both an exciting and formidable challenge. We hope that readers of this volume are stimulated by the work of the volume contributors and join them in meeting these challenges.

REFERENCES

Alessandro, F., Vincenzo, Z. G., Marco, S., Marcello, G., & Enrica, R. (1994). Compliance with pharmocologic prophylaxis and therapy in bronchial asthma. *Annals of Allergy, 73*, 135–140.

Anderson, B. J., Auslander, W. F., Jung, K. C., Miller, J. P., & Santiago, J. V. (1990). Assessing family sharing of diabetes responsibilities. *Journal of Pediatric Psychology, 15*, 477–492.

Anderson, B. J., Wolf, F. M., Burkhart, M. T., Cornell, R. G., & Bacon, G. E. (1989). Effects of peer-group intervention on metabolic control of adolescents with IDDM: Randomized outpatient study. *Diabetes Care, 3*, 179–183.

Bandura, A. (1997). *Self-efficacy: The exercise of control.* New York: Freeman.

Berg, J. S., Dischler, J., Wagner, D. J., Raia, J., & Palmer-Shevlin, N. (1993). Medication compliance: A health care problem. *The Annals of Pharmacotherapy, 27* (Suppl.), 2–21.

Bobrow, E. S., AvRuskin, T. W., & Siller, J. (1985). Mother–daughter interaction and adherence to diabetes regimen. *Diabetes Care, 8*, 146–151.

Boer, H., & Seydel, E. R. (1996). Protection motivation theory. In M. Conner & P. Norman (Eds.), *Predicting health behaviors* (pp. 95–120). Philadelphia, PA: Open University Press.

Bond, G. G., Aiken, L. S., & Somerville, S. (1992). The health belief model and adolescents with insulin-dependent diabetes mellitus. *Health Psychology, 11,* 190–198.

Brown, S. J., Lieberman, D. A., Germeny, B. A., Fan, Y. C., Wilson, D. M., & Pasta, D. J. (1997). Educational video game for juvenile diabetes: Results of a controlled trial. *Medical Informatics, 22,* 77–89.

Brownlee-Duffeck, M., Peterson, L., Simonds, J. F., Goldstein, D., Kilo, C., & Hoette, S. (1987). The role of health beliefs in the regimen adherence and metabolic control of adolescents and adults with diabetes mellitus. *Journal of Consulting and Clinical Psychology, 55,* 139–144.

Charney, E., Bynum, R., Eldredge, D., Frank, D., MacWhinney, J. B., McNabb, N., Scheiner, A., Sumpter, E. A., & Iker, H. (1967). How well do patients take oral penicillin: A collaborative study in private practice. *Pediatrics, 40,* 188–195.

Charron-Prochownik, C., Becker, M. H., Brown, M. B., Liang, W. M., & Bennett, S. (1993). Understanding young children's health beliefs and diabetes regimen adherence. *Diabetes Educator, 19,* 409–418.

Clark, N. M., Rosenstock, I. M., Hassan, H., Evans, D., Wasilewski, Y., Feldman, C., & Mellins, R. B. (1988). The effect of health beliefs and feelings of self-efficacy on self-management behavior of children with a chronic disease. *Patient Education and Counseling, 11,* 131–139.

Chmelik, F., & Doughty, A. (1994). Objective measurements of compliance in asthma treatment. *Annals of Allergy, 73,* 527–532.

Colland, V. T. (1993). Learning to cope with asthma: A behavioral self-management program with children. *Patient Education and Counseling, 22,* 141–152.

Conley, S. B., & Salvatierra, O. (1996). Noncompliance among adolescents: Does it impact the success of transplantation? *Nephrology News & Issues, 10,* 18–19.

Conrad, P. C. (1985). The meaning of medications: Another look at compliance. *Social Science and Medicine, 20,* 29–37.

Corcoran, K. J. (1995). Understanding cognition, choice, and behavior. *Journal of Behavioral Therapy and Experimental Psychiatry, 206,* 201–207.

Coutts, J. A., Gibson, N. A., & Patton, J. Y. (1992). Measuring compliance with inhaled medication in asthma. *Archives of Diseases in Children, 67,* 332–333.

Czajkowski, D. R., & Koocher, G. P. (1987). Medical compliance and coping with cystic fibrosis. *Journal of Child Psychology and Psychiatry, 28,* 311–319.

Deaton, A. V. (1985). Adaptive noncompliance in pediatric asthma: The parent as expert. *Journal of Pediatric Psychology, 10,* 1–14.

Delamater, A. M., Bubb, J., Davis, S. G., Smith, J. A., Schmidt, L., White, N. H., & Santiago, J. V. (1990). Randomized prospective study of self-management training with newly diagnosed diabetic children. *Diabetes Care, 13,* 492–498.

Diabetes Control and Complications Trial Research Group. (1993). The effect of intensive treatment of diabetes on the development and progression of long-term complications in insulin-dependent diabetes mellitus. *New England Journal of Medicine, 329,* 977–986.

Dolgin, M. J., Katz, E. R., Doctors, S. R., & Siegel, S. E. (1986). Caregivers' perceptions of medical compliance in adolescents with cancer. *Journal of Adolescent Health Care, 7,* 22–27.

Donovan, J. L., & Blake, D. R. (1992). Patient noncompliance: Deviance or reasoned decision making? *Social Science and Medicine, 34,* 507–513.

Dressler, W. W., & Oths, K. S. (1997). Cultural determinants of health behavior. In D. S. Gochman (Ed.), *Handbook of health behavior research: I. Personal and social determinants* (pp. 357–378). New York: Plenum.

Dunbar-Jacob, J., Dunning, E. J., & Dwyer, K. (1993). Compliance research in pediatric and adolescent populations: Two decades of research. In N. A. Krasnegor, L. Epstein, S. B. Johnson, & S. J. Yaffe (Eds.), *Developmental aspects of health compliance behavior* (pp. 29–51). Hillsdale, NJ: Lawrence Erlbaum Associates.

Ettenger, R. B., Rosenthal, J. T., Marik, J. L., Malekzadeh, M., Forsythe, S. B., Kamil, E. S., Salusky, I. B., & Fine, R. N. (1991). Improved cadaveric renal transplant outcome in children. *Pediatric Nephrology, 5,* 137–142.

Epstein, L. M., & Cluss, P. A. (1982). A behavioral medicine perspective on adherence to long-term medical regimens. *Journal of Consulting and Clinical Psychology, 50,* 950–971.

Erickson, S. R., Ascione, F. J., Kirking, D. M., & Johnson, C. E. (1998). Use of a paging system to improve medication self-management in patients with asthma. *Journal of the American Pharmaceutical Association, 38,* 767–769.

Feldman, H. M., Ploof, D., & Cohen, W. J. (1999). Physician–family partnerships. The adaptive practice. *Journal of Developmental Behavioral Pediatrics, 20,* 111–116.

Festa, R. S., Tamaroff, M. H., Chasalow, F., & Lanzkowsky, P. (1992). Therapeutic adherence to oral medication regimens by adolescents with cancer: I. Laboratory assessment. *Journal of Pediatrics, 120,* 807–811.

Finney, J. W., Hook, R. J., Friman, P. C., Rapoff, M. A., & Christophersen, E. R. (1993). The overestimation of adherence to pediatric medical regimen. *Children's Health Care, 22,* 297–304.

Flynn, M. F., Lyman, R. D., & Prentice-Dunn, S. (1995). Protection motivation theory and adherence to medical treatment regimens for muscular dystrophy. *Journal of Social and Clinical Psychology, 14,* 61–75.

Freund, A., Johnson, S. B., Silverstein, J., & Thomas, J. (1991). Assessing daily management of childhood diabetes using 24-hour recall interviews: Reliability and stability. *Health Psychology, 10,* 200–208.

Glasgow, R. E., McCaul, K. D., & Schafer, L. C. (1986). Barriers to regimen adherence among persons with insulin-dependent diabetes. *Journal of Behavioral Medicine, 9,* 65–77.

Golden, M. D., Herold, A. J., & Orr, D. P. (1985). An approach to prevention of recurrent diabetic ketoacidosis in the pediatric population. *Journal of Pediatrics, 93,* 195–200.

Greinder, D. K., Loane, K. C., & Parks, P. C. (1995). Reduction in resource utilization by an asthma outreach program. *Archives of Pediatric and Adolescent Medicine, 149,* 415–420.

Greenan-Fowler, E., Powell, C., & Varni, J. W. (1987). Behavioral treatment of adherence to therapeutic exercise by children with hemophilia. *Archives of Physical Medicine and Rehabilitation, 68,* 846–849.

Hampson, S. E., Glasgow, R. E., & Toohert, D. J. (1990). Personal models of diabetes and their relation to self-care activities. *Health Publication, 9,* 632–646.

Hanson, C. L. (1992). Developing systemic models of the adaptation of youths with diabetes. In A. M. La Greca, L. J. Siegel, J. L. Wallander, & C. E. Walker (Eds.), *Stress and coping in child health* (pp. 212–241). New York: Guilford.

Hanson, C. L., Henggeler, S. W., & Burghen, G. A. (1987). Social competence and parental support as mediators of the link between stress and metabolic control in adolescents with insulin-dependent diabetes mellitus. *Journal of Consulting and Clinical Psychology, 55,* 529–533.

Hauser, S. T., Jacobson, A. M., Lavori, P., Wolfsdor, J. I., Herskowitz, R. D., Milley, J. E., Bliss, R., Wertlieb, D., & Stein, J. (1990). Adherence among children and adolescents with insulin-dependent diabetes mellitus over a four-year longitudinal follow-up: II. Immediate and long-term linkages with the family milieu. *Journal of Pediatric Psychology, 15,* 527–542.

Hazzard, A., Hutchinson, S. J., & Krawiecki, N. (1990). Factors related to adherence to medication regimens in pediatric seizure patients. *Journal of Pediatric Psychology, 15,* 543–555.

Hentinen, M., & Kyngas, H. (1992). Compliance of young diabetics with health regimens. *Journal of Advanced Nursing, 17,* 530–536.

Horan, P. P., Yarborough, M. C., Besigel, G., & Carlson, D. R. (1990). Computer-assisted self-control of diabetes by adolescents. *The Diabetes Educator, 16,* 205–211.

Jacobson, A. M., Hauser, S. T., Lavori, P., Wolfsdorf, J. I., Herskowitz, R. D., Milley, J. E., Bliss, R., Gelfand, E., Wertlieb, D., & Stein, J. (1990). Adherence among children and adolescents with insulin-dependent diabetes mellitus over a four-year longitudinal follow-up: I. The influence of patient coping and adjustment. *Journal of Pediatric Psychology, 15,* 511–526.

Jamison, R. N., Lewis, S., & Burish, T. G. (1986). Cooperation with treatment in adolescent cancer patients. *Journal of Adolescent Health Care, 7,* 162–167.

Janz, N. K., & Becker, M. H. (1984). The Health Belief Model: A decade later. *Health Education Quarterly, 11,* 1–47.

Johnson, S. B. (1994). Health behavior and health status: Concepts, methods and applications. *Journal of Pediatric Psychology, 19,* 129–141.

Johnson, S. B., Silverstein, J., Rosenbloom, A., Carter, R., & Cunningham, W. (1986). Assessing daily management in childhood diabetes. *Health Psychology, 5,* 545–564.

Johnson, S. B., Freund, A., Silverstein, J., Hansen, C. A., & Malone, J. (1990). Adherence-health status relationships in childhood diabetes. *Health Psychology, 9,* 606–631.

Johnson, S. B., Tomer, A., Cunningham, W. R., & Henretta, J. C. (1990). Adherence in childhood diabetes: Results of a confirmatory factor analysis. *Health Psychology, 9,* 493–501.

Kaplan, R. M., Chadwick, M. W., & Schimmel, L. E. (1985). Social learning intervention to promote metabolic control in type I diabetes mellitus: Pilot experiment results. *Diabetes Care, 8,* 152–155.

Kaplan, R. M., & Simon, H. J. (1990). Compliance in medical care: Reconsideration of self-predictions. *Annals of Behavioral Medicine, 12,* 66–71.

Kasi, S. V. (1983). Social and psychological factors affecting the course of disease: An epidemiological perspective. In D. Mechanic (Ed.), *Handbook of health, health care, and the health professions* (pp. 683–708). New York: The Free Press.

Kibby, M. Y., Tyc, V. L., & Mulhern, R. K. (1998). Effectiveness of psychological intervention for children and adolescents with chronic medical illness: A meta-analysis. *Clinical Psychology Review, 18,* 103–117.

Kleinman, A. (1980). *Patients and healers in the context of culture.* Berkeley: University of California Press.

Klerman, L. V. (1985). Interprofessional issues in delivering services to chronically ill children and their families. In N. Hobbs & J. M. Perrin (Eds.), *Issues in the care of children with chronic illness* (pp. 420–440). San Francisco: Jossey-Bass.

Koocher, G. P., McGrath, M. L., & Gudas, L. J. (1990). Typologies of nonadherence in cystic fibrosis. *Journal of Developmental and Behavioral Pediatrics, 11,* 353–358.

Kuhthau, K., Walker, D. K., Perrin, J. M., Bauman, L., Gortmaker, S. L., Newacheck, P. W., & Stein, R. E. K. (1998). Assessing managed care for children with chronic conditions. *Health Affairs, 17,* 42–52.

La Greca, A. M. (1990a). Issues in adherence with pediatric regimens. *Journal of Pediatric Psychology, 15,* 423–436.

La Greca, A. M. (1990b). Social consequences of pediatric conditions: Fertile area for future investigations and intervention? *Journal of Pediatric Psychology, 15,* 285–308.

La Greca, A. M., & Schuman, W. B. (1995). Adherence to prescribed medical regimens. In M. C. Roberts (Ed.), *Handbook of pediatric psychology* (2nd ed., pp. 55–83). New York: Guilford.

Lasagna, L., & Hutt, P. B. (1991). Health care, research, and regulatory impact of noncompliance. In J.A. Cramer & B. Spilker (Eds.), *Patient compliance in medical practice and clinical trials* (pp. 393–403). New York: Raven.

Liptak, G. S. (1996). Enhancing patient compliance in pediatrics. *Pediatric Review, 17,* 128–134.

Littlefield, C. H., Daneman, D., Craven, J. L., Murray, M. A., Rodin, G. M., & Rydall, A. C. (1992). Relationship of self-efficacy and bingeing to adherence to diabetes regimen among adolescents. *Diabetes Care, 15,* 90–94.

Liss, D. S., Waller, D. A., Kennard, B. D., McIntire, D., Capra, P., & Stephens, J. (1998). Psychiatric illness and family support in children and adolescents with diabetic ketoacidosis: A controlled study. *Journal of the American Academy of Child and Adolescent Psychiatry, 37,* 536–544.

Lowe, K., & Lutzker, J. R. (1979). Increasing compliance to a medical regimen with a juvenile diabetic. *Behavior Therapy, 10,* 57–64.

Maddux, J. E., & DuCharme, K. A. (1997). Behavioral intentions in theories of health behavior. In D. S. Gochman (Ed.), *Handbook of health behavior researcher: I. Personal and social determinants* (pp. 133–152). New York: Plenum.

Matsui, D. M. (1997). Drug compliance in pediatrics. Clinical and research issues. *Pediatric Clinics of North America, 44,* 1–14.

Mathews, J. R., & Christophersen, E. R. (1988). Measuring and preventing noncompliance in pediatric health care. In P. Karoly (Ed.), *Handbook of child health assessment* (pp. 519–557). New York: Wiley.

Meyers, K. E., Thomson, P. D., & Weiland, H. (1996). Noncompliance in children and adolescents after renal transplantation. *Transplantation, 62,* 186–189.

Meyers, K. E., Weiland, H., & Thomson, P. D. (1995). Pediatric renal transplantation noncompliance. *Pediatric Nephrology, 9,* 189–192.

Newacheck, P. W., & Taylor, W. R. (1992). Childhood chronic illness: Prevalence, severity, and impact. *American Journal of Public Health, 82,* 364–371.

Newfeldt, V., & Guralnik, D. B. (1988). *Webster's New World Dictionary of American English* (3rd ed.). New York: Simon & Schuster.

Norman, P., & Conner, M. (1996). The role of social cognition models in predicting health behaviors: Future directions. In M. Conner & P. Norman (Eds.), *Predicting health behaviors* (pp. 197–225). Philadelphia, PA: Open University Press.

Olson, R. A., Holden, E. W., Friedman, A., Faust, J., Kenning, M., & Mason, P. J. (1989). Psychological consultation in a children's hospital. An evaluation of services. *Journal of Pediatric Psychology, 13,* 479–482.

Orme, C. M., & Binik, Y. M. (1989). Consistency of adherence across regimen demands. *Health Psychology, 8,* 27–43.

Palardy, N., Greening, L., Ott, J., Holderby, A., & Atchison, J. (1988). Adolescents' health attitudes and adherence to treatment for insulin-dependent diabetes mellitus. *Journal of Developmental and Behavioral Pediatrics, 19,* 31–37.

Passero, M. A., Remor, B., & Salomon, J. (1981). Patient-reported compliance with cystic fibrosis therapy. *Clinical Pediatrics, 20,* 264–268.

Patterson, J. M., Budd, J., Goetz, D., & Warwick, W. J. (1993). Family correlates of a 10-year pulmonary health trend in cystic fibrosis. *Pediatrics, 91,* 383–389.

Pedersen, S., & Moller-Petersen, J. (1984). Erratic absorption of a slow-release theophylline sprinkle product. *Pediatrics, 74,* 534–538.

Prochaska, J. L., & DiClemente, C. C. (1984). *The transtheoretical approach: Crossing traditional boundaries of change.* Homewood, IL: Dorsey.

Prochaska, J. O., & DiClemente, C. C. (1983). Stages and processes of self-change of smoking: Toward an integrative model of change. *Journal of Consulting and Clinical Psychology, 51,* 390–395.

Prochaska, J. O., DiClemente, C. C., & Norcross, J. C. (1992). In search of how people change: Applications to addictive behaviors. *American Psychologist, 47,* 1102–1114.

Prochaska, J. O., Velicer, W. F., Rossi, J. S., Goldstein, M. G., Marcus, B. H., Rakowski, W., Fiore, C., Harlow, L. L., Redding, C. A., Rosenbloom, D., & Rossi, S. R. (1994). Stages of change and decisional balance for 12 problem behaviors. *Health Psychology, 13,* 39–46.

Quittner, A. L., DiGirolamo, A. M., Michel, M., & Eigen, J. (1992). Parental response to CF: A contextual analysis of the diagnosis phase. *Journal of Pediatric Psychology, 17,* 683–704.

Radius, S. M., Becker, M. H., Rosenstock, I. M., Drachman, R. H., Schuberth, K. C., & Teets, K. C. (1978). Factors influencing mothers' compliance with a medication regimen for asthmatic children. *The Journal of Asthma Research, 15,* 133–149.

Rand, C. S. (2000). "I took the medicine like you told me doctor": Self report of adherence with medical regimens. In A. Stone, J. S. Tukkan, C. M. Bachrael, J. B. Jobe, H. J. Kurtzman, & V. S. Cain (Eds.), *The science of self report* (pp. 257–276). Mahwah, NJ: Lawrence Erlbaum Associates.

Rapoff, M. A. (1999). *Adherence to pediatric medical regimens.* New York: Kluwer Academic/Plenum.

Rapoff, M. A., Lindsley, C. B., & Christophersen, E.R. (1985). Improving compliance with medical regimens: Case study with juvenile rheumatoid arthritis. *Archives of Physical Medicine and Rehabilitation, 65,* 267–269.

Reynolds, L. A., Johnson, S. B., & Silverstein, J. (1990). Assessing daily diabetes management by 24-hour recall interview: The validity of children's reports. *Journal of Pediatric Psychology, 15,* 493–509.

Riekert, K. A., Wiener, L., Drotar, D., & Sprunk, K. (1999, April). *Medication use among adolescents with HIV.* Paper presented at the 7th Florida conference of Child Health Psychology, Gainesville, FL.

Rogers, R. W., & Prentice-Dunn, S. (1997). Protection Motivation Theory. In D. S. Gochman (Ed.), *Handbook of health behavior researcher: I. Personal and social determinants* (pp. 113–132). New York: Plenum.

Roter, D. L., Hall, J. S., Merisca, B., Nordstrom, B., Cretin, D., & Suarstad, B. C. (1998). Effectiveness of interventions to improve patient compliance. *A Meta-Analysis, 36,* 1138–1161.

Rudd, P. (1993). The measurement of compliance: Medication taking. In M. A. Krasnegor, L. Epstein, S. B. Johnson, & S. J. Yaffe (Eds.), *Developmental aspects of health compliance behavior* (pp. 185–213). Hillsdale, NJ: Lawrence Erlbaum Associates.

Ruggiero, L., & Prochaska, J. O. (1993). Readiness for change: Application of the transtheoretical model to diabetes. *Diabetes Spectrum, 6,* 21–60.

Satin, W., La Greca, A. M., Zigo, M. A., & Skyler, J. S. (1989). Diabetes in adolescence: Effects of multifamily group intervention and parent simulation of diabetes. *Journal of Pediatric Psychology, 14,* 259–276.

Sclar, D. A., Skaer, T. L., Chin, A., Okamoto, M. P., & Gill, M. A. (1991). Utility of a transdermal delivery system for antihypertensive therapy: Part 1. *American Journal of Medicine, 91,* 50S–56S.

Schafer, L. C., Glasgow, R. E., & McCaul, K. D. (1982). Increasing the adherence of diabetic adolescents. *Journal of Behavioral Medicine, 5,* 353–362.

Schafer, L. C., Glasgow, R. E., McCaul, K. D., & Dreher, M. (1983). Adherence to IDDM regimen: Relationship to psychosocial variables and metabolic control. *Diabetes Care, 6,* 493–498.

Schoni, M. H., Horak, E., & Nikolaizik, W. H. (1995). Compliance with therapy in children with respiratory diseases. *European Journal of Pediatrics, 154,* S77–S81.

Sergis-Deavenport, E., & Varni, J. W. (1982). Behavioral techniques in teaching hemophilia factor replacement procedures to families. *Pediatric Nursing, 8,* 416–419.

Sergis-Deavenport, E., & Varni, J. W. (1983). Behavioral assessment and management of adherence to factor replacement therapy in hemophilia. *Journal of Pediatric Psychology, 8,* 367–377.

Shope, J. T. (1988). Compliance in children and adults: Review of studies. *Epilepsy Research* (Suppl. 1), 23–47.

Sly, R. M. (1988). Mortality for asthma in children 1979–1984. *Annals of Allergy, 60,* 433–443.

Smith, N. A., Ley, P., Seale, J. P., & Shaw, J. (1987). Health beliefs, satisfaction, and compliance. *Patient Education and Counseling, 10,* 279–286.

Stein, M. T. (1999). An adolescent who abruptly stops his medication for attention deficit hyperactivity disorder. *Journal of Developmental and Behavioral Pediatrics, 20,* 106–110.

Strecher, V. J., Champion, V. L., & Rosenstock, I. M. (1997). The health belief model and health behavior. In D. S. Gochman (Ed.), *Handbook of health behavior research: I. Personal and social determinants* (pp. 71–91). New York: Plenum.

Stroebe, W., & Stroebe, M. S. (1995). *Social psychology and health.* Belmont, CA: Brooks/Cole.

Swanson, M., Hull, D., Bartus, S., & Schweizer, R. (1992). Economic impact of noncompliance in kidney transplant recipients. *Transplantation Proceedings, 24,* 27–32.

Tamaroff, M. A., Festa, R., Adesman, A. R., & Walco, G. (1992). Therapeutic adherence to oral medication regimens by adolescents with cancer: II. Clinical and psychologic correlates. *Journal of Pediatrics, 120,* 812–817.

Taylor, W. R., & Newacheck, P. W. (1992). Impact of childhood asthma on health. *Pediatrics, 90,* 657–662.

Tebbi, C. K. (1993). Treatment compliance in childhood and adolescence. *Cancer, 71* (Suppl.), 3441–3449.

Tebbi, C. K., Cummings, K. M., Zeron, M. A., Smith, L., Richards, M., & Mallon, J. (1986). Compliance of pediatric and adolescent cancer patients. *Cancer, 58,* 1179–1184.

Tebbi, C. K., Richards, M. D., Cummings, K. M., Zevon, M. A., & Mallon, J. C. (1988). The role of parent–adolescent concordance in compliance with cancer chemotherapy. *Adolescence, 23,* 599–611.

Vernazza, P. L., Gilliam, B., Dyer, M., Fiscus, S., Eron, J., Frank, A., & Cohen, M. (1997). Quantification of HIV in semen. Correlation with anti-retroviral treatment and immune states. *AIDS, 11,* 987–993.

Wade, S. L., Islam, S., Holden, G., Kruszon-Moran, D., & Mitchell, H. (1999). Division of responsibility for asthma management between caregivers and children in the inner city. *Journal of Developmental and Behavioral Pediatrics, 20,* 93–98.

Weinstein, A. G., & Faust, D. (1997). Maintaining theophylline compliance/adherence in severely asthmatic children: The role of psychologic functioning of the child and family. *Annals of Allergy, Asthma & Immunology, 29,* 311–318.

Weisberg-Benchell, J., Glasgow, A. M., Tynan, W. D., Wirtz, P., Turek, J., & Ward, J. (1995). Adolescent diabetes management and mismanagement. *Diabetes Care, 18,* 77–82.

Wood, P. R., Casey, R., Kolski, G. B., & McCormick, M. C. (1985). Compliance with oral theophylline therapy in asthmatic children. *Annals of Allergy, 54,* 400–404.

Wysocki, T., Meinhold, P. A., Abrams, K. C., Barnar, M. U., Clarke, W. L., Bellando, B. J., & Bourgeois, M. J. (1992). Parental and professional estimates of self-care independence of children and adolescents with IDDM. *Diabetes Care, 15,* 43–52.

PART II

HISTORICAL FOUNDATIONS

The contributors to this section consider historical foundations and evolution of the concept of *treatment adherence* and trends in research and practice. Trostle (chap. 2) begins with an interesting historical and anthropological account of compliance and adherence as definitions and research topics. He points out that the terms *compliance* and *adherence* reflect ideologies that support the authority of medical professionals, overemphasize the patient's response to the treatment regimen, and underemphasize the multiple competing tasks faced by individuals with chronic illness. Trostle registers concern that clinical care and research guided by concepts of adherence/compliance have generally neglected the broader context of illness management. Potentially important elements of this context includes patients' assumptions, motivations, and understandings of chronic illness and its treatment, and the changing context of prescribing and consuming medication, which is heavily influenced by managed care and pharmaceutical companies that advertise medications directly to consumers. Trostle considers reasons that the concepts of compliance/adherence continue to be so compelling to physicians and clinical researchers and articulates conceptual flaws of these concepts.

At the core of Trostle's analysis is that definitions of words such as *adherence* and *compliance* reflect ideologies—that is, systems of shared belief that legitimize behavioral norms and values. Such ideologies may serve to maintain the perception that health professionals are in control of health and health-related behavior. Along with his strong critique of the concepts of compliance and adherence, Trostle recognizes that taking medication according to an established routine can be productive for patients.

Tracing the historical foundations of *compliance* in the development of professional medicine and pharmaceutical industries in the United States, Trostle reminds readers that the newer term *adherence* may moderate the judgmental overtones of *compliance*, but does not really offer a new definition of behavior. Current health care trends relevant to this analysis include that physicians have less direct authority than previously compared with hospitals, HMOs, and pharmaceutical companies. At the same time, there is more emphasis on direct advertising to patients and their families in which compliance with medical treatment is proclaimed as a positive attribute.

One of the important features of this chapter is the description of the implications of a critical analysis of adherence for research and clinical practice, especially in understanding contextual influences on why medications are sought and taken. Important but as yet unanswered research questions are also raised by the impact of direct advertising to consumers on patient and provider behavior and the reported accuracy of medication use by patients.

In her discussion of pediatric compliance from a patient–family perspective in chap. 3, Korsch describes her pioneering research concerning the doctor–patient relationship in light of modern changes in patient care and consumer attitudes. Korsch's pioneering research describes a specific link between patient satisfaction and compliance, such that highly satisfied patients tend to comply with medical advice more than those who are not satisfied. Moreover, the quality of physician–parent communication is also correlated with patient satisfaction. Patients' perceptions of physicians as friendly and having elicited and understood their main concerns and expectations are strong predictors of satisfaction. Korsch's early findings have been replicated by many others.

Another line of Korsch's early research documents significant problems in compliance to immunosuppressive treatment among adolescents with renal transplants. This work also underscores the difficulty of communication with such patients, including the ineffectiveness of certain communication strategies (e.g., fear tactics) to motivate patients to comply with prescribed treatments.

One contribution of Korsch's chapter is to consider the potential implications of the changing role of the patient in modern health care—in particular, the fact that patients have become increasingly aware of their own rights and autonomy. Consistent with these trends, Korsch cites innovative research that has successfully intervened to improve health status and patient satisfaction. This is done by coaching patients to focus their questions and concerns and thus enhance their interactions with their physicians.

Korsch describes her current collaboration with the Bayer Institute for Health Communication and the Bayer model of patient–physician communication, which includes four sets of interrelated communication tasks to be accomplished in a medical consultation: (a) engaging patients in the relationship, (b) empathizing with the patients' concerns, (c) educating patients about their health and illness or concerns, and (d) enlisting patients in a therapeutic regimen. Korsch's recent work has centered on a practical examination of the doctor–patient relationship and the implications for medical education.

CHAPTER TWO

The Ideology of Adherence: An Anthropological and Historical Perspective

James A. Trostle
Trinity College, Hartford, CT

The focal point of the shrine is a box or chest which is built into the wall. In this chest are kept the many charms and magical potions without which no native believes he could live. These preparations are secured from a variety of specialized practitioners. The most powerful of these are the medicine men, whose assistance must be rewarded with substantial gifts. . . . The charm is not disposed of after it has served its purpose, but is placed in the charm-box of the household shrine. As these magical materials are specific for certain ills, and the real or imagined maladies of the people are many, the charm-box is usually full to overflowing. The magical packets are so numerous that people forget what their purposes were and fear to use them again. While the natives are very vague on this point, we can only assume that the idea in retaining all the old magical materials is that their presence in the charm-box, before which the body rituals are conducted, will in some way protect the worshipper.

—Miner (1956, p. 504, "Body Ritual Among the Nacirema")

Miner paid specific attention to what Americans (*Nacirema* spelled backward) do with unused medicines, thereby revealing our culture to ourselves. In fact, what people do with prescribed medicines has received extensive research attention since Miner published his essay. Almost 16,000 English-language articles on how people take medicines have been published in the past two decades. Yet one of the best-known researchers in the field recently lamented that few rigorous intervention trials have been published, concluding that "strategies tested in these studies for improving adherence with long-term medication prescriptions were not very effective despite the amount of effort and resources that they consumed" (Haynes, McKibbon, & Kanani, 1996, p. 382).

I argue that medication taking (or rather *not taking* in the context of this volume) is poorly understood and that this is so at least partly because the concept and definition of *medication taking* has been flawed from the start. The reason for this is that researchers and clinicians alike have failed to pay adequate attention to history, meaning, and the social context surrounding the taking of pills. Better understanding of this context can yield more accurate descriptions of what people do with the medicines they are prescribed and, more important, yield more complete pictures of the multiple determinants of pill taking. In turn, a more complete understanding of determinants can potentially lead to more effective interventions.

Since the 1970s, the range of ways that pills, medications, and other prescribed treatments have been taken has most often been called *medical compliance*, although many other words and definitions have been suggested (e.g., adherence, self-medication, self-regulation, medication consumption, concordance; see Riekert & Drotar, chap. 1, this volume; Bauman, chap. 4, this volume; Creer, chap. 5, this volume). A major book in the late 1970s provided what came to be the accepted definition of *medical compliance*: "the extent to which the patient's behavior (in terms of taking medications, following diets, or executing other lifestyle changes) coincides with medical or health advice" (Haynes, 1979, p. 2). Although the word *compliance* continues to predominate in research and advertising two decades later, the word *adherence* is now jockeying for position. According to one proponent of the term, *adherence* refers to following a plan more than it does following a professional's advice, and therefore is less judgmental and more descriptive (Fawcett, 1995).

Compliance as a research topic has attracted a great deal of contemporary attention both in clinical and social science journals. As of mid-May 1999, 16,658 English-language research and review articles on the topic had been included in the *Index Medicus* and other bibliographic collections since 1943. A 1979 cumulative bibliography on the subject listed only 22 articles in English published before 1960 and 850 published by 1978 (Haynes, Sackett, & Taylor, 1979). Production of articles about compliance increased dramatically between 1966 and 1995 (see Fig. 2.1). It increased almost six-fold between 1971–1975 and 1976–1980 and then grew by 56% in the next 5 years (1981–1985), 30% between 1986 and 1990, and 17% between 1991 and 1995. This illustrates the dramatic and

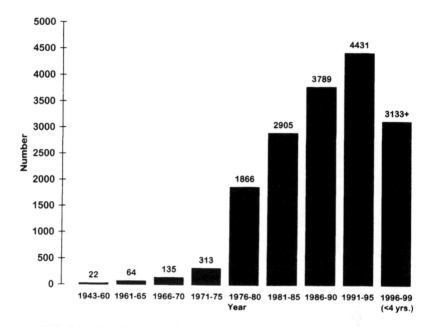

FIG. 2.1. Compliance articles published by grouped year of publication. Adapted from Haynes (1979), Figure 1.1, and *Index Medicus* postings from 1978 to 1999 (last period incomplete).

continuing growth of research interest in this aspect of patient–doctor relationships.

This chapter explores why therapeutic compliance—and, more recently, adherence—have received such attention over the past three decades. It employs Horace Miner's strategy of taking what is familiar and trying to make it strange. I have previously contended that compliance is not a productive topic for behavioral research in medicine and should instead be analyzed primarily as an ideology supporting the authority of medical professionals (Trostle, 1988). In this chapter, I argue that the concept of *patient adherence* maintains this problem because it offers a new word but continues many of the problematic assumptions of the old one. Adherence emphasizes fidelity to a medical regimen over the many other concerns facing people with illnesses. Its primary focus on treatment regimen reduces our ability to see that managing illness is just one of the multiple competing but ongoing tasks facing an individual with a treatable disease. Like leaving a hospital against medical advice, refusing to wear seatbelts, or engaging in high-risk behavior, nonadherence is one of those behaviors resistant to understanding from a health-centered perspective, at least in part because it contravenes professional notions of rational (health-seeking or health-maintaining) behavior.

Anthropology contributes to the study of compliance/adherence[1] by showing that pills have symbolic power in addition to active ingredients (Nichter & Vuckovic, 1994; Van der Geest, Whyte, & Hardon 1996). Pill taking is just one of a range of things people do to take care of themselves, and pill prescribing just one way that healers can potentially reduce suffering. Anthropology broadens our frame of reference, emphasizing that the context of pill taking matters as much as the behavior. To understand the multiple determinants of pill taking, we must expand beyond the existing emphasis on patients to include more and better attention to health personnel, researchers, and pharmaceutical companies.

It is easy to understand why patients—those closest to the act of taking a pill—are commonly seen as primarily responsible for noncompliance/adherence. However, we too often forget the many other sources of influence: Physicians help create or sustain expectations of rapid cure (Quirt et al., 1997), but often fail to explore patient assumptions, motivations, and understandings (Braddock, Fihn, Levinson, Jonsen, & Pearlman, 1997; Makoul, Arntson, & Schofield, 1995); they resort to medications rather than other disease management or healing strategies (Colley & Lucas 1993). Researchers also pay excessive attention to the patient-based side of compliance/adherence. For example, they neglect how advertising influences the cost and attractiveness of medications to physicians and patients alike (Ferner & Scott, 1994; Zuger, 1999). They have failed to adequately study the dramatically changing context of prescribing and consuming medications in the United States, where managed care companies influence the length of doctor–patient encounters (Gordon, Baker, & Levinson, 1995) and pharmaceutical companies advertise medications directly to consumers (Hollon, 1999). Finally, pharmaceutical companies are implicated in the problem of compliance/adherence through pressuring physicians to prescribe medications rather than look for other treatment options (Nyquist, Gonzales, Steiner, & Sande, 1998; Schwartz, Mainous, & Marcy, 1998; Zuger, 1999). This creates impossibly high expectations about the efficacy of medications among patients (Brody, 1998; Ferriman, 1999) or, as I show later, transforms compliance from a behavioral issue into an attribute of pills.

Instead of repeating a series of criticisms of compliance that have been articulated for three decades (e.g., Conrad, 1985; Haug & Lavin 1983; Hayes-Bautista, 1976; Lerner, Gulick, & Dubler, 1998; Morris & Schulz, 1993; Stimson, 1974; Trostle, Hauser, & Susser, 1983; Weintraub, 1976; Zola, 1981), I instead ask why the concepts of compliance/adherence continue to be so compelling to physicians and clinical researchers. Second, I

---

[1]Because the concepts *compliance* and *adherence* are so similar, I use the phrase *compliance/adherence* when I wish to refer to the overlapping domains they represent. I separate the two words when I want to pay more specific attention to one or the other.

look more carefully to prove that adherence and compliance both suffer from the same conceptual handicaps. Finally, and most fundamentally, I ask how the consumption of medicine (the behavioral base for most acts of compliance or adherence) is likely to change in the future as television and the Internet make medical knowledge more available and pharmaceutical companies again advertise directly to patients.

WHY ARE COMPLIANCE AND ADHERENCE SO COMPELLING?

I explore three answers to this question: (a) because the concepts are ideologies; (b) although compliance and adherence are ideologies, medicines matter because they have both curative and symbolic power; and (c) because compliance is about relationships between professional healers and sufferers. As those relationships change over time, so do research models, intervention designs, and other attempts to influence the distribution and use of medications.

Because Compliance and Adherence Are Ideologies

The continuing popularity of adherence and compliance can be better understood if they are analyzed as ideologies—that is, systems of "shared beliefs that legitimize particular behavioral norms and values at the same time that they claim and appear to be based in empirical truths. Ideologies help to transform power (potential influence) into authority (legitimate control)" (Trostle, 1988, p. 1300). Most theories about compliance and adherence transform the behavior of people who are sick into a series of research strategies, research results, and potentially coercive interventions that appear appropriate and reinforce professional authority over health care. Most compliance research defines and evaluates patient behavior in terms of imposed professional expectations. Most adherence research, even when it pays closer attention to a regimen mutually negotiated between health professionals and patients, also defines fidelity to that regimen as the central component of proper care. Both compliance and adherence as research topics still generally ignore other health-related behaviors and practices (saving medications at home, re-using prescriptions or sharing medications with others, using antibiotics in animal feed) that contradict the common perception of health professionals that they are central to all health care. The topics of adherence and compliance help physicians make sense of the world and the dilemmas of patient care. Ideas like these develop in professional training, get reinforced through personal experience, and maintain the perception that health professionals rightfully control health and health-related behavior.

Because Taking Medication Matters

This strong critique of *compliance* and *adherence* should not be interpreted to mean that taking medication according to some established routine is an impossible or unreasonable goal. Taking pills at irregular intervals, or at consistently reduced or excessive levels, can cause health problems or extend the illnesses of individuals or groups, although it does not always do so. Directly observed therapy for tuberculosis was developed partly to ensure that therapeutic levels of medications were reached and maintained through time, and the increased compliance under these conditions has led to dramatically higher rates of control or cure (Lerner et al., 1998).

Both consumption that varies from professional expectations and prescription that varies from accepted standards can cause a medication's therapeutic effectiveness to be reduced and/or misjudged both in individuals and large-scale clinical trials. Unfortunately, research on compliance/adherence generally neglects to wonder whether prescribing has been appropriate in the first place, although this was one of the ethical standards mentioned in the early days of the field (Jonsen, 1979) and was one of the reasons for emphasizing quality improvement or developing treatment plans and practice guidelines. The goal of most adherence research is to help patients take medications, not to help physicians decide whether or how to prescribe them. Such research appears to assume that medication consumption, and underlying illness management, is always a person's first priority.

Failure to take medications is becoming more damaging to the public health because of the increased risk of developing drug-resistant strains of bacteria (see e.g., Wise et al., 1998). Under these circumstances, complete and timely consumption of medicines is becoming a more important component of treatment strategies. This also means that those whose medication taking is least predictable are at greatest risk of being denied treatment (Lerner et al., 1998). Under these circumstances, mere risk of poor adherence can be detrimental to an individual's welfare. A distinction between compliance and adherence is largely academic here.

Medications also matter because they are a large and profitable portion of the economy. The total value of shipments of pharmaceutical preparations in the United States in 1996 was $61.5 billion, or about .8% of the nation's gross domestic product in that year (U.S. Department of Commerce, 1998). Pharmaceutical companies use the word *compliance* in their advertisements to promote therapeutic effects and more: Compliance is part of a promotional strategy to increase market share and product sales. Increased compliance is a positive attribute like low cost, short course, few side effects, or therapeutic efficacy.

Because History Shows Us That Compliance and Adherence Are About Relationships Between Healers and Sufferers (This section is a revised and condensed version of the historical argument in Trostle, 1988)

Most compliance researchers have explained the growth of their literature by linking it to the development of antibiotics in the 1950s and the subsequent wide availability of these effective treatments. They mistakenly assume that scientific measures of efficacy are the foundation of professional beliefs about clinical efficacy. However, medical anthropologists and historians have shown that most healers in any historical period (be they physicians, bonesetters, barbers, surgeons, or shamans) believe in and help reinforce the curative powers of their treatments (Etkin, 1991; Temkin, 1964; Unschuld, 1991). Physicians are part of a historically and geographically bounded profession that was organized within the past century to provide health care. Yet people everywhere consume substances to cure illness and have apparently been doing so since recorded history began (Temkin, 1964). What one era called *effective treatments* become labeled as *outmoded therapies* in later times, but at each of those historical moments the healers would insist that their treatments are effective and that their patients should do as they have been told.

To explain the popularity of compliance, we must go beyond the efficacy of pharmaceuticals measured in biomedical terms to cultural beliefs in curative substances and the history of medicine. The history of compliance as an ideology can be uncovered by looking at texts that address and reveal the self-image of the medical profession. Such a history portrays the origins and growth of concerns about compliance. Rather than resulting solely from medical advances in the past three decades, contemporary concern for compliance also grew out of the monopoly of physicians over health care in the United States from the early 1900s to the late 1980s.

The growing concern for medication compliance/adherence can be explained in part by pointing to the developing consolidation of the profession of medicine and the growth and sales strategies of the pharmaceutical and proprietary drug industries. In the early 1900s, U.S. physicians were still struggling for prestige and market control. This was a time when patent medicine companies advertised their products directly to the general public and touted them as cheap alternatives to medical care. The federal government fought against this practice with the Pure Food and Drugs Act of 1906, where it set initial standards for labeling drug ingredients and claims of efficacy. In 1938, it passed the Food, Drug, and Cosmetic Act with further restrictions and additional enforcement provisions. The American Medical Association (AMA) stopped accepting patent medicine advertisements in its Journal in 1905, and in 1924 it reserved the right to reject advertising for approved drugs from companies that derived earnings from other unapproved drugs. Although physicians and politicians both campaigned against misrepresentation of health products, they did so with somewhat different goals: The government meant to make consumer information more accurate, whereas the AMA wanted to make information accurate as well as control the amount of health product information consumers received. It could thereby increase physician control over medicines and other health-related products (Apple, 1982, 1987; Starr, 1982).

At this time of increasing government regulation, infant formula companies took preparation directions and feeding schedules off containers of infant formulas and directed advertising at physicians rather than the lay public. (This is called the *ethical push* route for advertising, whereas the *consumer pull* strategy is to advertise in the mass media directly to the public.) Physicians would be more respectable and profitable salesmen than the company sales force; as time passed, physician control over the distribution of certain health-related products began to appear natural and even necessary. (See Apple's [1982] recounting of the history of the formula-marketing decision.) The sales strategy was expanded to vitamin supplements and became the model for marketing prescription pharmaceuticals until the past decade. The strategy was forthrightly articulated in the advertising section of the *Journal of the American Medical Association*, where one full-page advertisement in 1931 concluded with the following paragraphs:

> When the physician reads this class of exploiting advertisement which patronizingly refers to his endorsement of the most ridiculous claims, and later hears his patients knowingly repeating these to him, he cannot help asking himself these questions:
> (1) Should the layman receive his medical education, including his vitaminmindedness, from the commercial house, or from his doctor?
> (2) Should the commercial house exploit vitamins in modern patent medicine style, or should the physician control their intelligent application?
> Mead Johnson & Company, for one, continue to feel that vitamin therapy, like infant feeding, should be in the hands of the medical profession, and consequently refuse to lend their aid to exploiting these valuable agents to the public. This house, for one, advertises its vitamin products exclusively to the medical profession and furnishes no directions to the public. (p. 46)

This deliberate company decision to advertise its marketing strategy was effective because it reflected and amplified a sentiment already common among U.S. physicians—namely, that the medical profession should maintain control over the distribution of infant formula. What is most interesting is that an ideology of *physician control itself* is being created and promoted here; an explicit announcement of support for physician control of patient behavior is used to sell products.

Mead Johnson had the most visible "No Laity Advertising" strategy used in its campaigns until the mid-1940s for products ranging from infant formula to fish liver oil. However, it was not the only company to extol this strategy. Similar claims were also made by the Corn Products Sales Company for its Karo syrup for infant feeding and by the Nestlé corporation for its Lactogen infant formula.

Patient control and physician self-interest were not the only advertising strategies used to emphasize compliance. Companies also raised concerns about patients' abilities to take medications reliably, suggesting that particular formulations would reduce patient forgetfulness. This strategy was used in the 1934 *Journal of the American Medical Association* in an advertisement promoting evaporated milk with cod-liver oil extract, part of which stated:

> YOU FORGOT again MOTHER. Yes . . . mothers *do* forget!
> How many mothers forget to give regularly the cod-liver oil you prescribe? Many doctors are now recommending DEAN'S so that the children under their care are assured a regular and definite supply of Vitamin "D." . . . (p. 33)

Taken together, these advertisements demonstrate that: (a) a concern for controlling patient behavior antedated the development of antibiotics; (b) the U.S. medical profession's interest in maintaining control over patients' behavior and access to information was recognized and reinforced from the 1920s to 1940s; (c) professional self-interest was a significant factor in the movement to limit popular advertising of infant feeding products and vitamins; and (d) the contemporary concern for compliance was openly articulated earlier in the 20th century as a concern for patient cooperation and physician control.

IS ADHERENCE A BETTER CONCEPT?

Even if adherence does moderate the judgmental overtones of compliance, it does not offer a new definition of behavior. Both adherence and compliance face a classificatory challenge: These words are really epithets—broad labels that mask and blend complex sets of actions into seemingly coherent and consistent categories.

Adherence is a particularly problematic concept for pediatric patients because taking medications is often not under a child's control. Worse yet, many of the assumptions about patient responsibility, rationality, and control inherent in the concept of adherence do not apply in the case of children. The literature on compliance, and what little predictive conclusions have emerged from it, have been based primarily on adult patients rather than pediatric patients or adult caregivers of children.

Adherence is also attracting increasing attention as a focus of clinical research. It is far harder to trace scientific production under this term, however, because the *Index Medicus*, the indexing system used by the U.S. National Library of Medicine, does not use patient adherence as a Medical Subject Heading (MeSH) on MedLine—its online index to its journal holdings. In contrast, *patient compliance* has been used since 1975 as a MeSH search term, defined as "voluntary cooperation of the patient in following a prescribed regimen" (U.S. Department of Health and Human Services and National Library of Medicine, 1998, p. 885). *Patient nonadherence* is not a MeSH term either, but the MedLine subject heading guide notes that "it is associated with the MeSH term 'Treatment Refusal.' " *Treatment refusal* has been a MeSH category only since 1991, defined as "refusal of a person to accept medical or psychiatric treatment or his unwillingness to comply with the physician's instructions or prescribed regimens" (U.S. Department of Health and Human Services and National Library of Medicine, 1998, p. 1198). The outcome of this categorization is that the National Library of Medicine appears to classify voluntary cooperation as compliance, but unwillingness to comply as treatment refusal.

Although the term *adherence* is thought by some to reduce some problematic assumptions within the term *compliance*, it is still practically invisible in the research literature. Because adherence is not a recognized MeSH term, it can only be searched as a text word in titles and abstracts. To get a rough sense of the growing popularity of this concept, the set of 16,114 English-language MedLine records categorized under the MeSH term *patient compliance* between 1976 and mid-1999 was searched to find titles using the word *adherence*. (The year 1976 was chosen because that is when the MeSH heading *patient compliance* was started.) It was found that 490 of these articles used the word *adherence* in their titles between 1976 and 1999, with 311 doing so between 1991 and 1999. Expressed as a percentage of total articles in English categorized under the MeSH heading *patient compliance*, those using the word *adherence* in their titles increased from 1.6% of the total in the 1976–1980 period to 2.2% of the total in 1981–1985, 2.2% again between 1986 and 1990, 3.5% between 1991 and 1995, and 5.0% between 1996 and 1999 (and this last is a 4- rather than 5-year period). The term *adherence* still occupies a relatively small proportion of the articles on compliance, although it is growing in popularity among contemporary researchers. The present concern to distinguish compliance from adherence can clearly be seen more than 20 years ago in an article by Steckel, Funnell, and Dragovan (1979) published by the American Nursing Association, entitled "How Nursing Care Can Increase Patient Adherence Rather Than Patient Compliance."

The concern for compliance is a cultural phenomenon intimately connected with the self-image of physicians and their organized (and often successful) attempts to define the limits of their own discipline. Yet the present respect and authority accorded physicians in the United States is of recent origin and has been diminishing over the past two decades (Balint & Shelton, 1996; Haug & Lavin, 1983; McKinlay & Arches, 1985; Mechanic & Scheslinger, 1996). Physicians have exercised their control over medical technology and pharmaceuticals only in the past century. Now for-profit hospitals, HMOs, and other types of medical groups are employing physicians as salaried workers; their growth is reducing physicians' monopolistic power. Physician control over the technology of medical care is also decreasing because pharmaceutical companies are again advertising directly to consumers, the Food and Drug Administration (FDA) is moving drugs from prescription to nonprescription categories, and HMOs are developing restricted formularies.

Some would argue that the preoccupation with compliance over the past two decades is partly a consequence of this declining authority of the medical profession. Since the 1980s, pharmaceutical companies have increasingly recognized patient power outside the examining room, most directly in the increasing trend of direct to consumer advertising. Even the ads they direct to physicians in medical journals acknowledge the dilemma posed by patients' power. For example, an ad for the cough suppressant Tessalon Perles™ announces that the product can "Balance the cough suppression doctors demand and the side-effect profile patients prefer." The explicit mention of patient preference reflects the research finding that side effects reduce medication compliance. Although the ad raises the delicate issue of patients' power here, note how adroitly it manages it for a physician audience. In addition to offering the alliteration of "doctors demand" and "patients prefer," the ad also grants doctors the greater power of demand over preference.

Advertisers proclaim compliance as an attribute to increase the visibility of their products and enhance their company's positive image among physicians and the lay public. Thus, in 1998, two-page advertisements in pediatric medical journals for the single-dose injectable antibiotic Rocephin™ proclaimed in large bold type that the product offered "Guaranteed 100% compliance." Is *compliance* a relevant category to use for a single injection? Not according to the Haynes definition because a single injection allows no variance between patient behavior (accepting an injection) and medical advice (if injecting a patient could be construed as advice). Furthermore, why combine the concepts of *guaranteed* and *100%* in describing compliance with a single injection unless the concept of

compliance raises compelling uncertainty? Could there be less than complete compliance with an injection? Not if it is given. The idea that compliance could be an issue and that a therapy guaranteeing 100% compliance is better than one offering, say, 65% compliance creates new routes
by which to convince physicians that Rocephin™ is a powerful product.
These advertising slogans show the rhetorical power that the concept of
compliance contains: Raised as a relevant benefit and strengthened by
guarantees and percentages, compliance becomes an important part of a
sales pitch.

This is not the only manifestation of this symbolic power of compliance.
For example, advertisements in pediatric journals in 1998 for the oral
antibiotic Suprax™ stated that it offered "compliance-enhancing features
that work against otitis media." Although its simplified regimen may
increase compliance, the treatment efficacy of Suprax™ for otitis media in
children does not appear to be dramatically better than that of other far
less expensive regimens. (Some clinical data increasingly support that
often no antibiotic at all is the best treatment for otitis media.) When once-
a-day dosing becomes a compliance-enhancing feature, we should be
aware that language is being manipulated toward some end.

Of course, this is nothing new. We have reviewed some of the ways professionals (and industries) have concerned themselves in the past with
patient consumption of vitamins, infant formula, and medications. We saw
images of forgetful mothers and weak patients in the 1930s and 1940s,
accompanied by sales strategies that increased physician control and
patient dependence. From the 1960s to the early 1980s, physician control
over patient medical regimes was almost taken for granted, and efficacy,
convenience, and safety became important themes in drug advertising. For
example, a full-page advertisement in 1984 for the cardiovascular agent
Lopressor™ had all three of its bold-faced claims emphasizing safety: "Safe
from diaretic-induced K-loss complications," "Excellent safety record," and
"A safe bet for compliance." The late 1980s and 1990s saw a growing
awareness of the limited power physicians have to change their patient's
behavior and the introduction in advertising of themes like patient
lifestyle. This is captured in the headline for a 1998 ad for a diabetes medication called GlucotrolXL™: "Since it's hard to change lifestyle, their first
diabetic agent should be easy." We can expect the rationale for medication
usage to continue to change in the future in response to changing perceptions of the doctor–patient relationship and changing constraints on
that relationship. If physicians increasingly become sources of prescriptions rather than sources of advice and care, we will see more pharmaceutical advertising directed at consumers and more emphasis on patient
lifestyle, convenience, and quality of life in pharmaceutical advertising
directed at physicians. In this new context, the financial power of phar-

maceutical companies will compel both patients and physicians to grapple with questionable claims about the efficacy, safety, and cost-effectiveness of medications. Additional strategies will be needed to evaluate this rapidly increasing flow of information and advice and to form credible sources of guidance.

Antibiotic resistance is a relatively new concern in prescribing and will form a growing part of arguments about both prescribing and taking medications. Poor compliance is one contributor to this resistance, especially remarked on at present in treatment for HIV and tuberculosis. Ironically, just as pharmaceutical companies are increasing their direct pressure on consumers to request medications, concerns about antibiotic-resistant strains of bacteria are moving researchers to inquire how to reduce inappropriate prescribing and inappropriate use of antibiotics in animal feed (Belongia & Schwartz, 1998). This may cause researchers in the future to pay more attention to patient, professional, and industrial contributions to inappropriate medication use.

RECOMMENDATIONS

I have not described the growth of the compliance/adherence ideology here merely for historical interest. It has pragmatic consequences for researchers, physicians, and patients because, like any ideology, it guides and justifies behavior. My recommendations for what to do about this ideology fall into two areas: First, investigate why medications are sought and taken; second, investigate how medications are used. Such investigations should be a task for both researchers and healers.

Why Medications Are Sought and Taken

The meaning of medication differs within different groups and for different conditions. More research and clinical inquiry must explore how people think medications work and where medications fit into patient definitions of quality of life. Questions should include whether medication effects might be manipulated for nonmedical purposes (skipping some medications to precipitate parental concern for an adolescent in crisis) or medical purposes other than those envisioned by the physician (a patient takes extra beta-blockers to calm nerves).

Researchers could hypothesize that all patients are potential noncompliers and that particular kinds of situations or expectations cause noncompliance. Instead, most compliance research hypothesizes that there are noncompliant types of people and that with sufficient ingenuity their traits can be identified. If we assume that all patients are potential noncompliers, we need more research and clinical attention paid to exactly what the margins of tolerance are for error among different drugs (which ones *must* be taken on schedule and which, because of half life or pharmacological pathway, tolerate more variability in dosage or frequency). The goal here is to tailor the prescription to the patient and drug, asking and expecting no greater adherence than is required.

Finally, we need to better understand what role prescriptions and medications play in doctor–patient interactions. If physicians see prescriptions as the best way to close a clinical encounter and patients expect good physicians to prescribe drugs, the power of medications is both symbolic and pharmacological. Interventions that ignore these and other aspects of the context of medication usage are less likely to be effective.

How Medications Are Used

To have a clinical effect, medications must be prescribed appropriately, taken appropriately, and therapeutically effective. Research on doctor–patient interaction can form one important part of this solution by increasing attention to the need to listen, explain, and explore patients' and physicians' motivations for their behavior and how they communicate together (see DiMatteo, chap. 10, this volume).

Compliance/adherence research can also pay far more attention to how medications are used by individuals, families, physicians, veterinarians, and even feedlots. For example, how do physician and patient beliefs about the efficacy of medications influence the probability that they will be consumed appropriately? Are specific strategies of pill taking (consistent excessive or reduced amounts, excessive amounts just before clinical appointments, sporadic consumption) associated with any qualities of a medication, illness, or expectations about the ways medications work within the body? Are they associated with specific intrafamily conflicts and relationships? Are different perceptions of side effects (desirable/undesirable; short-term/long-term; physiological vs. emotional) associated with different patterns of medication consumption? Are different types of regimens tolerable to different (age/sex/ethnicity/disease) groups of patients? At present these questions are largely unanswerable because we do not know enough about how people use medications when they depart from clinical prescriptions.

This chapter has emphasized that compliance/adherence is one component of the relationship between patients and physicians. How do other aspects of that relationship (e.g., ease of communication, familiarity, level of mutual understanding, frequency of contact) influence this aspect of medication consumption? Other aspects of the context of medication taking must also receive more detailed research attention: How are leftover prescriptions disposed of? What causes compliance with placebos to produce better clinical results than noncompliance with placebos?

With the advent of Internet prescribing, direct advertising to consumers, managed care, and increased newspaper and media attention to the newsworthiness of health issues, new forces are influencing the doctor–patient relationship. Does medication use change when people obtain medications directly from Internet sites? Does it change when they request and get specific medications from their physicians or when they obtain medications from other types of healers? Are people more compliant/adherent to their own pill-taking regimens (e.g., when taking vitamins) than they are to regimens suggested by others? These questions about medication use require more attention and research.

The issue of reporting accuracy is related to medication use. Existing research on medications pays too little attention to the accuracy and method of recall and estimation processes. What mental processes do people use to reconstruct how accurately they take their pills? Do they calculate from a hypothetical average number of pills missed? Count the number of days containing errors? Extrapolate from an overall judgment about the nature of their ability to follow instructions? How often are electronic monitoring devices useful to patients and how often are they used without a patient's knowledge (see Drotar et al., chap. 20, this volume)?

Finally, the therapeutic power of medications rests partly on their clinical efficacy, but we can no longer take this efficacy for granted. It is likely that some uses of medications (e.g., poor prescribing for otitis media or diarrheal diseases or distribution to animals to promote weight gain) actually promote the growth of antibiotic-resistant bacteria. It does little good to urge greater adherence to medications that are unneeded in the first place or are losing their clinical efficacy in the population at large.

CONCLUSION

Compliance and adherence are popular topics among health care workers because they provide a focus to their interactions with *problem* patients, reflect their ideas about how patients should behave, and address their notions about the determinants of proper patient behavior. A number of factors have combined to bring noncompliance to clinical attention within the past four decades: Increasing numbers of prescription drugs made noncompliance more possible and thus more visible, drug companies often mentioned compliance in their advertising, social scientists and clinicians convinced the growing biomedical research industry to examine the behavioral correlates of the problem, and health educators designed interventions. None of these should be singled out as the most important influence, but all have combined to create and sustain a long period of research on the topic.

Analyzing compliance as an ideology is useful because it helps explain why the more than 16,600 English-language articles on the topic form a literature so contradictory and incomplete, yet so repetitive. Looking at patient behavior in terms of medical compliance/adherence perpetuates the notion that health care is (and should be) centered around proper use of physicians. The causes of problems in the patient–physician relationship are usually sought in patient behavior and beliefs.

In essence, my argument is that we (researchers, patients, health care workers, pharmaceutical companies) have come to act as if compliance/adherence and noncompliance/nonadherence are specifiable categories of behavior capable of being analyzed as discrete attributes of individuals. However, we only know what compliance/adherence is: faithfulness to a particular regimen. The actions falling under the rubric *noncompliant/nonadherent* range broadly from stopping medications too early to taking them infrequently, sporadically, or excessively. Keeping unused medications in the medicine cabinet, as described in Miner's earlier quote, could also be labeled *noncompliance*. Thus, although we can specify what compliance/adherence is, it is not particularly easy to specify what noncompliance/nonadherence is. Second, compliance is thought to be a discrete behavior because it is too often analyzed separately from its (historical, social, relational) context and because behavior called *compliance* is assumed to be a primary objective of people receiving treatment. When medication taking is seen in context, it can be shown to fulfill many other motivations at once, ranging from a desire to satisfy a physician or family members or peers to a work-related need or a desire to enhance or diminish specific side effects.

Descriptions of patient behavior and interventions designed to influence it have come full circle during this century. Early in the 1900s, there was a struggle in the United States between companies that sought to influence patients directly and physician organizations that sought to consolidate their professional control. Patient education became accepted practice somewhat later, accompanied by attempts to increase patient responsibility and self-control, as well as attempts to bring patients subtly around to adopting physician desires as their own. More recently, we can again see attempts by advertisers to directly influence patients to request and use prescription medications. At the same time, regimens are being simplified with long-acting medications increasingly marketed and injectable forms recommended. These interventions can be effective, but they risk turning patients from responsible subjects to responsive objects, with information about the appropriateness of treatment again becoming the primary domain of people other than patients. When medicines become more powerful and their delivery guaranteed (through injection, for example), it becomes even more important to balance the attention compliance/adherence researchers have paid to patients. Given recent estimates of the death toll from adverse drug reactions (Stolberg, 1999), we must work as hard to ensure that a medication is prescribed correctly as we do to ensure that it is taken correctly.

ACKNOWLEDGMENT

This chapter is a substantially revised version of J. Trostle (1988), "Medical Compliance as an Ideology," *Social Science & Medicine 27*(12), 1299–1308, used here with permission from Pergamon Press. The original article was supported by the Epilepsy Foundation of America, the Wenner-Gren Foundation for Anthropological Research, the U.C. Berkeley Rennie Endowment, and the National Institute of Mental Health (MH09039-01 to -03.) I am grateful to Andrew Noymer for his bibliographical assistance.

REFERENCES

Apple, R. D. (1982). To be used only under the direction of a physician: Commercial infant feeding and medical practice, 1870–1940. *Bulletin of the History of Medicine, 54*, 402–417.

Apple, R. D. (1987). *Mothers and medicine: A social history of infant feeding, 1890–1950* (Wisconsin Publications in the History of Science and Medicine, Number 7). Madison, WI: University of Wisconsin Press.

Balint, J., & Shelton W. (1996). Regaining the initiative. Forging a new model of the patient–physician relationship. *Journal of the American Medical Association, 275*, 887–891.

Belongia, E. A., & Schwartz, B. (1998). Rethinking adherence: Historical perspectives on triple-drug therapy for HIV disease. *Annals of Internal Medicine, 129*, 573–578.

Braddock, C. H. III, Fihn, S. D., Levinson, W., Jonsen, A. R., & Pearlman, R. A. (1997). How doctors and patients discuss routine clinical decisions. Informed decision making in the outpatient setting. *Journal of General Internal Medicine, 12*, 339–345.

Brody, J. E. (1998, December 15). Drug ads lure patients into jargon-strewn territory. *The New York Times*, p. D7.

Colley, C. A., & Lucas, L. M. (1993). Polypharmacy: The cure becomes the disease. *Journal of General Internal Medicine, 8*, 278–283.

Conrad, P. (1985). The meaning of medications: Another look at compliance. *Social Science & Medicine, 20*, 29–37.

Etkin, N. (1991). Cultural constructions of efficacy. In S. Van der Geest & S. R. Whyte (Eds.), *The context of medicines in developing countries: Studies in pharmaceutical anthropology* (pp. 299–326). Amsterdam: Het Spinhuis.

Fawcett, J. (1995). Compliance: Definitions and key issues. *Journal of Clinical Psychiatry, 56* (Suppl. 1), 4–8.

Ferner, R. E., & Scott, D. K. (1994). Whatalotwegot—the messages in drug advertisements. *British Medical Journal, 309*, 1734–1736.

Ferriman, A. (1999). Drug companies criticised for exaggeration. *British Medical Journal, 318*, 962.

Gordon, G. H., Baker, L., & Levinson, W. (1995). Physician–patient communication in managed care. *Western Journal of Medicine, 163*, 527–531.

Haug, M., & Lavin, B. (1983). *Consumerism in medicine: Challenging physician authority.* Beverly Hills, CA: Sage.

Hayes-Bautista, D. (1976). Modifying the treatment: Patient compliance, patient control and medical care. *Social Science & Medicine, 10*, 233–238.

Haynes, R. B. (1979). Introduction. In R.B. Haynes, D.L. Sackett, & D.W. Taylor (Eds.), *Compliance in health care* (pp. 1–10). Baltimore: Johns Hopkins University Press.

Haynes, R. B., McKibbon, K. A., & Kanani, R. (1996). Systematic review of randomised trials of interventions to assist patients to follow prescriptions for medications. *Lancet, 348*, 383–386.

Haynes, R. B., Sackett, D. L., & Taylor, D. W. (Eds.). (1979). *Compliance in health care.* Baltimore: Johns Hopkins University Press.

Hollon, M. F. (1999). Direct-to-consumer marketing of prescription drugs: Creating consumer demand. *Journal of the American Medical Association, 281*, 382–384.

Jonsen, A. R. (1979). Ethical issues in compliance. In R. B. Haynes, D. L. Sackett, & D. W. Taylor (Eds.), *Compliance in health care* (pp. 113–120). Baltimore: Johns Hopkins University Press.

Lerner, B. H., Gulick, R. M., & Dubler, N. N. (1998). Rethinking nonadherence: Historical perspectives on triple-drug therapy for HIV disease. *Annals of Internal Medicine, 129*, 573–578.

Makoul, G., Arntson, P., & Schofield T. (1995). Health promotion in primary care: Physician–patient communication and decision making about prescription medications. *Social Science and Medicine, 41*, 1241–1254.

McKinlay, J. B., & Arches, J. (1985). Towards the proletarianization of physicians. *International Journal of Health Services, 15*, 161–195.

Mechanic, D., & Schlesinger, M. (1996). The impact of managed care on patients' trust in medical care and their physicians. *Journal of the American Medical Association, 275*, 1693–1697.

Miner, H. (1956). Body ritual among the Nacirema. *American Anthropologist, 58*, 503–507.

Morris, L. S., & Schulz, R. (1993). Medication compliance: The patient's perspective. *Clinical Therapeutics, 15*, 593–606.

Nichter, M., & Vuckovic, N. (1994). Agenda for an anthropology of pharmaceutical practice. *Social Science & Medicine, 39*, 1509–1525.

Nyquist, A. C., Gonzales, R., Steiner, J. F., & Sande, M. A. (1998). Antibiotic prescribing for children with colds, upper respiratory tract infections, and bronchitis. *Journal of the American Medical Association, 279*, 875–877.

Quirt, C. F., Mackillop, W. J., Ginsburg, A. D., Sheldon, L., Brundage, M., Dixon, P., & Ginsburg, L. (1997). Do doctors know when their patients don't? A survey of doctor–patient communication in lung cancer. *Lung Cancer, 18*, 1–20.

Schwartz, B., Mainous, A. G. III, & Marcy, S. M. (1998). Why do physicians prescribe antibiotics for children with upper respiratory tract infections (Editorial)? *Journal of the American Medical Association, 279*, 881–882.

Starr, P. (1982). *The social transformation of American medicine.* New York: Basic Books.

Steckel, S. B., Funnell, M. M., & Dragovan, A. (1979). How nursing care can increase patient adherence rather than patient compliance. *American Nursing Association Publication (NP-59)*, 345–349.

Stimson, G. V. (1974). Obeying the doctor's orders: A view from the other side. *Social Science & Medicine, 8*, 97–104.

Stolberg, S. G. (1999, June 3). The boom in medications brings rise in fatal risks. *New York Times*, p. A1.

Temkin, O. (1964). Historical aspects of drug therapy. In P. Talalay (Ed.), *Drugs in our society* (pp. 3–16). Baltimore: Johns Hopkins University Press.

Trostle, J. A. (1988). Medical compliance as an ideology. *Social Science & Medicine, 27,* 1299–1308.

Trostle, J. A., Hauser, W. A., & Susser, I. S. (1983). The logic of non-compliance: Management of epilepsy from the patient's point of view. *Culture, Medicine, & Psychiatry, 7,* 35–56.

U.S. Department of Commerce. (1998). *Statistical Abstract of the United States.* Washington, DC: U.S. Government Printing Office.

U.S. Department of Health and Human Services and National Library of Medicine. (1998). *Medical subject headings—Annotated alphabetic listing, 1999.* Bethesda, MD: National Library of Medicine.

Unschuld, P. U. (1991). Culture and pharmaceutics: Some epistemological observations on pharmacological systems in ancient Europe and Medieval China. In S. Van der Geest & S. R. Whyte (Eds.), *The context of medicines in developing countries: Studies in pharmaceutical anthropology* (pp. 179–197). Amsterdam: Het Spinhuis.

Van der Geest, S., Whyte, S. R., & Hardon, A. (1996). The anthropology of pharmaceuticals. *Annual Review of Anthropology, 25,* 153–178.

Weintraub, M. (1976). Intelligent noncompliance and capricious compliance. In L. Lasagna (Ed.), *Patient compliance* (pp. 39–47). Mt. Kisco, NY: Futura.

Wise, R. A., Hart, T., Cars, O., Streulens, M., Helmuth R., Huovinen P., & Sprenger, M. (1998). Antimicrobial resistance is a major threat to public health (Editorial). *British Medical Journal, 317,* 610–611.

Zola, I. K. (1981). Structural constraints in the doctor–patient relationship: The case of non-compliance. In L. Eisenberg & A. Kleinman (Eds.), *The relevance of social science for medicine* (pp. 241–252). Dordrecht: Reidel.

Zuger, A. (1999, January 11). The fever pitch: Getting doctors to prescribe is big business. *New York Times,* p. A13.

CHAPTER THREE

Pediatric Compliance From a Patient and Family Perspective

Barbara M. Korsch
Stephanie N. Marcy
Children's Hospital of Los Angeles, Los Angeles, CA

Pediatric compliance has been one of my interests for many years. Not that I am as preoccupied with having patients do what doctors tell them as many of my colleagues. Being a therapeutic minimalist and having a profound faith in *the wisdom of the body*, with the *tincture of time* as my preferred prescription for self and others, I have often thought that some patients who elected to refuse or modify the advice they got were quite wise. Having become aware of the doctor–patient relationship dilemma, I was interested in subjecting this broad and important issue to scientific inquiry and quantitative analysis, with hopes that the ensuing body of scientific information would be applied to pediatric education and practice.

In our first large-scale study of over 1,000 patient visits carried out in the 1960s (Francis, Korsch, & Morris, 1969; Freemon, Negrete, Davis, & Korsch, 1971; Korsch, Gozzi, & Francis, 1968), there was a high incidence of noncompliance. Although the quality of care was not one of the foci of study, we could not avoid noticing that a great many prescriptions given were unnecessary and that some of the advice offered was open to question.

Yet we, like so many other investigators, used compliance as one of our outcome measures because the physicians we interviewed all stated that one of their goals in every medical encounter was to have the patient follow the advice he or she was given. In those days, no one would have said the advice was *offered* or *negotiated*. It was given with the expectation that it would be faithfully followed, and those patients who did not were labeled *uncooperative* (then and unfortunately even now).

Because my specific assignment was to discuss pediatric compliance from the patient and parent point of view, I summarize my own limited work on this topic and my current views, which are based in part on the work of others as well as my own work, experience, and reason.

I briefly summarize the incidence and distribution of noncompliance in our original study (Francis, Korsch, & Morris, 1969). In our first sample of 587 patient visits, there were 247 patient visits rated as *high compliance*, 224 rated as *moderate compliance*, and 67 rated as *noncompliance*. The remaining 49 patients received no specific treatment and are not included in the ratings. It was noted that, in those patients who were highly dissatisfied with their visits, compliance was significantly reduced. Less than one quarter of the highly dissatisfied patients were compliant, whereas among the highly satisfied more than one half complied with all the advice they received. Satisfaction was consistently correlated with specific findings from our interaction analysis, such as increased patient participation, less negative and more positive affect, and more nontask-oriented psychosocial content. In analysis of the interview responses about patients' perceptions of the interaction, perceiving the physician as friendly and having elicited and understood the patient's main concerns and expectations were strong predictors of patient satisfaction. Because we had no idea what our study would reveal and, in fact, whether there would be any attributes of the communication that would make a detectable difference and what these attributes might be, we analyzed for a great many other variables. These have been summarized in some of our papers, but are not presented here. Strikingly the communication variables were the strongest predictors.

These findings were historically significant especially from two viewpoints. First, no one had realized before now that most of the patients' compliance was influenced by communication issues. Second, I believe we were the first to document high correlation between compliance and satisfaction. When we interviewed physicians before our studies, some of them were not interested in satisfying their patient. Diagnoses and treatment were their task; "find it and fix it" (or "F2") is the Bayer Health Communication Institute formula for this model (Carroll & Korsch, 1996).

In our original quantitative research, we were faced with the challenge that you all know only too well—namely, that when you work with human beings, no matter how simple your research design, you are promptly faced with a host of variables, controlling or otherwise, that get between you and your research question. In our research, we needed to come up with outcomes that were relevant and as *hard* and compelling to the skeptics (which were ubiquitous at that time) as we could find them (Francis, Korsch, & Morris, 1969).

Because it would have complicated the issue, we elected not to include the child's own health behavior in our analysis. Therefore, we only included patients below 10 years of age because we assumed that in these families the compliance would measure the parents' response to the encounter. Hence, our results from the study reflect pediatrician–parent communication and cooperation. The occasional report that a child had refused the medicine did not prove a significant obstacle to the analysis.

All our original findings have held up amazingly well throughout succeeding decades of research. There has been consistent confirmation that, although satisfaction relates (always) strongly to communication skills (e.g., Lewis, Pantell, & Sharp, 1991; Worchel, Prevatt, Miner, Allen, Wagner, & Nation, 1995), compliance is also independently related to doctor-patient communication (Bartlett, Grayson, Barker, Levine, Golden, & Libber, 1984; Lewis, Pantell, & Sharp, 1991).

The main issue in patient–clinician communication that has truly changed in the decades since I became interested has been the recognition of the patient's role (e.g., Keller & Carroll, 1994; Rifkin, Wolf, Lewis, & Pantell, 1988). The patients used to accept their assigned role—more or less—in a sense, passive victims in the doctor's office. It was the patient community that first motivated drastic changes in this paradigm. Over the last few decades, patients have become increasingly aware of their rights and autonomy. More important, they have become much more educated about their own bodies in health and disease. They have demanded that health care workers respect patients' rights to information, and they expect clinicians to participate directly in patients' health education. This in turn has resulted in more joint decision making and in negotiating treatment advice instead of *giving it*.

For many years now, research on this subject has flourished. When I started investigating the subject, the general view was that it was unresearchable and unteachable. There were just a few studies of noncompliant patients, dominantly from the psychiatric community, where noncompliance was equated with patients' resistance. Now there are literally thousands of articles, many of which are research based.

STUDIES OF TREATMENT COMPLIANCE
FOR RENAL TRANSPLANTATION

In brief review, my own early studies emphasized that the doctor–patient relationship and the nature of the communication were the strongest predictors of compliance and satisfaction in the presence of acute illness. Our later studies of chronically ill children were confirmatory and additionally identified certain patient groups who constituted high-risk patients for noncompliance.

In our longitudinal study of patients with end stage renal disease (Korsch, Fine, & Negrete, 1977), we amazed the nephrologists who had in all innocence condemned a number of immunosuppressive agents as being less effective without ever considering the possibility that the patient might simply not have taken the drug.

I briefly summarize our results from this study (Korsch, Fine, & Negrete, 1977): To our dismay, of the 80 patients on whom we had 10-year follow-up data, 14 (13 of them adolescents) interrupted their immunosuppressive treatment to the extent that their kidney function or general health was impaired. Twelve of the 14 patients were girls and 2 were boys. Available psychosocial data obtained by extensive but simple personality testing and semistructured interviews over time reveal that families of those patients who interrupted their therapy had lower incomes, more fatherless households, and more communication difficulties within the family and with the medical staff. The personality attributes most significantly associated included poor social adaptation and low self-esteem. These were the two most significant predictors of noncompliance.

Because ours were chronic patients who were seen over time and by many health professionals, it was difficult to tease out those communication aspects of their care that may have contributed to their behavior. Still we have enough documented visits to know that the seriousness of their condition was continuously emphasized and that fear tactics were freely used *to motivate them* and to know that these were ineffective in our high-risk patients (especially in adolescents), just leading to more denial (e.g., "When they told you that you might lose your kidney or you might even die if you do not take your medicine, how did that make you feel?" "I just put it out of my mind").

The highest risk patients in this study were female adolescents who were depressed, had little family support, and had disorganized families. They also had low self-esteem, external locus of control, and poor social support. Demography was not distinguishing. Side effects and complexity of regimen were mentioned, but were not the most important determinants.

Patients who had lost one kidney with noncompliance were given psychosocial interventions. However, to the indignation of the treatment team, in isolated instances, patients repeated their behavior after they received another transplant, although intellectually they certainly knew the seriousness of the consequences. As you all know, these findings are not surprising, although the high incidence of noncompliance was not anticipated in this particular situation.

In general, over time most investigators have confirmed the cardinal role played by the reemphasized doctor–patient relationship in eliciting patient compliance (Silverman, Kurtz, & Draper, 1998). However, they have also documented high-risk situations such as complex treatment regimens, long-lasting illness, undesirable side effects from the treatment regimen, and many others with which we are all familiar.

RECENT WORK ON PATIENT-BASED INTERVENTIONS TO PROMOTE TREATMENT COMPLIANCE

When it comes to strategies to elicit patient cooperation, the changed role of the patient has increasingly prompted patient-based interventions. A number of recent studies have been prompted by the recognition that, although it is traditionally hard to change physician behavior (not to speak of attitudes), patients tend to be highly motivated to engage in behavior aimed at improving the medical encounter and leading to improved satisfaction and services for themselves.

Traditionally, efforts addressed to the patient consisted largely of health education and the communication of cognitive messages about health-related topics. Sometimes these addressed basic issues of hygiene (dental floss, a device traditionally associated with noncompliance until 2 days before the visit to the dentist) or preventive measures (immunizations, participating in screening procedures, etc.). Often they focused on specific diseases such as diabetes, hypertension, heart disease, and so on. Until recently, such efforts consisted primarily of printed matter, brochures, instruction sheets, and the like. More recently, other media are increasingly utilized (e.g., CD-ROMs, videotapes). Unfortunately, these informational messages were not tailored to the individual patient's needs, tastes, personality, and culture. The printed diet sheets for 800-calorie diets that were available to patients who needed to lose weight and who came from different cultures and widely varied socioeconomic status (SES) in the inner city might as well have been in Greek for all the sense they made in the context of the daily life of the patients. The research with which I am familiar suggests that, in general, most patients did not use these printed educational materials. In our own studies, we found many of them on the floor of the consultation rooms and even in the trash.

Results are slightly better when these materials can be individualized, if the clinician highlights relevant portions, and, more important, if the clinician discusses the message with the patient. When this type of literature is used outside the context of the patient–clinician communication, it is rarely effective.

We taped encounters in one pediatric office where, as soon as the patient uttered a problem (e.g., "and he is still wetting the bed at night"), the pediatrician would cut him or her off with, "well my nurse will give you a brochure on your way out that will tell you all about it and what to do about the problem." He had a whole rack of brochures dealing with enuresis, temper tantrums, speech problems, and so on.

In some instances, when a clinician asks a patient whether he or she would like some relevant material to read or, better yet, if the patient requests the material, it is much more likely to be used. Moreover, when the physician actually writes out instructions for the particular patient that are tailored to that patient's needs, these are likely to be referred to and valued.

All of these materials were intended to give patients knowledge about health care and the disease for which they were being treated. In fact, they usually did not change the patients' role in the medical encounter, although at times they prompted them to ask certain questions. At present, those patients who quote the Internet do not necessarily elicit more positive responses from the physician. In many cases, clinicians are irritated or even threatened by the extra questions. An early study by Debra Roter in which patients were actually encouraged to ask more questions did not have the desired result. The resulting increase in patients' questions can sometimes be perceived by the clinician as an annoyance or a lack of trust.

In the last couple of decades, there have actually been some new developments, including some promising ones (Roter & Hall, 1992). Greenfield and Kaplan (Greenfield, Kaplan, & Ware, 1985; Greenfield, Kaplan, Ware, Yano, & Frank, 1988), in their impressive studies originally begun in California and then continued in Boston, made a successful intervention by coaching patients before the encounter with the physician to help them focus their questions and concerns. They were successful in demonstrating actual improvement in biological function as well as improved patient satisfaction as a consequence of this intervention. Dr. Robert Pantell, in San Francisco, has been working for some time on communication interventions in a pediatric practice (Lewis, Scott, Pantell, & Wolf, 1986). His theme has been *it takes two to tango*. Thus, in a study of the efficacy of a brief educational intervention program for parents and children during pediatric office visits, he has addressed both clinician and, in this case, the pediatric patient as well as the parent with excellent results (Lewis, Pantell, & Sharp, 1991). More specifically, Pantell and colleagues found that physicians in the intervention group more often included children in discussions of medical recommendations compared with controls, that children in the intervention group recalled significantly more medication recommendations than their counterparts in the control group, and that children in the intervention group reported greater satisfaction and preference for an active health role than did the children in the control group.

NEW DIRECTIONS

Recently, I have been working closely with the Bayer Institute for Health Communication. In fact, I just finished my term as chair of their advisory board after 7 years. These were exciting and formative years in relation to our field. Most of you are probably familiar with the impressive series of educational ventures initiated by Bayer with physicians and other clinicians that have (at least in short-term follow-up) proved amazingly effective in improving clinicians' communication skills and, in fact, sometimes improving outcomes for patients. The "E4" model of physician–patient communication is one of the major contributions of clinicians at the Bayer Institute to the ongoing educational aims of the Bayer Institute. The model describes four sets of interrelated communication tasks to be accomplished in a typical medical consultation: engaging patients in doctor–patient relationships; empathizing with patients' concerns; educating patients about their health, illness, or concerns; and enlisting patients in a therapeutic regimen (Keller & Carroll, 1994).

Based on my own experience (personally as well as in my role at Bayer), it originally seemed reasonable to assume that it was the physicians' responsibility and that it is they who need to be taught to communicate effectively, just as other aspects of the health care process are learned and practiced by clinicians for the benefit of their patients. Bayer has emphasized that doctor–patient communication is the most frequently used procedure in medical practice (an average number of such communications in a lifetime of practice has been estimated to be 100,000). I still believe that it is morally up to clinicians to reach out to patients in the interaction no matter how difficult the patient, how complex the situation, or how unsupportive the system is in which one practices.

However, with the accumulated evidence of patient potential to participate in their own health care at all levels, I became convinced that it would also be productive to address educational efforts directly to the patient and teach the patient as well as the doctor specifically concerning their communication with the clinician and the health care system.

It was to this end, and in response to this need and patients' request that after years of addressing the communication skills of health professionals at different stages of their education and in different venues, I decided to focus also on the patient. My book, *The Intelligent Patient's Guide to Doctor-Patient Communication*, is my most elaborate such effort (Korsch & Harding, 1997). This literary work provides a practical examination of the complex doctor–patient relationship. Although answering most of the common questions that patients have regarding treatment and interactions with physicians, this book also offers insight into the doctor's side of the relationship, showing how doctors are trained to be task oriented and how their natural human sympathy is often discouraged throughout the course of their training and practice. Responses of various patients and community groups have suggested that such material is utilized and felt to be helpful by many patients. We also have a patient-directed initiative at Bayer now that is being implemented and studied carefully at a medical center in California as we speak.

If you read newspapers and journals and watch the media, it quickly becomes evident that efforts to educate patients to communicate more effectively and, in general, to get better health care for themselves are being made all over the place, especially in the United States. Our former Surgeon General, Everett Koop, has pronounced the need for improved communication to be a primary goal to improve medical care in the next few years. No one could be more delighted than I with the current multifaceted interest and efforts to develop knowledge in my long-time favorite subject (i.e., the doctor–patient relationship).

Some of the support for these efforts comes from surprising directions. The pharmaceutical community has always had a special interest in patient compliance, but interest also comes from patient support groups—especially populations destined to have more communication problems. These include those with complex, long-lasting, or psychosomatic illnesses; the geriatric group; women; and those who are especially concerned with wellness and preventive care—a subject in which physicians have never demonstrated sufficient interest. Groups interested in alternative and complementary health care are always articulate about weaknesses in so-called *scientific medical practice* especially in relation to communication and relationship problems with patients.

Finally, the most important support in increasing focus on the clinician–patient relationship and communication are the representatives of managed care. Although they often limit the time allotted to patient visits, to such an extent that communication becomes almost impossible, they have learned and recognized that from the point of view of health economics effective communication is absolutely essential. Managed health care is responsible for more quality control, more patient satisfaction surveys, and focusing on wellness and prevention more than almost any other system. Their motives are mixed between humanism and good business. They support a great many continuing education activities in the field because effective communication has increasingly shown to be related to successful marketing as well as to malpractice litigation.

In looking back on all this activity and progress, I am truly pleased. However, my one caveat in this mushrooming educational effort directed at the patient relates to the need to design such efforts in a manner that the patient feels truly reempowered. I do not like the phrase *empowering patients* because I think originally patients had all the power, but over the years we have made them feel that they do not have any independent power. In fact, we have taken their power away, and current interventions should be aimed at reempowering patients who basically have all the rights.

REFERENCES

Bartlett, E. E., Grayson, M., Barker, R., Levine, D. M., Golden, A., & Libber, S. (1984). The effects of physician communication skills on patient satisfaction, recall, and adherence. *Journal of Chronic Disease, 37*, 755–764.

Carroll, J. G., & Korsch, B. M. (1996). *Medical discourse: "Difficult" patients and frustrated doctors.* Paper presented at the Oxford Conference on Teaching about Communication in Medicine, Oxford, England.

Francis, V., Korsch, B. M., & Morris, M. J. (1969). Gaps in doctor–patient communication: Patient's response to medical advice. *New England Journal of Medicine, 288*, 535–540.

Freemon, B., Negrete, V. F., Davis, M., & Korsch, B. M. (1971). Gaps in doctor–patient communication: Doctor–patient interaction analysis. *Pediatric Research, 5*, 298–311.

Greenfield, S., Kaplan, S., & Ware, J. E., Jr. (1985). Expanding patient involvement in care: Effects on patient outcomes. *Annals of Internal Medicine, 102*, 520–528.

Greenfield, S., Kaplan, S. H., Ware, J. E., Jr., Yano, E. M., & Frank, H. J. L. (1988). Patients' participation in medical care: Effects on blood sugar control and quality of life in diabetes. *Journal of General Internal Medicine, 3*, 448–457.

Keller, V. F., & Carroll, J. G. (1994). A new model for physician–patient communication. *Patient Education and Counseling, 23*, 131–140.

Korsch, B. M., Fine, R. N., & Negrete, V. F. (1977). Noncompliance in children with renal transplants. *Pediatrics, 61*, 872.

Korsch, B. M., Gozzi, E., & Francis, V. (1968). Gaps in doctor–patient communications: Doctor–patient interaction and patient satisfaction. *Pediatrics, 42*, 855.

Korsch, B. M., & Harding, C. (1997). *The intelligent patient's guide to the doctor–patient relationship.* Oxford University Press: New York.

Lewis, C. C., Pantell, R. H., & Sharp, L. (1991). Increasing patient knowledge, satisfaction, and involvement: Randomized trial of a communication intervention. *Pediatrics, 88*, 351–358.

Lewis, C. C., Scott, D. E., Pantell, R. H., & Wolf, M. H. (1986). Parent satisfaction with children's medical care. Development, field test, and validation of a questionnaire. *Medical Care, 24*, 209–215.

Rifkin, L., Wolf, M. H., Lewis, C. C., & Pantell, R. H. (1988). Children's perceptions of physicians and medical care: Two measures. *Journal of Pediatric Psychology, 13*, 247–254.

Roter, D. L., & Hall, J. A. (1992). *Doctors talking with patients/patients talking with doctors.* Westport, CT: Auburn House.

Silverman, J., Kurtz, S., & Draper, J. (1998). *Skills for communicating with patients.* Abington, England: Radcliffe Medical Press.

Worchel, F. F., Prevatt, B. C., Miner, J., Allen, M., Wagner, L., & Nation, P. (1995). Pediatrician's communication style: Relationship to parents' perceptions and behaviors. *Journal of Pediatric Psychology, 20*, 633–644.

PART III

CONCEPTUAL MODELS OF ADHERENCE AND COMPLIANCE FOR CLINICAL CARE AND RESEARCH

In this section, authors contribute new conceptual models that promise to enhance understanding of adherence. In chap. 4, Bauman presents a patient-centered model of treatment adherence that broadens our understanding of the factors that influence treatment adherence and the factors that may affect treatment compliance. Arguing convincingly that treatment nonadherence is a common problem and in many ways more the exception than the rule, she critically evaluates the assumptions of conceptual models that have been utilized to understand patient behavior in response to medical advice. Bauman questions the major assumptions that underlie the traditional adherence/compliance model (e.g., that patients with health problems should comply with treatment to reduce symptoms and should be motivated to initiate and maintain treatment). Bauman contrasts these assumptions with those that underlie the Health Belief Model, which does not assume that treatment adherence is expected and focuses on patients' perceptions of beliefs to treatment.

Bauman also describes the need to consider and understand different types of adherence, such as volitional adherence (in which the patient has heard and understood a provider's advice but makes an informed choice not to comply with treatment) versus inadvertent nonadherence (in which patients accept their providers' advice and attempt to implement the treatment, but for a variety of reasons do not do what was prescribed). She considers the multitude of risk factors that can affect treatment compliance, including patient-related factors (e.g., concerns about side effects, costs of care, physician prescribing practices, and provider system characteristics such as inadequate doctor–patient communication).

Bauman's cogent analysis suggests several strategies to reduce risk for nonadherence, such as identifying key risk factors, targeting them for intervention, and improving patient education and patient–provider communication. Bauman also recommends that providers consider patients' needs for ongoing support for medical treatment adherence.

In his description of patient self-management concerning chronic pediatric illness, Creer (chap. 5) contrasts the management of acute illnesses, which are often self-limiting and/or involve intensive treatment from a health care professional versus that of a chronic illness, where the primary emphasis of clinical care shifts toward control of the illness rather than cure. To develop and implement effective self-management programs for chronic illnesses, Creer advocates putting the patient at the center of his or her treatment. He contributes a useful working definition of *self-management* in pediatric chronic illness: the performance of a set of procedures by children and their caregivers to help control a chronic disorder. Examples of self-management include selective treatment goals, information collection, and processes such as decision making, actions, and self-reactions. Creer identifies the key variables that impact self-management, including task demands such as the effort and time involved in managing a chronic illness, rhythm or course of the disorder, child and family treatment expectations, uncertainty in the illness course and response to treatment, ages and abilities of children with chronic illness, and the specific contexts (e.g., school, home, etc.) in which treatment-related actions are supposed to be taken.

One of Creer's contributions is to identify potentially effective ingredients of the application of the self-management model in pediatric chronic illness. These ingredients include health providers' abilities to accept patients with a chronic illness as active participants in their own health care, improving communication skills between providers and families, working to build the trust of patients and families, using established guidelines of treatment, and preparing patients to engage in effective self-management of their condition by improving their communication skills, their ability to seek information about health and illness, and training in self-management and skill development.

Creer's description of the key components of self-management is instructive. For example, the specific components of one important dimension of self-management of chronic illness—goal selection—include the following: discussing treatment options, selecting a treatment option, negotiating a schedule for treatment, writing of contracts, and introducing cues and reminders.

The conceptual framework of self-management has significant implications for the application of self-management techniques to chronic illness in children, the outcome variables that are assessed in illness management, and especially performance of self-management procedures over time. New research directions suggested by this model include charting the development and course of self-management for different chronic conditions across time and settings.

CHAPTER FOUR

A Patient-Centered Approach to Adherence: Risks for Nonadherence

Laurie J. Bauman
Albert Einstein College of Medicine, Bronx, NY

The two dominant theoretical approaches used in adherence research—Adherence/Compliance and the Health Belief Model—have provided a rich and important foundation for understanding patient behavior. However, despite the huge investment in compliance research and over 10,000 articles published, patient noncompliance remains high, with more than half of patients failing to take medications properly (Donovan, 1995). A new approach needs to incorporate the strengths of existing frameworks but enhance our ability to guide interventions. This new approach begins with three observations: (a) Noncompliance is common, therefore models that treat nonadherence as unexpected or deviant are of limited utility. (b) There are different kinds of nonadherence that have different risk factors, pose different clinical problems, and require different interventions. (c) The assumption by providers that patients should and will comply with provider advice leads to defining the problem of nonadherence in a limited, static way: "Why don't patients comply?" This chapter presents a different way of looking at adherence—by conceptualizing it from the patient view rather than the provider view.

From the provider perspective, it is puzzling and frustrating to have successful medical treatments available for a patient's serious health condition only to have them ignored. In the provider's mind, the patient came for care and sought his or her advice, and therefore should comply with the prescribed medical regimen. From patients' points of view, providers are an important source of needed information about their health and what is wrong with them. However, the advice providers give is often complex, anxiety provoking, and challenging to implement. It may be incompatible with personal and cultural beliefs, may contradict what other providers say, and be inconsistent with the admonitions of family and friends. Therefore, patients use the information providers give as only one source of input into a complicated decision about whether to accept medical advice and how much of it to incorporate into their daily life.

The patient-centered approach to adherence asks a different question than "Why don't patients comply?" Instead, it asks "Under what circumstances can adherence be improved?" Rather than assuming that something has *gone wrong* when patients do not comply, the patient-centered approach assumes that adherence is a complex human behavior that is facilitated or hindered by many factors. These include patient personal, cultural, and personality characteristics; characteristics of the interaction or exchange between provider and patient; provider personal and professional characteristics; and characteristics of the regimen. Providers can influence many but not all of these factors. Thus, adherence seen through the patient-centered lens becomes part of the routine challenge of providing medical care—a focus of attention and intervention, rather than an assumed outcome of the provider–patient interaction.

This chapter begins with a brief distinction between adherence and compliance. It then reviews the literature on rates of noncompliance, describes the two dominant theoretical approaches to adherence/compliance research, draws a distinction between two kinds of nonadherence (volitional and inadvertent), introduces a new way to look at nonadherence (risks for nonadherence), and reviews strategies to reduce nonadherence.

ADHERENCE VERSUS COMPLIANCE

Before proceeding, it is important to address the difference between *adherence* and *compliance* (see Riekert & Drotar, chap. 1, this volume; Trostle, chap. 2, this volume). *Compliance* assumes that one person conforms or adapts to another's agenda. It has come to have a negative connotation because it assumes that the patient is a passive participant in his or her care and should simply follow medical advice. It is rooted in the deviance models that put doctors in authority and consider noncompliance a puzzling deviation from the expected. *Adherence* assumes an active, voluntary, and mutual relationship in which both patient and provider collaborate to produce a desired or therapeutic outcome (Huss, Travis, & Huss, 1997).

Although adherence and compliance are different in the process by which a medical regimen is prescribed, they are not different in the most important way the concepts are used. That is, the expected result is the same—to increase the extent to which patients comply with medical advice. Adherence differs from compliance in that it is a process of joint decision making that is hypothesized to enhance patients' willingness and ability to comply. However, there is little empirical research that describes the proportion of the time actual provider–patient interactions fit either an adherence or a compliance model or evaluates which is associated with better patient adherence with medical advice.

RELEVANCE TO CHILDHOOD CHRONIC ILLNESS

Because this chapter presents a new approach to conceptualizing adherence to treatment in general, it is not limited to pediatric chronic illness. Although most of the discussion applies to both child and adult adherence problems, there are several special issues that are most relevant when a child has a chronic illness. First, the *patient* in pediatric settings is both the child and the parent. Many potential adherence barriers can emerge for either the child or the parent, in effect doubling the risk for nonadherence. Second, the interaction between the child and parent as well as the larger family dynamics affect child behavior. Parent–child conflict can emerge for the first time because of the child's illness and/or adherence problems, or they may already characterize the parent–child relationship and adherence offers just one more venue for the conflict to emerge. Third, developmental issues are especially relevant in pediatric chronic illness. Developmental stages pose different adherence challenges. Toddlers can be oppositional especially when adherence imposes activity restrictions, painful procedures, or distasteful medication. School-age children may not comply if they feel different from other children or are teased because of their need, for example, to take an asthma inhaler to school. Adolescents are at risk for nonadherence as they struggle for independence from parents. Many experiment with medication to exert some control over their bodies or to prove to themselves whether they really need the medication—or as a result of their feelings of invulnerability, which lead to denying their health problem. Related adherence challenges are to (a) assess how developmental changes in children affect their willingness and ability to adhere over time, and (b) evaluate when children have acquired sufficient cognitive skills and maturity to share the responsibility for their own care.

NONADHERENCE IS COMMON

It is critically important to emphasize that nonadherence is a common, even typical response to medical advice (see Riekert & Drotar, chap. 1, this volume). It is not aberrant, unusual, or deviant: It is the norm and occurs regardless of age, race, gender, and disease. For example, it was estimated that between 30% and 60% of patients are totally nonadherent (Ley, 1988; Masek, 1982), between half and three quarter of patients fail to take medications properly (Haynes, Taylor, & Sackett, 1979; Stimson, 1974), and one half of prescriptions are adhered to partly or not at all (Buckalew & Sallis, 1986). Levels of adherence for asthma vary from 3% to 88% (Adams, Pill, & Jones, 1997; Bosely, Parry, & Cochrane, 1994; Brooks et al., 1994; Dompeling et al., 1992; Kelloway, Wyatt, & Adlis, 1994; Kinsman, Dirks, & Dahlem, 1980; Kleiger & Dirks, 1979; Mawhinney et al., 1991; Tashkin, 1995; Van Sciver, D'Angelo, Rappaport, & Woolf, 1995), with an average level of 50%. The rate of adherence in pediatric asthma is similar to that in adults, with the average rate about 50% in both populations (Alessandro, Vincenzo, Marco, Marcello, & Enrica, 1994; Baum & Creer, 1986; Cochrane, 1992; Coutts, Gibson, & Paton, 1992; Gong, Simmons, Clark, & Tashkin, 1988; Rand & Wise, 1994; Spector, 1985; Tettersell, 1993; Yeung, O'Connor, Parry, & Cochrane, 1994).

Clearly most people are unable or unwilling to accept and adhere to medical advice. If research had demonstrated that most people comply, then the goal of adherence research and interventions would be to identify the kinds of patients who cannot fulfill expectations or management protocols that pose special difficulties. However, because most people do not comply with expectations, we must look elsewhere for explanations.

TWO THEORETICAL APPROACHES: ADHERENCE TO TREATMENT VERSUS ADOPTION OF PREVENTIVE HEALTH PRACTICES

Two dominant theoretical approaches have been used to understand patient behavior when medical advice is given—Adherence/Compliance and the Health Belief Model and its variations. Adherence/Compliance approaches have emphasized patient adherence with therapy for a diagnosed condition. The Health Belief Model is more typically used in research to understand adherence with medical advice to prevent or reduce risk for a condition that is not yet present.

Adherence/Compliance Approach

The Adherence/Compliance approach has traditionally guided research when patients are prescribed a treatment regimen for an existing health problem. There are unstated assumptions that underlie this approach: (a) when a person has a diagnosed health problem, the need to initiate and maintain treatment is necessary, not optional; (b) if a patient has a health problem, he or she will want to initiate and maintain the recommended treatment; (c) patients who are symptomatic should be motivated to comply with treatment that provides symptom relief; and (d) if a patient seeks out care for a problem, he or she should be motivated to accept prescribed treatment. In summary, if a patient comes to a doctor with a symptom, is diagnosed with a condition, and is instructed to take medication and/or change health practices, then of course—from the provider's perspective—the patient should comply with treatment advice. In this model, the puzzle is why patients would not comply with the solution they sought out in the first place.

Unfortunately, the Adherence/Compliance approach is faulty if the assumptions underlying it do not apply. For example, it assumes that an existing health problem presents real and present danger, not a theoretical or possible harm in the future. However, many patients are diagnosed through routine screening tests with a condition in an early stage before it is symptomatic, and the goal of treatment is to prevent long-term serious sequelae (e.g., hypertension, obesity, early stage cancer). These mainly asymptomatic patients often require treatment regimens that incur side effects (e.g., chemotherapy, hypertension medication that can result in impotence). Symptomatic patients may indeed be motivated to comply with treatment if it provides relief, but when symptoms disappear (e.g., either spontaneously or with initiation of treatment) the motivation to continue with treatment may also disappear. This may explain premature termination of antibiotic therapy for infection and difficulty maintaining preventive daily oral steroid use in patients with asthma.

Even when patients have a symptomatic condition and seek relief, there are many barriers to perfect compliance, that are often rooted in the nature of the treatment. These include degree of difficulty, pain (e.g., needle stick to check blood sugar), need for ongoing change in lifestyle (e.g., dialysis), intrusiveness (e.g., blood sugar monitoring, diet in diabetes, daily radiation therapy for cancer), complexity (e.g., HIV triple therapy), expense (e.g., growth hormone treatment), length of time (e.g., 10 days? 6 weeks? all your life?), purpose of treatment (e.g., to cure the underlying condition, simply manage symptoms, or prevent future consequences of the illness), or lack of perceived effectiveness (e.g., it does not make you feel better). Adherence is less likely when the clinical course of the disease varies in severity, with acute episodes punctuating long intervals of no overt disease activity (e.g., asthma).

The conclusion is that the Adherence/Compliance approach, which has guided much research on patient acceptance of medical advice, rests on assumptions that often do not apply. In fact, these assumptions may not be true of patients with a diagnosed illness any more than they are for those prescribed a regimen to prevent a condition or reduce risk. Prevention research on how to persuade people to adopt health-promoting and disease-preventing behaviors has been guided by a different tradition.

Health Belief Model

When a regimen is prescribed to prevent a health problem or lower risk for a condition in the future (e.g., eat healthy, exercise, use condoms, do not do drugs, plan pregnancies), the models used to guide research on patient acceptance of advice do not use compliance assumptions or language. Instead, most often we find variants of theoretical models using cognitive-behavioral approaches such as the Health Belief Model (Becker, 1974; Becker & Janz, 1984; Becker & Maiman, 1975; Rosenstock, 1974). This different conceptual approach is used rather than Adherence/Compliance because the regimen prescribed is to prevent a future harm rather than fix or manage a current problem (see Riekert & Drotar, chap. 1, this volume). The model does not assume that adherence is expected. Instead, it acknowledges that patients are autonomous not passive, that there should be a partnership between provider and patient in choosing a prevention strategy, and that the patient chooses to adhere with a prevention regimen.

The Health Belief Model posits that people are more likely to act on advice to initiate preventive health practices if they understand that (a) they are at risk (that there is a threat or susceptibility of illness and consequences of that threat are serious), (b) there is an effective action that can be initiated (i.e., the intervention suggested will reduce the risk or severity of the consequences), and (c) the barriers or costs of adopting the preventive practice are lower than the benefits. A cue or stimulus to change must occur to trigger the process. This model has been modified for use in studying compliance with medical advice when an illness is diagnosed to include health concerns and beliefs, especially general beliefs about illness susceptibility, faith in provider, and regimen characteristics.

The approaches share some similarities. Both give a great deal of attention to patient motivation as a factor in adherence to advice and the predictors of high motivation, such as the severity of the condition and accompanying prognosis; the degree to which adherence with the regimen will reduce discomfort; the degree that adherence will improve or cure the underlying condition; and the degree to which the condition interferes with daily activity. Both also focus on barriers to adherence/compliance: If patients choose to accept medical advice, what factors interfere with their ability to follow it, such as patient characteristics (poor sight or forgetfulness), regimen characteristics (e.g., complexity or side effects), and provider–patient relationship?

The models differ mainly in the assumption of the provider and patient. The Adherence/Compliance model assumes that providers decide what treatment is best and most appropriate and patients should implement the medical treatment prescribed. The Health Belief Model acknowledges that patients are autonomous *decision makers* who follow a suggested regimen based on their health beliefs, the degree to which the diagnosis and treatment make sense to them, and the barriers and costs associated with compliance. The conclusion we draw from reviewing the dominant models of research on adherence is that patients do not fail to comply, rather, they choose another course of behavior (Donovan, 1995). The doctor's advice is just one input among many in how to handle health and illness. Providers may consider the decisions that patients make irrational, but they may be quite rational from the patients' perspective.

TWO TYPES OF NONADHERENCE

Studies that document nonadherence monitor and report several kinds of behaviors (Meichenbaum & Turk, 1987): missed appointments (Sackett & Snow, 1979); dropping out of treatment or stopping treatment prematurely (Goldman, Holcomb, & Perry, 1982; Caldwell, Cobb, & Dowling, 1971; Agras, Taylor, & Kraemer, 1987); errors in medication use (both too much and too little), including failing to fill prescriptions, taking incorrect doses of medications, taking medication at the wrong times, and missing doses; and erratic or nonimplementation of other behavior changes, such as avoidance of allergens among people with asthma or following a diet for those with diabetes.

It is crucial to distinguish between two different types of nonadherence: inadvertent and volitional. They are not mutually exclusive, although it is likely that most of the time a patient will only exhibit one kind. We posit that different factors predict the two kinds and that different interventions may be needed to manage each type. Further, the reporting biases accompanying each may be different: Those not adhering by choice may deliberately misrepresent their degree of adherence to providers and researchers, whereas those who are not adherent inadvertently may fail to report nonadherence because they believe they are in compliance with medical advice. The solutions to limit these sources of reporting error would be expected to differ as well.

In *volitional nonadherence*, patients heard and understood the provider's advice but make a reasoned choice not to comply. These patients are fully aware that they are not following the provider's advice; they may openly acknowledge their nonadherence or go to some lengths to deceive the provider about that decision. Patients may choose not to follow provider advice because their treatment goals are different than the provider's goals, they may have lifestyles that affect acceptability of treatment, or their health beliefs may interfere with adherence (Mellins, Evans, Zimmerman, & Clark, 1992). *Inadvertent nonadherence* is probably more common. These patients accept treatment advice and believe that they are adhering to provider advice either perfectly or well enough that it is considered to be sufficient.

There are three different kinds of inadvertent nonadherers. The first are *satisficers*. They acknowledge missing doses occasionally, but few are concerned about it; if asked, they will say they are compliant. These patients believe that the extent of their compliance is *good enough* to accomplish treatment goals and that there is elasticity around adherence boundaries. Their motivation to improve adherence tends to be low. The second type of patient wants to be compliant and is working hard at being compliant. They understand the demands of the protocol and want to follow it, but face obstacles to adequate adherence (e.g., parents whose children refuse medication, cost). This type of patient has high motivation to adhere to treatment. The third type is the patient who has misunderstood what is expected or has been given incorrect instruction about his or her treatment regimen. They are following the advice they heard or remembered, which is not what the provider intended. These patients believe they are compliant and report this to providers and researchers alike.

RISKS FOR NONADHERENCE

It appears that a more fruitful way to conceptualize the problem of adherence is to avoid the underlying assumption of the Adherence/Compliance approach—that patients should or will accept medical advice. Instead, we should assume that patients are decision makers who face complex challenges in choosing a course of action based on the explanation of the health problem or risk by the provider. The advantage of shifting expectations is that we reframe the problem from a deviance model—why don't patients do what they are supposed to do—to a constructive approach— under what conditions will adherence be improved? This shift in expectations changes the ground rules. Instead of assuming that compliance should occur (and therefore will occur), we assume that compliance is a problematic outcome that needs to be negotiated, planned, evaluated, and reassessed over time. This focuses attention on understanding the various conditions associated with patient nonadherence—what we now introduce as *risk factors* for nonadherence. We hypothesize that some risk factors are typical of volitional nonadherence, some characterize inadvertent nonadherence, and a few are risks for both kinds of nonadherence.

RISK FACTORS FOR VOLITIONAL NONADHERENCE

I have categorized risk factors for volitional nonadherence into eight groups described herein.

Difficulty and Disruptiveness of Medical Regimen

Patients may decide that some kinds of treatment regimens are simply too much trouble, too hard to do, or too intrusive (Turk & Spears, 1984). Although the patients accept the need for the treatment, they choose not to act on it because the task posed by the provider is beyond their will or ability. For these patients, taking medication is more than a nuisance—it imposes activity restrictions, disrupts lifestyle, causes family conflict, or increases perceived vulnerability. Examples of nonadherence in this category are: (a) need to make lifestyle changes, such as parents of an asthmatic child being asked to quit smoking or obese children being asked to reduce levels of fat consumption and increase physical exercise; (b) erratic medication dosing when a child refuses medication or refuses needle sticks for blood glucose monitoring; and (c) missing doses because a child is embarrassed to take medication in public. For example, children with asthma and their caregivers may not adhere to a therapeutic program because inhaled medication may make the child feel different, unpopular, or less accepted among peers.

Skepticism About Efficacy

Some patients are skeptical about treatment efficacy and do not believe the proposed regimen is effective or helpful. Some experiment with medication or stop taking it to evaluate whether the treatment is helping (Adelman & Taylor, 1986; Conrad, 1985) or to see whether the treatment was needed. This problem is less likely when the benefit of the medication is experienced soon after dosing. For example, pain medication has a contingency benefit—when taken properly, pain subsides and the benefit of the medication is clear. However, many medications have invisible effects to the child and parent, such as long-term steroid use for asthma. Further, some medications do not have any short-term experienced benefit—the benefit is in the long-term future (e.g., chemotherapy for early stage cancers). Some patients may decline to take medication that incurs immediate difficult side effects for a theoretical benefit in the future. Patients in pain may discontinue medication when no relief is evident (Haynes et al., 1979).

Experienced Side Effects

Many medications cause side effects ranging from mild (e.g., dry mouth) to severe (e.g., nausea, immunosuppression from chemotherapy). The actual experience of side effects may result in patients reducing the dose of their medication until side effects are manageable or disappear, but the reduced dose may be less effective. Similarly, some medications may be painful to give or distasteful. Injections and needle sticks to monitor blood glucose are painful, and patients may seek ways to reduce this burden. Often patients may run a series of *experiments* with their medication dosing to see how little they can take and still receive benefit (or minimize side effects). They balance the negative aspects of adherence with the benefits. Although they believe that the medication is effective, if the benefits are invisible and costs direct and immediate, the decision to curtail or drop out of treatment is much more likely (Donovan, Blake, & Fleming, 1989).

Patient Beliefs, Fears, and Concerns

People come to a health care provider with a set of experiences with medical care in the past, with beliefs (correct or not) about illness and death, and with cultural practices and expectations about illness in general and their role as patients in particular. People rely on these expectations, beliefs, and meanings in each exchange with providers. The problem comes when the provider's definition, explanation, or prescription is inconsistent or in contradiction to the patient's belief system. Misunderstandings about health and illness contribute to noncompliance (Leventhal, Zimmerman, & Gutmann, 1984; Taylor, 1986). When the patient's model of how illness occurs differs from the providers' model, adherence tends to be lower. Patient beliefs about medications also may play a large role in their decision making. Many patients have fantasies regarding the power and danger of drugs (Brody, 1997; Van Sciver et al., 1995). They may fear medications and try to avoid taking them at all. Others may try to wean themselves from them so that they do not become *accustomed* to the medication because it might lose its effectiveness. Many parents worry about side effects to the extent that this anticipatory fear results in parents neglecting to give children the medication they need (Meichenbaum & Turk, 1987).

Cost of Treatment

Rising health care costs have led to many changes in insurance programs. In particular, the costs of prescription medications have risen dramatically. In an effort to contain costs, few insurance plans cover prescription medication. Children with chronic health conditions often require ongoing expensive medications, averaging hundreds of dollars per month. Children who live in households that qualify for Medicaid usually have access to the medications they need, but near-poor children who may not have any health insurance are rarely able to benefit from expensive therapies. Recent policy initiatives, such as the Child Health Insurance Plan (CHIP), assist such parents to afford medications, equipment, and ancillary therapies. However, it is already apparent that there is substantial state variation in the implementation of this federal program, and the package of services covered by CHIP may be inadequate to assist children with special needs. Even in more affluent homes, the ongoing burden of expensive drug therapies or ancillary services such as speech or physical therapy can result in attenuation of adherence over time. There may be other more subtle costs incurred by adhering to medical regimens, including costs of glucose strips (diabetes), inhalers (asthma), and special diets. When the medication or protocol prescribed is too expensive and the family cannot afford it, the risk for nonadherence is high (Stockwell & Schulz, 1992).

Denial of Diagnosis

Some patients question the accuracy of the diagnosis they have been given or deny that they have the condition (Donovan et al., 1989). When a diagnosis does not explain inconsistent symptoms, does not fit the patient's knowledge or beliefs about the disease, or is made by a physician who is not known to the patient, there is some danger that the patient will not accept it because it does not make sense to him or her (Donovan, 1995). In some instances, children are diagnosed with a condition such as asthma, which parents believe will be outgrown. If children are well managed and become asymptomatic, some parents may discontinue therapy in the belief that the asthma is cured. Among adults with asthma, patients who adhere have been characterized as *acceptors* of their diagnosis, whereas the nonadherent population or *deniers* refuse to accept the diagnosis and the impact the disease has on their lives (Adams et al., 1997).

Physician Prescribing Practices

Another reason for volitional noncompliance by patients is errors by providers in treatment. Prescription practices are not always rational or neutral (Donovan, 1995). Doctors do not always make correct diagnoses and treatment decisions and sometimes fail to offer the most effective treatment with the least complexity. There is heterogeneity in prescribing practices among physicians (Garattini & Garattini, 1993), which reflects their own knowledge, training, and experience; this generates idiosyncratic practices based on their own spectrum of patients. Two patients with the same diagnosis may be given different treatments based only on which physician they see. The result is that individual patients may engage in *therapeutic experimentation* to find the right medication and optimum dose level for them (Steiner, Fihn, Blair, & Inui, 1991), or they may seek care from several providers.

RISK FACTORS FOR INADVERTENT NONADHERENCE

The literature on nonadherence also has identified factors that are associated with inadvertent nonadherence. These are conceptualized as falling into three categories: patient characteristics, child characteristics, and provider/system characteristics.

Patient Characteristics

Nonadherence appears unrelated to race, gender, disease diagnosis, and personality type (O'Brien, Petrie, & Raeburn, 1992). Patient-related factors that may result in inadvertent noncompliance include: forgetfulness (Annals, 1993; Buchholz, 1990), poor hearing or eyesight, poor mental and functional capabilities, poor quality of life, stress, lack of resources (Antonovsky, 1987; Eraker, Dirscht, & Becker, 1984; Nehemkis & Gerber, 1986; Taylor, 1986), lack of social support (Bloom, 1990; Dakof & Taylor, 1990; Martin & Dubbert, 1986; Melamed & Brenner, 1990; Rees, 1985; Sarason, Sarason, & Pierce, 1988), presence of multiple caregivers, apathy about health, pessimism (Mayer & Kellogg, 1989; Robbins, 1980; Rosenstock, 1985), poor understanding of the provider's instructions (Brody, 1997; Creer & Levstek, 1996; Donovan, 1995; Huss et al., 1997; Rand, Nides, Cowles, Wise, & Connett, 1995; Turner, Wheaton, & Lloyd 1995), low literacy, and language barriers.

Developmental Characteristics

When the child is the patient, a new set of adherence problems occurs. Although parents may be willing and able to implement even complex regimens on behalf of their child's welfare, several barriers may apply. First, child medication refusal can turn adherence into a daily struggle that becomes a dreaded time for parent and child. Parents may simply choose to not adhere at all. However, many do the best they can, but give in on occasion to their children's pleas or reduce the frequency of dosing to reduce the conflict. Second, children's cognitive abilities change with age and can affect adherence. Further, children with chronic conditions grow older with time and achieve the developmental maturity and skills to take on some or most of the responsibility for their own medical regimen. However, data suggest that premature transition of responsibilities for managing a health problem may result in increased nonadherence. Third, many adolescents may become noncompliant as a way to test for independence and autonomy. Compared to the well-developed literature on adult compliance, adherence among child populations is less well studied.

Provider/System Characteristics

One of the most frequently cited reasons for noncompliance is poor patient–doctor communication (Annals, 1993; Kessler, 1991; Proos et al., 1992). Studies have found that patients fail to remember between one third and one half of doctors' statements (Annals, 1993; DiMatteo, 1994; Ley & Spelman, 1981), and a majority of patients forget some doctor instructions (Donovan, 1991; Sarafino, 1990). Studies have shown that most physicians do not give clear instructions about how patients should take their medications (Svarstad, 1976).

Sometimes providers fail to teach patients to comply properly so that the instructional role of the provider is compromised. For example, several studies have documented that physicians do not demonstrate proper inhaler technique for delivering asthma medications (Chapman, Hanania, & Kesten, 1995), with only about 10% accurately demonstrating all the steps required (Kelling, Strohl, Smith, & Altose, 1983; Mas, Resnick, Firschein, Feldman, & Davis, 1992). There are other examples of improper patient education about use of preventive asthma medications that were inappropriately used for an acute episode (Bone, 1995; Finkelstein, 1994). Patients may also be prescribed incorrect medications or incorrect dosages so that proper adherence would not result in therapeutic benefit (Altman, 1993). Incomplete or inadequate instruction by providers to patients means patients cannot be adherent to prescribed regimens—they have not been properly taught what to do. Providers are increasingly suggesting that part of the blame for noncompliance rests with providers themselves (Creer & Levstek, 1996; Dunbar-Jacob, 1993).

RISK FACTORS FOR BOTH INADVERTENT AND VOLITIONAL NONADHERENCE

Characteristics of the provider and regimen can result in both types of nonadherence as considered next.

Provider/System Factors

Specific communication skills of practitioners are associated with improved adherence, including clarity of explanation, willingness to listen, asking patients their opinion, and avoiding medical jargon or overly simple words (Francis, Korsch, & Morris, 1969; Hall, Roter, & Katz, 1988; Korsch, Gozzi, &

Francis, 1968; Ley, 1988; Taylor, 1986). In addition, patient dissatisfaction with the medical consultation or physician are associated with low adherence (Francis et al., 1969; Hoelscher, Lictenstein, & Rosenthal, 1986; Korsch et al., 1968; Scott, 1981; Taylor, 1986; Whitcher-Alagna, 1983). Satisfaction with care is associated with increased memory about provider instructions as well as better communication (Ley, 1988). Some have demonstrated that a participatory style (more consistent with an adherence model than a compliance model) is associated with better adherence (Francis et al., 1969; Hall et al., 1988; Heszen-Klemens & Lapinska, 1984).

Medical system characteristics that have been associated with adherence include long waiting time (Dunbar & Agras, 1980), uncomfortable waiting area, unfriendly staff (Brownell, Cohen, Stunkard, Felix, & Cooley, 1984; Fielding & Breslow, 1983), and geographic distance between facilities (Meichenbaum & Turk, 1987).

Regimen Characteristics

Overall, adherence behavior appears more sensitive to the characteristics of the regimen, including properties of the medications used and the complexity of the regimen, than individual patient characteristics (Blackwell, 1979; Creer & Levstek, 1996; Donovan, 1995; Haynes et al., 1979; Huss et al., 1997). Factors associated with the medical regimen include medication taste; need to take many medications with multiple dosing intervals (Reichgott & Simons-Morton, 1983; Stone, 1979), need to take medicine over a long period (Garfield, 1982; Haynes et al., 1979; Nehemkis & Gerber, 1986), demanding or stressful treatment regimens, and incorrect prescriptions given by clinicians (Brody, 1997; Creer et al., 1996; Huss et al., 1997). Especially problematic is the risk of drift in skill level of patients over time. For example, it is hard for patients with asthma to remember how to properly use an inhaler during an asthma attack because its use is intermittent and complex, requiring multiple steps to use it correctly (Creer et al., 1996; Renne, Dowrick, & Wasek, 1983).

STRATEGIES TO REDUCE RISK FOR NONADHERENCE

Interventions to reduce nonadherence may benefit by applying a patient-centered conceptual model of adherence, particularly one that focuses on risk factors. It is possible for providers to assess patient risks for nonadherence on a routine basis. If providers assume that the patient is a decision maker rather than a passive advice taker, they would be more likely to examine patient, provider, system, and regimen characteristics that might interfere with adoption of medical therapy. When risk factors are identified, they can be intervened on.

We have developed a measure of risk for nonadherence among children with asthma. It is used to count up the number of risk factors for nonadherence (including regimen complexity, concerns, and beliefs about medications). This measure is strongly related to subsequent asthma morbidity (Bauman et al., 1999).

Second, it is important that providers begin to develop ways to distinguish the two different types of nonadherence. *Volitional nonadherers—*those who reject medical advice—need a different kind of intervention than *inadvertent nonadherers—*those who believe they are adherent or face obstacles to compliance. Even the degree of accuracy that patients report in terms of their own adherence behavior differs depending on whether they choose to not adhere.

Third, patient education is clearly necessary. Providers need to find ways to provide better quality information, perhaps through written instructions, to help patients retain the information they need to comply properly (Annals, 1993; Bond & Hussar, 1991; Rotar & Hall, 1994; Schlar, 1991; Stockwell & Schulz, 1992). However, although patient education is necessary (they cannot comply with recommended treatment without understanding what is expected), it is not sufficient to result in adherence. For example, doctors' adherence with their own medical regimens is very low, suggesting that only a small part of the problem is lack of knowledge.

Fourth, we should look for every opportunity to improve patient–doctor communication, including building a patient–provider partnership, increasing provider friendliness, making the provider more approachable, encouraging more cooperation between provider and patient, and improving physician communication skills (Annals, 1993; Bartlett et al., 1984; Heszen-Klemens & Lapinska, 1984). Specific communication issues include how to describe risk from illness and treatment to avoid framing effects (Malenka, Baron, Johansen, Wahrenberger, & Ross, 1993; Redelmeier, 1993), ability to connect cause with effect for the patient (Morrison, 1993), taking an active role in providing information and teaching (Wright, 1993), and treating patients with warmth and respect (Korsch, Freeman, & Negrete, 1971). Physician accuracy of diagnosis and treatment approach is also associated with improved compliance (Starfield et al., 1981).

Complexity of regimen is always an issue. Providers should actively seek ways to reduce the number of medications prescribed and the frequency of dosing (Annals, 1993; Rudd, Ahmed, Zachary, Barton, & Bonduelle, 1992; Schlar, 1991). They should also incorporate aids to adherence such as patient organizers, calendars, blister packs, and so on (Bond & Hussar, 1991; Rivers, 1992; Stockwell & Schulz, 1992). For example, if a dosing schedule requires a dose of medication during school hours, but the child is not permitted to take medication in school, noncompliance is impossible to avoid.

CONCLUSIONS

Over several decades, thousands of compliance studies have assumed that patients should adhere; they have asked the question, Why don't patients adhere? We need to turn the problem of nonadherence on its head. The data suggest that it is the exceptional patient who adheres—and we need to withdraw the expectation. Clinicians should reframe their expectations of patients. Many risk factors for nonadherence can be addressed by clinicians who approach their task of patient care as one of persuasion rather than assumed compliance. Providers need to consider moving away from the Adherence/Compliance approach, which focuses only on their goal of patient adherence, to a patient-centered model—the patient makes the decision about goals for treatment and how to fit treatment into the his or her schedule (Mellins et al., 1992). This means talking with patients about their health beliefs, eliciting fears and concerns, and giving patients not just a sense of control but the actual control over decision making (Mellins et al., 1992).

Providers need to be sure that when people make treatment choices, they are not influenced by misinformation, erroneous beliefs, fear, or costs and barriers that could be removed. Clearly part of the clinician's obligation is health education at multiple levels. Facts are what people need to know what to do—what to take, how often, what to do if side effects occur, and what drug interactions are possible. People also need help to integrate the meaning of their disease and treatment into their system of beliefs and knowledge. They may use nonscientific models to challenge the diagnosis, change their treatment, and terminate early. They may assume that taking more of a drug will increase its benefit or that it is a sign of health if they can *wean* themselves from the medication. This kind of education is not factual; it means identifying health beliefs that can interfere with medication adherence and uncovering fears that patients have about their condition that would lead to voluntary noncompliance.

Clinicians need to look to their own prescribing practices and the nature of the task presented to patients. The vast majority of studies treat the problem of noncompliance as the patient's fault. Few identify the *problem* to be inherent in the task (e.g., the complexity or level of demand of the treatment protocol), although many acknowledge that this makes compliance more difficult.

Providers also need to examine their own behavior and style of interacting with patients. For many parents, communication patterns of providers contribute to noncompliance. As Donovan (1995) pointed out, we assume that doctors know what is best for their patients; that they are able to impart medical information clearly and neutrally; that they prescribe effective treatments rationally; and that they are the principal (or only) contributors to decisions about medications and other treatments. (p. 444)

Clinicians should assume that everyone needs assistance in taking advantage of the medical miracles that are routinely prescribed. Consequently, the health care system needs to (a) provide universal, ongoing adherence support to patients so they have the information they need to implement the therapy, (b) help them devise strategies to use medications appropriately, (c) help them maintain behaviors as long as necessary, and (d) help them adjust to changing needs. All patients who have medical regimens, particularly those with chronic conditions requiring chronic therapies, should have ongoing access to expert medical and psychological advice on adherence. We cannot continue to define adherence as a failure of patients, but as our failure of care.

Patients need access to ongoing assistance to identify and overcome the barriers they experience to adherence. Those with a chronic condition may need their regimens altered frequently to respond to changes in disease, their overall health status, individual maturation and developmental changes over time, new treatment options, and the changing family situation of the patient. Adherence is not a static behavior. We cannot assume that a patient who is adherent at one point in time will always be adherent or that someone who is routinely adherent to some prescriptions will be adherent to others. Children who are adherent to treatment at one developmental stage may not continue to be adherent as they mature. Therefore, ongoing professional advice is needed to help patients adapt to change and minimize nonadherence. Developmental check-ups by providers with parents and patients can help assess child readiness to assume treatment responsibilities and ensure a smooth transition from family-based to more autonomous care during adolescence.

Some of this ongoing support should come from the patient's own provider. The impetus to adhere with complex, difficult, or worrisome treatment regimens must come from the provider, who can provide the rationale for its need and reassure patients about their concerns. However, most patients with chronic conditions also need access to a professional who is an expert in behavior and in helping patients understand how their own beliefs and fears interfere with their health behavior. They also need to consult these professionals for advice on how to integrate treatment adherence into a child's routine in a way that is developmentally appropriate; these professionals can help families overcome adherence barriers posed by family conflict, oppositional child behaviors, cost, and regimen complexity.

Need for Research

The patient-centered approach leads to a new and different set of research questions. First, how often do providers use an adherence model compared with a compliance model? When an adherence model is used, are providers more likely to identify barriers to compliance? Are they successful in removing those barriers? Are patients more adherent compared with a compliance approach? The philosophical shift from compliance to adherence is more ideological than empirical—we need good research to examine the consequences of each approach for quality patient care. Second, providers need specific techniques and/or measures that will help assess patient health beliefs. Few clinicians have been trained in strategies to understand the ways individual patients think about their disease and its treatment and how these beliefs increase or reduce the risk for non-adherence. Third, how can providers assess the two kinds of nonadherence—volitional and inadvertent? Good clinical interviewing style, combined with an acceptance of the validity of patient choices, may encourage patients to openly acknowledge their reservations about specific protocols and medications. However, research is needed to identify methods to help clinicians assess volitional and inadvertent nonadherence so that appropriate interventions can be initiated. Fourth, which risk factors for nonadherence are amenable to intervention? Which types of interventions fit which types of nonadherence? Can we begin to develop a systematic empirical strategy to assess the reasons for noncompliance? Can we match these with the most effective intervention for each? Finally, in pediatric chronic illness, both parents and children can introduce independent risk factors for nonadherence. How do developmental stage and change, parent–child conflict, parental beliefs, and child behaviors increase or reduce risk for nonadherence?

Scientific progress in medical research has made many potential therapies available to people with health problems, but many are not used to their potential because we have failed in our responsibility to provide systematic routine assistance to those asked to adopt these therapies. Part of medical treatment needs to include this assistance or we will continue to have high rates of nonadherence, unnecessary morbidity, and potentially avoidable mortality.

REFERENCES

Adams, S., Pill, R., & Jones, A. (1997). Medication, chronic illness and identity: The perspective of people with asthma. *Social Science and Medicine, 45,* 189–201.
Adelman, H., & Taylor, L. (1986). Children's reluctance regarding treatment: Incompetence, resistance, or an appropriate response. *School Psychology Review, 15,* 91–99.

Agras, W., Taylor, C., & Kraemer, H. (1987). Relaxation training for essential hypertension at the worksite: II. The poorly controlled hypertensive. *Psychosomatic Medicine, 49,* 264–273.

Alessandro, F., Vincenzo, Z. G., Marco, S., Marcello, G., & Enrica, R. (1994). Compliance with pharmacologic prophylaxis and therapy in bronchial asthma. *Annals of Allergy, 73,* 135–140.

Altman, J. (1993, May 4). Rise in asthma deaths is tied to ignorance of many physicians. *New York Times,* p. B8.

Annals. (1993). Patient compliance. *Annals of Pharmacotherapy, 27*(Editorial), s5–s24.

Antonovsky, A. (1987). *Unraveling the mystery of health how people manage stress and stay well.* San Francisco: Jossey-Bass.

Bartlett, E., Grayson, M., Barker, R., Levine, D., Golden, A., & Libber, S. (1984). The effects of physician communication skills on patient satisfaction, recall and adherence. *Journal of Chronic Disease, 37,* 755–764.

Baum, D., & Creer, T. L. (1986). Medication compliance in children with asthma. *Journal of Asthma, 23,* 49–59.

Bauman, L. J., Wright, L., Leickly, F., Crain, E., Kruszon-Moran, D., & Wade, S. L. (1999, May). *Relationship of asthma morbidity among inner-city children to nonadherence.* Paper presented at the annual meeting of the Ambulatory Pediatrics Association, San Francisco, CA.

Becker, M. (1974). The Health Belief Model and personal health behavior. In M. Becker (Ed.), *Health education monographs* (pp. 324–473). San Francisco, CA: Society for Public Health Education.

Becker, M., & Janz, N. (1984). The Health Belief Model: A decade later. *Health Education Quarterly, 11,* 1–47.

Becker, M., & Maiman, L. (1975). Sociobehavioral determinants of compliance with health and medical care recommendations. *Medical Care, 13,* 1–24.

Blackwell, B. (1979). The drug regimen and treatment compliance. In R. Haynes, D. Taylor, & D. Sackett (Eds.), *Compliance in health care* (pp. 144–156). Baltimore, MD: Johns Hopkins University Press.

Bloom, J. (1990). The relationship of social support and health. *Social Science and Medicine, 30,* 635–637.

Bond, W., & Hussar, D. (1991). Detection methods and strategies for improving medication compliance. *American Society of Hospital Pharmacists, 48,* 1978–1987.

Bone, R. (1995). Another word of caution regarding a new long-acting bronchodilator. *Journal of the American Medical Association, 273,* 967.

Bosely, C., Parry, D., & Cochrane, G. (1994). Patient compliance with inhaled medicine: Does combing betaagonists with corticosteroids improve compliance? *European Respiratory Journal, 7,* 504–509.

Brody, J. (1997). Bait poisoning and why kids complain about their medication. *Journal of Child and Adolescent Psychopharmacology, 7,* 71–72.

Brooks, C. M., Richards, J. M., Kohler, C. L., Swoong, S., Martin, B., Windsor, R. A., & Bailey, W. C. (1994). Assessing adherence to asthma medication and inhaler regimens: A psychometric analysis of adult self-report scales. *Medical Care, 32,* 298–307.

Brownell, K., Cohen, R., Stunkard, A., Felix, M., & Cooley, N. (1984). Weight loss competitions at the work site: Impact on weight, morale, and cost-effectiveness. *American Journal of Public Health, 74,* 1283–1285.

Buchholz, W. (1990). When competent patients make irrational choices (letter). *New England Journal of Medicine, 323,* 1354.

Buckalew, L., & Sallis, R. (1986). Patient compliance and medication perception. *Journal of Clinical Psychology, 42,* 49–53.

Caldwell, J., Cobb, S., & Dowling, M. (1971). The dropout problem in antihypertensive treatment: A pilot study of social and emotional factors influencing a patient's ability to follow antihypertensive treatment. *Journal of Chronic Disease, 22,* 572–579.

Cochrane, G. (1992). Therepeutic compliance in asthma; its magnitude and implications. *European Respiratory Journal, 5*, 122–124.

Conrad, P. (1985). The meaning of medications: Another look at compliance. *Social Science and Medicine, 20*, 29–37.

Coutts, J., Gibson, N., & Paton, J. (1992). Measuring compliance with inhaled medication in asthma. *Archives of Diseases of Childhood, 67*, 332–333.

Creer, T., & Levstek, D. (1996). Medication compliance and asthma: Overlooking the trees because of the forest. *Journal of Asthma, 33*, 203–211.

Dakof, G., & Taylor, S. (1990). Victims' perceptions of social support: What is helpful from whom. *Journal of Personality and Social Psychology, 58*, 80–89.

DiMatteo, M. (1994). Enhancing patient adherence to medical recommendations. *Journal of the American Association of Medicine, 271*, 79–83.

Dompeling, E., Van Grunsven, P., Van Schayck, C., Folgering, H., Molema, J., & Van Weel, C. (1992). Treatment with inhaled steroid in asthma and chronic bronchitis: Long-term compliance and inhaler technique. *Family Practice, 9*, 161–166.

Donovan, J. (1991). Patient education and the consultation: The importance of lay beliefs. *Annals of Rheumatic Disease, 50*, 418–421.

Donovan, J. (1995). Patient decision making: The missing ingredient in compliance research. *International Journal of Technological Association in Health Care, 11*, 443–455.

Donovan, J., Blake, D., & Fleming, W. (1989). The patient is not a blank sheet: Lay beliefs and their relevance to patient education. *British Journal of Rheumatology, 28*, 58–61.

Dunbar, J., & Agras, W. (1980). Compliance with medical instructions. In J. Ferguson & C. Taylor (Eds.), *Comprehensive handbook of behavioral medicine* (Vol. 3, pp. 115–145). New York: Spectrum.

Dunbar-Jacob, J. (1993). Contributions to patient adherence: Is it time to share the blame? *Health Psychology, 12*, 91.

Eraker, S., Dirscht, J., & Becker, M. (1984). Understanding and improving patient compliance. *Archives of Internal Medicine, 100*, 258–268.

Fielding, J., & Breslow, L. (1983). Health promotion programs sponsored by California employers. *American Journal of Public Health, 73*, 538–542.

Finkelstein, F. (1994). Risks of salmeterol. *New England Journal of Medicine, 331*, 1314.

Francis, V., Korsch, B. M., & Morris, M. J. (1969). Gaps in doctor–patient communication: Patients' response to medical advice. *New England Journal of Medicine, 280*, 535–540.

Garattini, S., & Garattini, L. (1993). Pharmaceutical prescriptions in four European countries. *Lancet, 342*, 1191–1192.

Garfield, E. (1982). Patient compliance: A multifaceted problem with no easy solution. *Current Comments, 37*, 5–14.

Goldman, A., Holcomb, R., & Perry, H. (1982). Can dropout and other noncompliance be minimized in a clinical trial? *Controlled Clinical Trials, 3*, 75–89.

Gong, H. J., Simmons, M. S., Clark, V. A., & Tashkin, D. P. (1988). Metered-dose inhaler usage in subjects with asthma: Comparison of nebulizer chronolog and daily diary recordings. *Journal of Allergy Clinical Immunology, 82*, 5–10.

Hall, J., Roter, D., & Katz, N. (1988). Meta-analysis of correlates of provider behavior in medical encounters. *Medical Care, 26*, 657–675.

Hanania, N. A., Wittman, R., Kesten, S., & Chapman, K. R. (1995). Medical personnel's knowledge of the ability to use inhaling devices. *CHEST, 107*, 290.

Haynes, R., Taylor, D., & Sackett, D. (1979). *Compliance in health care.* Baltimore, MD: Johns Hopkins University Press.

Heszen-Klemens, I., & Lapinska, E. (1984). Doctor–patient interactions, patients' health behavior and effects of treatment. *Social Science and Medicine, 19*, 9–18.

Hoelscher, T., Lictenstein, K., & Rosenthal, T. (1986). Home relaxation practice in hypertension treatment: Objective assessment and compliance induction. *Journal of Consulting Clinical Psychology, 54,* 217–221.

Huss, K., Travis, P., & Huss, R. (1997). Adherence issues in clinical practice. *Primary Care Practice, 1,* 199–206.

Kelling, J., Strohl, K., Smith, R., & Altose, M. (1983). Physician knowledge in use of canister nebulizers. *CHEST, 83,* 612.

Kelloway, J. S., Wyatt, R. A., & Adlis, S. A. (1994). Comparison of patients' compliance with prescribed oral and inhaled asthma medications. *Archives of Internal Medicine, 154,* 1349–1352.

Kessler, D. (1991). Communicating with patients about their medications. *New England Journal of Medicine, 325,* 1650–1652.

Kinsman, R. A., Dirks, J. F., & Dahlem, N. W. (1980). Noncompliance to prescribed-as-needed (PRN) medication use in asthma: Usage patterns and patient characteristics. *Journal of Psychosomatic Research, 24,* 97–107.

Kleiger, J. H., & Dirks, J. F. (1979). Medication compliance in chronic asthmatic patients. *Journal of Asthma Research, 16,* 93–96.

Korsch, B., Freeman, B., & Negrete, V. (1971). Practical implications of the doctor–patient interaction analysis for pediatric practice. *American Journal of Diseases of Childhood, 121,* 11–14.

Korsch, B., Gozzi, E., & Francis, V. (1968). Gaps in doctor–patient communication: I. Doctor–patient interaction and patient satisfaction. *Journal of Pediatrics, 42,* 855–871.

Leventhal, H., Zimmerman, R., & Gutmann, M. (1984). Compliance: A self-regulation perspective. In W. Gentry (Ed.), *Handbook of behavioral medicine* (pp. 369–423). New York: Guilford.

Ley, P. (1988). *Communicating with patients, improving communication, satisfaction, and compliance.* London: Croom Helm.

Ley, P., & Spelman, M. (1981). *Communicating with the patient.* London: Staples Press.

Malenka, D., Baron, J., Johansen, S., Wahrenberger, J., & Ross, J. (1993). The farming effect of relative and absolute risk. *Journal of General Internal Medicine, 8,* 543–548.

Martin, J., & Dubbert, P. (1986). Exercise and health: The adherence problem. *Behavioral Medicine Update, 4,* 16–24.

Mas, J., Resnick, D., Firschein, D., Feldman, B., & Davis, W. (1992). Misuse of metered dose inhalers by house staff members. *American Journal of Diseases of Childhood, 146,* 783.

Masek, B. (1982). Compliance and medicine. In D. Doyleys, R. Meredith, & A. Ciminero (Eds.), *Behavioral medicine: Assessment and treatment strategies* (pp. 527–545). New York: Plenum.

Mawhinney, H., Spector, S. L., Kinsman, R. A., Siegel, S. C., Rachelefsky, G. S., Katz, R. M., & Rohr, A. S. (1991). Compliance in clinical trials of two nonbronchodilator, antiasthma medications. *66,* 294–299.

Mayer, J., & Kellogg, M. (1989). Promoting mammography appointment making. *Journal of Behavioral Medicine, 12,* 605–611.

Meichenbaum, D., & Turk, D. (1987). *Facilitating treatment adherence.* New York: Plenum.

Melamed, B., & Brenner, G. (1990). Social support and chronic medical stress: An interaction-based approach. *Journal of Social and Clinical Psychology, 9,* 104–117.

Mellins, R. B., Evans, D., Zimmerman, B., & Clark, N. M. (1992). Patient compliance: Are we wasting our time and don't know it? *American Review of Respiratory Diseases, 146,* 1376–1377.

Morrison, R. (1993). Medication non-compliance. *Canadian Nurse, 98,* 15–18.

Nehemkis, A., & Gerber, K. (1986). Compliance and the quality of survival. In K. Gerber & A. Nehemkis (Eds.), *Compliance: The dilemma of the chronically ill.* New York: Springer.

O'Brien, M. K., Petrie, K., & Raeburn, J. (1992). Adherence to medication regimens: Updating a complex medical issue. *Medical Care Review, 49*, 435–454.

Proos, M., Reiley, P., Eagan, J., Stengrevics, S., Castile, J., & Arian, D. (1992). A study of the effects of self-medication on patients: Knowledge of and compliance with their medication regimen. *Journal of Nursing Care Quarterly*, 18–26.

Rand, C. S., Nides, M., Cowles, M. K., Wise, R. A., & Connett, J. (1995). Long-term metered-dose inhaler adherence in a clinical trial. *American Journal of Respiratory and Critical Care Medicine, 152*, 580–588.

Rand, C. S., & Wise, R. A. (1994). Measuring adherence to asthma medication regimens. *American Journal of Respiratory and Critical Care Medicine, 149*, s69–s76.

Redelmeier, D. (1993). Understanding patients' decisions. *Journal of the American Medical Association, 270*, 72–76.

Rees, D. (1985). Health beliefs and compliance with alcoholism treatment. *Journal of Studies on Alcohol, 46*, 517–524.

Reichgott, M., & Simons-Morton, B. (1983). Strategies to improve patient compliance with antihypertensive therapy. *Primary Care, 10*, 21–27.

Renne, C., Dowrick, P., & Wasek, G. (1983). Considerations of the participant in video recordings. In P. Dowrick & S. Biggs (Eds.), *Using video psychological and social applications* (pp. 23–32). New York: Wiley.

Rivers, P. (1992). Compliance aids: Do they work? *Drugs and Aging, 2*, 103–111.

Robbins, J. (1980). Patient compliance. *Primary Care, 7*, 703–711.

Rosenstock, I. (1974). Historical origins of the health belief model. *Health Education Monographs, 2*, 328.

Rosenstock, I. (1985). Understanding and enhancing patient compliance with diabetic regimens. *Diabetes Care, 8*, 610–616.

Rotar, D., & Hall, J. (1994). Strategies for enhancing patient adherence to medical recommendations. *Journal of the American Medical Association, 271*, 80–81.

Rudd, P., Ahmed, S., Zachary, V., Barton, C., & Bonduelle, D. (1992). Issues in patient compliance: The search for therapeutic sufficiency. *Cardiology, 80*, 2–10.

Sackett, D., & Snow, J. (1979). The magnitude of compliance and noncompliance. In R. Haynes, D. Taylor, & D. Sackett (Eds.), *Compliance in health care* (pp. 11–22). Baltimore: University Press.

Sarafino, E. (1990). *Health psychology: Biopsychosocial interactions*. New York: Wiley.

Sarason, I., Sarason, B., & Pierce, G. (1988). Social support, personality, and health. In S. Maes, C. Spielberger, P. Darafes, & I. Sarason (Eds.), *Topics in health psychology* (pp. 245–256). New York: Wiley.

Schlar, D. (1991). Improving medication compliance: A review of selected issues. *Clinical Therapeutics, 13*, 436–440.

Scott, C. (1981). Patient compliance. In J. Braunstien & R. Taister (Eds.), *Medical application of the behavioral sciences* (pp. 470–482). Chicago: Yearbook Medical Publishers.

Spector, S. L. (1985). Is your asthmatic patient really complying. *Annals of Allergy, 55*, 552–555.

Starfield, B., Wray, C., Hess, K., Gross, R., Birk, P., & D'Lugoff, B. (1981). The influence of patient–practitioner agreement on outcome of care. *American Journal of Public Health, 71*, 127–131.

Steiner, J. F., Fihn, S., Blair, B., & Inui, T. (1991). Appropriate reductions in compliance among well-controlled hypertensive patients. *Journal of Clinical Epidemiology, 44*, 1361–1377.

Stimson, G. V. (1974). Obeying doctor's orders: A review from the other side. *Social Science and Medicine, 8*, 97–104.

Stockwell, M., & Schulz, R. (1992). Patient compliance: An overview. *Journal of Clinical Pharmacy and Therapeutics, 17*, 283–295.

Stone, G. (1979). Patience compliance and the role of the expert. *Journal of Social Issues, 35,* 34–59.

Svarstad, B. (1976). Physician–patient communication and patient conformity with medical advice. In D. Mechanic (Ed.), *The growth of bureaucratic medicine: An inquiry into the dynamics of patient behavior and the organization of medical care.* New York: Wiley.

Tashkin, D. P. (1995). Multiple dose regimens. *CHEST, 107,* 176–182.

Taylor, S. (1986). Patient–practitioner interaction. In S. E. Taylor (Ed.), *Health psychology* (pp. 240–263). New York: Random House.

Tettersell, M. J. (1993). Asthma patients' knowledge in relation to compliance with drug therapy. *Journal of Advanced Nursing, 18,* 103–113.

Turner, R. J., Wheaton, B., & Lloyd, D. A. (1995). The epidemiology of social stress. *American Sociological Review, 60,* 104–125.

Van Sciver, M. M., D'Angelo, E. J., Rappaport, L., & Woolf, A. D. (1995). Pediatric compliance and the roles of distinct treatment characteristics, treatment attitudes, and family stress: A preliminary report. *Developmental and Behavioral Pediatrics, 16,* 350–358.

Whitcher-Alagna, S. (1983). Receiving medical help: A psychosocial perspective on patient reactions. In A. Nadler, J. Fisher, & B. DePaulo (Eds.), *New directions in helping* (pp. 51–84). New York: Academic Press.

Wright, E. C. (1993). Non-compliance: Or how many aunts has Matilda? *Lancet, 342,* 909–913.

Yeung, M., O'Connor, S., & Parry, D. (1994). Compliance with prescribed drug therapy in asthma. *Respiratory Medicine, 88,* 31–35.

CHAPTER FIVE

Self-Management and the Control of Chronic Pediatric Illness

Thomas L. Creer
Ohio University, Athens, OH

In his seminal work, Kuhn (1996) described how science does not advance in an evolutionary manner, but as a series of peaceful interludes punctuated by crises and revolutions. The crises generate revolutions because existing paradigms—what members of a scientific community share—are unable to manage anomalies or confounding information. The result is a rejection of the existing paradigm and the development of a new one. Because new paradigms emerge from old ones, there is a period of transition from abandonment of the traditional paradigm to adoption of the new paradigm. This period—often tumultuous—allows a number of events to occur. For example, new paradigms generally incorporate much of the vocabulary and apparatus, both conceptual and manipulative, of the traditional paradigm. Because these borrowed elements are not used in quite the same way within a new paradigm, there is a transition period during which there is a shift in allegiance from one paradigm to another. The period is marked by resistance from those loyal to the old paradigm to advances made by proponents of the new paradigm; this transition is necessary because the transfer of allegiance from paradigm to paradigm is a conversion experience that cannot be forced. It is only through scientific research that the professional community of scientists succeeds, first, in establishing the scope and limitations of the older paradigm and, second, in confirming the need and rationale of a new paradigm.

A revolution in paradigms, analogous to what Kuhn described as occurs in science, is currently taking place in two areas: providing health care

services and shifting priorities in disease management. These paradigmat-
ic crises and revolutions, in turn, have consequences that affect both medication compliance and self-management. This becomes apparent in
briefly describing the two emerging paradigms.

PROVIDING HEALTH CARE SERVICES

Describing all of the changes currently taking place in the health care system is beyond the purview of this chapter. Basically what is occurring is a
revolution with respect to the paradigm by which we receive health care.
The move is away from the traditional paradigm of health care—what
some call an *unmanaged system*—toward managed care (Fox, 1997). At
the heart of the debate is whether to keep a system that relies on sole
practitioners and traditional fee-for-service toward what proponents
characterize as an integrated delivery system that offers more potential
benefits to consumers (Abbey, 1997).

Proponents of each model claim victories. Fox (1997) declared that
managed care is rapidly dominating the health care financing and delivery
system in the United States. He based his argument on the fact that there
are an increasing number of Americans enrolled in health maintenance
organization (HMO) plans, preferred provider organizations (PPO), and
public sector programs, such as Medicare and Medicaid. Advocates of
managed care add that economic forces, such as the projection by the
Health Care Financing Administration that national health spending will
reach $2.1 trillion by 2007 (Smith et al., 1998), will continue to fuel man-
aged care. Chronic illness will continue to account for most of these costs.
Hoffman, Rice, and Sung (1996) found that, in the United States alone,
over 45% of the population, including children, have one or more chronic conditions. Their direct health care costs consume three fourths of U.S.
health care expenditures. Total costs for people with chronic conditions
amounted to $659 billion—$425 billion in direct health care costs and
$234 billion in indirect costs—in 1990.

Those who advocate the traditional model of providing health care also
make compelling arguments for their cause. For example, most physicians
reportedly do not like managed care. A recent survey of 30,000 physicians
conducted by the MEDSTAT Group and J.D. Power and Associates (1998)
revealed that 7 out of 10 respondents characterized themselves as *anti-
managed care*. They cited a desire for independence from health plans as
the primary reason for their position. Patients, too, are frustrated with
managed care. The majority of the respondents in a recent survey in the
United States—53%—said they think veterinarians typically spend more
time with animals than HMO doctors do with patients (Luntz Research

Company, 1998). More than 60% of those surveyed expressed little or no confidence that their health insurer would do everything within its power to provide the best medical care for an individual or member of his or her family. Little faith was expressed that the government would resolve the problem: Only 28% said legislation would improve the health care system, whereas 60% said personal initiative by patients was the best solution.

In the long run, whatever health care system emerges will depend on the role we are willing to accept as patients. In her classic essay, *Illness as Metaphor*, Susan Sontag (1976) noted that:

> Illness is the night-side of life, a more onerous citizenship. Everyone who is born holds dual citizenship in the kingdom of the well and in the kingdom of the sick. Although we all prefer to use only the good passport, sooner or later each of us is obliged, at least for a spell, to identify ourselves as citizens of that other place. (p. 3)

What occurs to us when we are *citizens of that other place* must be a major factor in determining which model of health care is eventually adopted in the United States.

SHIFTING PRIORITIES OF DISEASE MANAGEMENT

Medicine—in terms of its institutions, pay mechanisms, goals, practices, technology, training, myths, and symbols—is a profession concerned primarily with acute disease (Cassell, 1997). It is a medicine modeled on the treatment of infectious diseases such as pneumonia or meningitis. Although well under control in the industrialized world, infectious diseases account for much of the mortality among children in developing nations (World Health Organization, 1998). For this reason, the World Health Organization (WHO), in conjunction with the United Nations (UN), launched a highly successful program entitled Integrated Management of Childhood Illness (IMCI). It addresses childhood illness at three levels: It promotes improvements in the health system, health workers' skills, and family and community practices. The latter point is important to self-management in that it is aimed at teaching children and their parents to take greater responsibility for their own health.

In addition, developing parts of the world are undergoing what is known as a *epidemiological transition*—they are beginning to inherit the problems of richer nations. It applies to children and adolescents in at least two respects. First, the World Health Organization (1998) pointed out that childhood and adolescence are prime times for unhealthy diets, unsafe sexual activity, and smoking, all of which provoke disease in adulthood but have their roots in these early formative years. Second, there is a disproportionate burden of different chronic diseases between industrialized and developing countries. For example, although a worldwide problem, childhood asthma is a greater problem in the more affluent and developed countries than in the less affluent and developing countries (e.g., Wiesch & Samet, 1998). However, the WHO (1998) noted that one of the biggest hazards to children in the 21st century will be the continuing spread of HIV/AIDS. In 1997, some 590,000 children under 15 years of age became infected with HIV; most of these children live in developing countries.

MANAGEMENT OF ACUTE
AND CHRONIC PEDIATRIC DISEASES

Acute diseases are treated by doctors, nurses, or other caregivers inside or outside the hospital or clinic. Although compliance rates by children to medications taken for acute illnesses have been estimated to be less than 50% (e.g., Wandstrat & Kaplan, 1997), compliance in acute disease is less a problem than it is in the case of chronic illness: Patients take what caregivers give them or, if they do not, either the disease is self-limiting or the patient receives intensive treatment from a health care professional. As noted, the medical system is oriented toward the treatment of acute disorders.

There are few, if any, cures for chronic illnesses and disorders. The emphasis shifts toward controlling rather than curing the disorder. Every case of chronic illness represents a burden thrust on an individual or, in the case of children, on every member of a child's family. The disease can have an impact on many facets of a family's life. These can range from purchasing equipment needed to monitor aspects of the child's condition, such as an instrument for assessing blood sugar in a youngster with juvenile diabetes, to setting the daily pattern of the family's life, such as providing daily medications and physiotherapy to a child with cystic fibrosis (CF). A chronic disorder may not be a major disruption to a family that only has to be certain that a child take daily medications to control epilepsy or asthma. However, the fabric of the family's existence can be affected by disorders such as juvenile rheumatoid arthritis (JRA), CF, cerebral palsy, HIV/AIDS, and, for that matter, almost any chronic disorder that is uncontrolled. Depending on circumstances, such as financial abilities, families may or may not have access to life-enhancing treatment or support. For example, most families in industrialized countries have health coverage to assist with the expenses of most chronic childhood disorders. This may not be an option for people with lower incomes in developed countries or for families in developing countries. Thus, although the IMCI program has been highly successful in teaching parents and their children to take more responsibility for acute conditions such as diarrhea, measles, and malaria, the prognosis for help with HIV/AIDS is poor in developing countries.

The health care crisis spawned by the movement of paradigms away from the treatment of acute diseases toward the management of chronic disorders has produced a medical revolution that is far from over. A factor giving rise to the revolution, succinctly summarized by Cassell (1997), is the fact that physicians have yet to make the transition from treating acute disease to treating chronic disorders. He pointed out that, in classical acute disease, the disease is central; patient actions with such diseases are peripheral. However, continued Cassell, the difficulty for medicine is the failure to recognize that if chronic disease is overwhelmingly personal, then the person, not the disease, is central. This means, concluded Cassell, "that the body of knowledge of medical science that has served medicine so well in acute disease, is only a part, albeit a crucial part, of the story in chronic disease" (p. 25). Putting the patient at the center of his or her treatment should give greater impetus to the development and application of self-management programs for various illnesses.

PERSPECTIVES OF PATIENT INVOLVEMENT IN CHRONIC ILLNESS

Patient involvement in chronic illnesses or disorders can be viewed from a number of perspectives. Callahan (1998) proclaimed that we need "to open up once again the ancient Greek struggle between *hygeia*, the belief that the body if well and prudently tended, can take care of and cure itself, and *aesculapius*, the contrasting belief that only a medical intervention can set the body straight" (p. 42). He made a persuasive argument for a return to the Greek tradition of *hygeia*. In doing so, Callahan explained that he is not arguing against medicine, but against the distortions introduced by scientific medicine that have often forgotten or ignored some of the strengths of older traditions and practices. Millenson (1997) quoted experts who saw the management of chronic disorders as a partnership between patients and their health care providers in which patients are empowered to be more responsible for their own care. To these experts, self-management by patients was a new movement that produced startlingly promising results.

A more operational perspective of the role of patient behaviors in illness was provided by Von Korff, Gruman, Schaefer, Curry, and Wagner (1997) in their description of the collaborative management of chronic illness. They noted that patients and their families are the primary caregivers in chronic illness. In particular, patients and their families provide self-care in the following ways: They (a) perform activities that promote health, build physiological strength, and prevent adverse consequences; (b) interact with health care providers and adhere to recommended treatment regimens; (c) monitor physical and emotional status and make appropriate decisions on the basis of self-monitoring; and (d) manage the effect of illness on the patient's ability to function in important roles and control emotions, acquire self-esteem, and develop relationships with others. More specifically, Von Korff and his colleagues suggested: "Collaborative management occurs when patients and care providers have shared goals, a sustained working relationship, mutual understanding of roles and responsibilities, and requisite skills for carrying out their roles" (p. 1097). This definition provides a strong conceptual basis for linking patient efforts with medical management.

SELF-MANAGEMENT OF CHRONIC
CHILDHOOD DISORDERS

Definition of Self-Management and Pediatric Illness

Different terminology has been introduced to describe skills that children and their families perform to help control chronic illness. Such terms include *self-regulation, self-management, self-directed behavior, self-control, self-change*, and *self-care*. Attempts have been made to define terms according to whether patients pursue goals set by others or goals set by themselves. In reality, however, there is no consensus of how the terms are used. At least with chronic illness, there is a strong and increasing trend to treat the terms *self-management, self-regulation, self-control, self-change, self-directed behavior*, and even *self-care* as synonymous (Creer, 2000). The term *collaborative management* can be added to this list. In addition, whatever terms are used with pediatric illness must consider not only chronically ill children, but their parents and other members of their families. This is especially important with younger children, who are not only dependent on their own skills, but on the action of their caregivers and other family members.

Considering the cooperation required between children and their caregivers, a working definition of *self-management* would read as follows:

> Self-management involves the performance of a set of procedures by children and/or their caregivers to help control a chronic disorder. Specific self-management skills performed are a function of task demands presented by different illnesses, the rhythm of the disorder, treatment expectations, beliefs of others, the problem of uncertainty, the age or abilities of a child,

and the contexts within which action is taken. Elements of self-management include: (a) goal selection; (b) information collection; (c) information processing and evaluation; (d) decision-making; (e) action; and (f) self-reaction. Successful mastery and performance of self-management skills, over time and across settings, should result in the following outcomes: (a) changes in mortality and morbidity indices of the illness; (b) improvement in the quality of life experienced by children, their caregivers, and members of their families; and (c) the development of self-efficacy beliefs on the part of patients and their caregivers that they can perform whatever skills are needed to contribute to the control of their disorder, in part through their becoming partners with health care providers to manage the chronic illness or disorder.

Several aspects of this definition are further described here or later in the chapter.

Treatment of a Chronic Illness

The definition recognizes that children do not treat their chronic illness by themselves. Successful self-management of chronic illness involves children, their parents or caregivers, and members of their families. It could be argued that this definition violates a pure conception of *self-management*; the latter would assume that we carry out all functions required to accomplish a goal, much like driving a car by ourselves. The argument is valid. However, as is the case with anyone afflicted with a chronic illness, all children need help in the management of their disorder. Younger children require assistance on a daily basis, but older children and adolescents occasionally require help from others. This aid should be provided within the framework of cooperation established by family members—children, parents, and siblings—with their physicians and other health care providers.

Impact of Other Variables on Self-Management

Whatever self-management skills are performed are a function of a number of variables, including task demands, rhythm of the disorder, treatment expectations, beliefs of others, problem of uncertainty, age or abilities of the child, and context within which action is required. Each of these variables merits a brief discussion.

Task Demands. Although elements of self-management are used across disorders (Creer & Holroyd, 1997), tasks involved in managing an illness vary from disorder to disorder. These tasks put dissimilar burdens on individual children and their families. This can be illustrated by comparing two childhood disorders: asthma and CF. Pediatric asthma can often be managed by children faithfully taking a daily controller medication to prevent asthma and, during exacerbations, using an inhaled quick relief drug (National Asthma Education and Prevention Program, 1997). The effort involved in performing these tasks is small; the tasks are more a nuisance than a disruption to the family. In contrast, the control of CF entails a number of tasks, including one to four chest physiotherapy treatments a day, exercise, prevention of bacterial infections, enzyme replacement, and consumption of a calorie-laden diet (Stark, Jelalian, & Miller, 1995). These tasks require considerable diligence and effort on the part of children and parents. Consequently, CF cannot help but be at the center of a family's daily existence.

Rhythm of the Disorder. Although patients and their families consistently deal with the condition on a regular basis, the rhythm of the disorder may wax and wane (Creer, 2000). This is the case with many pediatric disorders including arthritis, asthma, diabetes, CF, and migraine headache. Periods of quiescence are interspersed with exacerbations of the condition; alleviation of these episodic flare-ups require extra medications, additional treatments, and, in severe cases, hospitalization. Attempting to reduce the impact of the disorder's rhythm is a key to successful management of any chronic illness; it is why degree of control over a chronic illness is so salient.

Treatment Expectations. The nature of chronic conditions influences the expectations of children and their families concerning a given disorder and its consequences. When a diagnosis is made, children and their families often think that if only located, there is a silver bullet that will cure a chronic disorder, much as an acute illness is cured. They may explore an array of treatment alternatives, including both traditional and alternative health options. The ultimate failure to find a panacea for the disorder may be accompanied by a feeling of hopelessness that no matter what children and their families do they will be limited by the illness of the child.

Beliefs of Others. Insidious factors in the control of a chronic disorder are the beliefs others have about particular illnesses. A child with juvenile rheumatoid arthritis may be told, "You can't have arthritis. That only comes with old age." Such statements do not alleviate the pain experienced by the child. A youngster with asthma may be told, "Hey, you're bringing this on yourself! Asthma is all in the head." These comments do not help the child with asthma breathe better. A child with recurring headaches may be told, "Why are you sick today? You were fine yesterday."

The remarks do little to assuage the child's pain.

Erroneous beliefs undermine any treatment strategy taken with a chronic illness. They are particularly deleterious when they drive a wedge between the parents of a chronically ill child. This was described by Creer (1979), who reported that in the case of pediatric asthma fathers often heard information about the disorder—particularly suggesting asthma is a psychological disorder—that directly confounds scientific knowledge of the disorder. These beliefs often shattered any attempt to create a cooperative strategy by parents. As repeatedly voiced by the mothers of children with asthma, there were the false perceptions of their mothers in law to the effect that the disorder results from the relationship a child has with his or her mother. When these beliefs and stereotypes are formed, they prove enduring. Consequently, they are counterproductive to generating a cohesive family approach to the treatment of pediatric asthma.

The Problem of Uncertainty. Uncertainty by physicians and health care professionals underlies the treatment received by children with a chronic illness. Because there is no cure for most conditions, physicians or health care professionals can only guess at the best treatment for a given child with a particular illness (Creer, 2000). If they select an appropriate option, great: The child's disorder—whether it be juvenile rheumatoid arthritis or childhood leukemia—may be controlled. If the disorder is not controlled, as is too often the case, physicians or health care professionals can only consider other treatment options. This launches a trial-and-error process to find the best treatment for a given child and his or her condition.

Cassell (1997) discussed two factors that contribute to uncertainty. First, there are defects in the knowledge of individual physicians. Second, there are inadequacies in the profession's knowledge. As Cassell lamented, "Even if I, impossibly granted, knew everything medicine knew, I would not know everything. There would still be uncertainties" (p. 70). There are two other factors of uncertainty that can never be eliminated (Gorovitz & MacIntyre, 1975). First, every decision—large or small—is made about the future and the future is always uncertain. Second, all of science—including medical science—is about generalities. Yet as explained by Cassell (1997), "By contrast, every patient is a particular individual and, therefore, necessarily different in some respect from the general. Thus, clinical judgments are always uncertain and medical knowledge necessarily involves uncertainties" (p. 70).

The concern, dislike of ambiguity, and fear of uncertainty that plague physicians are present in patients. Their stakes, however, are higher (Cassell, 1997). Even increasing their knowledge of treatment options for a given chronic pediatric illness fails to extinguish their uncertainty and, ultimately, the disillusionment experienced by many parents and their chronically ill children.

Age and Abilities of Children. How much responsibility children can take for their own disorder depends on their age and abilities. Most self-management programs for pediatric asthma, for example, are aimed at those 7 years of age or older (Wigal, Creer, Kotses, & Lewis, 1990). This is because, in part, many of the materials used to teach self-management require some ability to talk, read, and write. Perhaps more important, developmental factors are involved in the evolvement of consciousness and its control (Kagan, 1998). Without these developmental changes, children are unlikely to learn how to contribute to their own health and well-being.

Other programs in asthma have been tailored for the parents of younger children. An example is Wee Wheezers—an asthma education program tailored for the parents of children under 7 years of age (Wilson et al., 1996). However, the deciding determinant in deciding which approach to take with an individual youngster are the abilities of that child. Often youngsters as young as 5 years of age are capable of self-monitoring their asthma with a peak flow meter. When this occurs, they can make the decision as to what action to take with an asthma exacerbation, even if it is nothing more than to inform a parent of a change in their breathing. It is unlikely, however, that the attention of many children is so developed as to permit them to distinguish the initial sign of an exacerbation, the subsequent analysis of the event, the initial interpretation, and the motor readiness required to establish control over the episode (Kagan, 1998). Research is required on the developmental aspects to determine when children can perform the set of behaviors sequentially to manage their condition.

Contexts Within Which Action Is Taken. Another reason school-age children are taught self-management skills is because they often need to perform these competencies at school or in other settings when away from parents and family members. This is true across pediatric disorders, including diabetes, CF, attention deficit hyperactivity disorder (ADHD), or asthma. Here it is the responsibility of individual children, perhaps with prompting by their teachers, to seek whatever help is available to manage an exacerbation of an existing chronic illness.

The rising tide of single-parent homes has also created different contexts for action for many chronically ill children. The change in families, in fact, was a major impetus for the development and application of self-management programs for pediatric asthma (Creer & Winder, 1986). A large number of children treated at the National Asthma Center in the 1960s and 1970s, for example, were discharged to return home to single-parent homes where the parent worked. Hence, it became imperative to teach children to help manage their asthma because they had no or limited assistance with their asthma attacks. This was also the basis for involving caregivers and siblings in some early asthma self-management programs (e.g., Creer et al., 1988). Only through such involvement, it was thought, could some fabric of support be created for the chronically ill child. This is not a universally accepted approach, particularly in managed care settings, to managing a pediatric illness, but it is imperative that consideration be given to strengthening the family context if a chronic illness is to be controlled (e.g., Kazak, Segal-Andrews, & Johnson, 1995).

Performance of Self-Management Skills Over Time and Across Settings

In the past, little attention has been focused on the continued performance of self-management skills after a particular educational or behavioral program has ended. If, as occurs in most clinical trials, pre- and postchanges were demonstrated, this was enough to validate the program. The approach is short-sighted in that a defining characteristic of chronic illness—some say the defining characteristic—is duration (Verbrugge & Patrick, 1995). This is certainly the case with most pediatric chronic illnesses, whether it be CF or diabetes. The children need to learn self-management strategies that can be adapted to fit changing contexts and performed for the remainder of their lives.

STRUCTURE FOR APPLICATION OF SELF-MANAGEMENT IN CHRONIC PEDIATRIC ILLNESS

Effective self-management of any health problem, particularly chronic pediatric illness, rests on the successful creation and maintenance of a viable structure composed of health care providers, children and their families, and education and performance variables. Like a complex puzzle, it is an intricate and constantly changing configuration that integrates components of the three sets of variables into some sort of pattern held together by the cooperative actions of medical personnel, patients and their families, and elements of the program. Under ideal conditions, the pattern can be of immense strength and subtlety. If this is to occur, however, certain factors must be present. Significant variables include the following.

Health Care Providers

A number of health care provider variables are relevant to the introduction and successful implementation of self-management. Prominent variables include the following.

Philosophy of Health Care.   Attempts to nudge health care providers
to accept patients with a chronic illness as active participants in their own
health care have yielded mixed results. On the one hand, the Center for
the Advancement of Health (1996) published an indexed bibliography on
self-management for people with chronic disease. They presented
abstracts of 439 articles or chapters published on the self-management of
chronic illness; of these abstracts, 30 concerned children. These studies
would not have been conducted without the encouragement and involvement of health care providers. On the other hand, Creer (1998) pointed
out that health care providers are often reluctant to share management of
a chronic disorder with their patients. Perhaps as if treating an acute infection, they ignore the basic autonomy of human actions and opt to use
other terms by saying patients are *co-managing* or using *guided self-management* in treating a chronic illness. Both terms are fallacious; they suggest that the mantle of medical treatment can be stretched far beyond the
boundaries of a health care worker's office to govern the behaviors of
chronically ill children and their parents over time and across settings.

The assumption ignores two major issues. First, once children and their
families receive medical instruction on how to manage a chronic pediatric
illness, they are on their own. Baring an exacerbation of a condition, families are responsible for 100% of the daily actions taken to manage a disease. For example, children with JRA and their families are responsible to
obtain and take antiinflammatory medications as prescribed. They also
determine where and when regular sessions of physical therapy occur. In
most cases, these independent actions are similar to those taken in the
management of diabetes, epilepsy, and asthma. This does not mean, as
long assumed by some health personnel, that patients will go their own
way and be totally autonomous (Creer, 1998). This would be as foolish as
if they failed to seek medical advice and treatment in the first place.

Second, use of the terms *co-management* or *guided self-management*
violate a basic assumption of self-management: Children and their families
have a greater stake in the management of a chronic illness than anyone
and, if trained appropriately, can make a significant difference in the control
of a youngster's illness. Treatment of a chronic condition requires that children and their families continuously engage in such self-directed behaviors
as monitoring a disorder, processing and evaluating gathered data, making
decisions on the basis of this information, and taking appropriate action.
Their skills, along with the self-confidence or self-efficacy they acquire about
executing these behaviors, are critical ingredients in the management of the
condition. A chronic illness will not be controlled as a result of health care
personnel solely applying techniques, effective in the treatment of acute
diseases, to the treatment of the condition. Only by adhering to a jointly
developed and agreed on treatment regimen—capitalizing on the optimal

utilization of the skills of both health care personnel and patients—can a chronic pediatric condition be successfully managed.

Improve Communication Skills. Perhaps because of time restrictions imposed by managed care, health care providers often fail to effectively communicate with patients and, in turn, teach them self-management skills. For example, treatment regimens in childhood asthma, including the distinction between preventive or controller drugs and quick relief medications, are often not explained to patients. Furthermore, techniques needed to properly use instruments for the dispensing of medications, such as inhalers, are not often demonstrated correctly (Creer & Levstek, 1996). These problems can be remedied through an improvement of the quality and quantity of doctor–patient interactions, particularly through the increased involvement of children (van Dulmen, 1998).

Work to Build Trust of Patients. The negative feelings patients have toward managed health care often generalize to their health care providers. Safran et al. (1998) described a study linking defining characteristics of primary care to treatment outcomes. It was found that patients' trust in their physicians and physicians' knowledge of patients were leading correlates of three important outcomes of care: adherence to physician's advice, patient satisfaction, and improved health status. Considering other aspects presented by a chronic pediatric illness, such as the problem of uncertainty regarding treatment options, the need to build and strengthen the trust of patients must be a priority in whatever health care system emerges from today's chaos.

Use Established Guidelines of Treatment. Evidence-based clinical guidelines are systematically developed statements to assist practitioners and patients to make decisions about appropriate health for specific clinical conditions and circumstances (Woolf, Grol, Hutchinson, Eccles, & Grimshaw, 1999). These guidelines are increasingly a familiar part of clinical practice. There are benefits to both patients and health care professionals inherent in the development and use of such directives. Woolf and his colleagues enumerated potential benefits to patients as improvements in health outcomes, consistency of care, and empowerment to consider personal needs in selecting the best treatment option and, therefore, to make informed health care choices. Benefits to health care professionals include potential improvement in the quality of clinical decisions, quality improvement activities, and provision of a common point of reference for prospective and retrospective audits of clinical or hospital practices.

Clinical guidelines are described because of their applicability to chronically ill children and their families in acquiring and performing self-management skills. Two potential benefits should be emphasized. First, the guidelines were prepared and issued to benefit health care workers and patients alike. This is a new twist in the treatment of pediatric disorders in that it recognizes that children and their families can play a leading role in the management of a chronic condition. Second, some guidelines have gone so far as to advocate that health care personnel and their patients jointly establish treatment goals, as well as ways to achieve these goals (e.g., National Asthma Education and Prevention Program, 1997). To develop and achieve treatment goals requires a cooperation hitherto lacking in the management of chronic disorders. It is for this reason that clinical guidelines should be the catalyst for mainstreaming self-management into health care, particularly in the management of chronic disorders.

Chronically Ill Children and Their Families

Several challenges are presented by patient variables.

Philosophy of Medical Care.   Patients are no better prepared for self-management than are health care professionals. For over half a century, Americans have been conditioned to see their physicians for everything ranging from whether to diet to what cough syrup to use. Self-management of chronic illness, however, calls for patients to become partners with their health care provider. The latter can advise and assist children and their families, but it is up to individual families to decide what actions are necessary in various contexts and then perform those actions. This is a radical departure from the management of acute diseases, but one required to establish control over a chronic condition within the boundaries set both by medical knowledge and economic reality.

Improve Communication Skills.   To become an ally with one's health provider means that children and their families assist in all aspects of their health care. They need to become knowledgeable regarding their condition, how it is treated, and steps to take to establish control over their condition. Children and their families should prepare for medical visits by not only assembling collected information on themselves and their condition, but by jotting down questions raised by their data. Finally, because communication underlies the relationship, children and their families must learn to communicate with their health care provider. Being a partner implies a *quid pro quo* arrangement, in that children and their families receive the health care services they require in return for providing the day-to-day care for their own condition.

Seek Information About Health and Disease.   Like their partners, the health care providers, children, and their families must constantly seek information about their condition and its treatment. There is evidence that this occurring. Not only do patients pay attention to pharmaceutical commercials regarding medications appropriate to their disorder, but they actively seek information. This was recently noted by data on MEDLINE searches by patients and their families. In 1997, the National Library of Medicine reported that 7 million MEDLINE searches were made in 1996. Today, by contrast, 7 million MEDLINE searches are made per month (National Library of Medicine, 1998). Almost one third of these searches are made by the general public.

Patient Education

A number of patient education variables affect the acquisition and performance of self-management skills. These variables include the following.

Mechanism of Introducing and Training in Self-Management.   A prudent view expressed in the Expert Panel Report 2 for asthma (National Asthma Education and Prevention Program, 1997) is that education for all patients should begin at the time of the diagnosis of a disease and be integrated into every step of a patient's care. This underlies the necessity that children and their families not only learn about a child's condition and its management, but have the opportunity to interact with their physician and other health care personnel. Whether this actually occurs given the brief amount of time physicians spend with their patients is questionable. It is difficult to teach basic techniques for managing a chronic disorder when the average patient visit with a physician is only 7 minutes and 12 minutes for new patients (Moeller, 1998). Rather, much of what patients learn about their condition comes from allied health care personnel, written handouts, or videotapes. As noted, patients also acquire knowledge about an illness on their own from the media, the Internet, or pharmaceutical commercials.

The approach currently taken often results in a hit-or-miss sequel, where patients and their families may or may not learn what they should about the management of a chronic illness. Regardless of learning situations, acquired knowledge must be translated into actual performance. All one need do is talk with chronically ill children, no matter their illness, and their families to recognize that the leap is easier said than done. What often happens is a failure to bridge the chasm between acquisition of knowledge to performance of the self-management skills needed to control a chronic illness (Creer, Levstek, & Reynolds, 1998).

Establishing a Working Relationship. Throughout most of the 20th century, physicians prided themselves on the relationship they forged with their patients. Callahan (1998) noted that, in the post-World War II West, the doctor–patient relationship remained at the center. However, it has been radically altered by technological developments, complex financial arrangements, and inroads of the surrounding culture. Herzlinger (1997) argued that the present health care system is not organized to provide convenient care to patients with a chronic disease. She concluded that, "In much of today's health care system, obtaining appropriate medical care for a chronic disease is like eating in a restaurant where you must bring in your own bread, entree, vegetables, dessert, and wine" (p. 19). Given this summation, it is surprising that patients form relationships with physicians, yet many do. The fact that they do is likely the result of patient skills being coupled with those of physicians who still care about their patients and the practice of medicine.

Teach Appropriate Patient Skills. Changing contexts requires that a variety of skills be taught and applied in self-management programs (Center for the Advancement of Health, 1996; Creer, 1997). Many of these skills are enumerated in Table 5.1. As noted, medication compliance or adherence is only one part, albeit a significant part, of self-management. Patients are not only taught prevention skills to control a chronic illness, but to apply other skills, as agreed on with their health care provider, to manage acute episodes of an illness. Other skills, such as self-directed behaviors and self-reinforcement, are used both to prevent acute episodes and manage them when they occur. The importance of these skills becomes clear in discussing essential elements of self-management.

Emphasis on Performance. Once children and their families have been taught self-management skills, the emphasis shifts to how they perform these skills in helping to control a chronic condition. This can be accomplished by teaching self-management skills over a period of time. There are three advantages to such an approach. First, when asthma self-management programs were taught over an 8-week period, the skills of individual families could be periodically monitored and evaluated (Creer et al., 1988). This permitted those conducting the program to assist individual families to close gaps in their performance or develop techniques that were appropriate for the distinct problems they faced. Second, there are emerging data that the part of the brain involved in behavior performance different from that involved in behavior acquisition (van Mier et al., 1998). By engaging in behaviors over and over again—a practice that occurs in the self-management of a chronic illness—children and their families develop the neural circuits necessary for continued performance

TABLE 5.1
Self-Management Skills Used With Chronic Illness

Skills	Description
I. Prevention	Adherence to medication advice as prescribed
	Take preventive or maintenance medications as prescribed
	Prevent acute episodes of illness
	Practice principles of good health
II. Acute episode management	Treat episode, as agreed on, in systematic manner
	Take as-needed medications in correct manner
III. Prevention and management of acute episodes	Self-directed behaviors
	Self-statements
	Self-induced response change
	Self-induced stimulus change
	Self-reinforcement
	Perform self-management skills
	Self-monitoring
	Gather, process, and interpret collected data
	Decision making
	Action
	Self-reaction or evaluation
	Perform coping skills
	Relaxation
	Imagery
	Skill rehearsal
	Self-desensitization

of specific behavioral tasks. Finally, the introduction and performance of behaviors over time permits skills to be gradually integrated into the behavioral repertoire of children and family members. They not only have the opportunity to practice self-management skills, but to adapt them to fit the unique needs of each family.

Needs of Individual Children and Their Families. Earlier it was noted that self-management programs, especially for pediatric asthma, came about because of the changing composition of patient families. In most instances, the day-to-day management of a pediatric illness falls on the shoulders of children, their parents, or other family members. Medications may be taken and other regularly scheduled treatments performed. When an exacerbation occurs, duties may be spread among all members of a family. For example, although mothers usually treat the child, fathers may help keep the stricken youngster and his or her siblings calm. Fathers may also be called on to review the quickest way to reach the nearest emergency room and, in the event of such a trip, arrange babysitting for other children in the family. Brothers or sisters may be given specific duties, such as packing their sibling's suitcase for a trip to hospital, as a way to assist the family manage a health care crisis (Creer, 1979).

COMPONENTS OF SELF-MANAGEMENT

There are components of self-management that are applied by children and their families across disorders, time, and contexts. These elements have been described in several sources (e.g., Creer, 1997, 2000; Creer & Holroyd, 1997; Ford, 1987; Karoly, 1993; Von Korff et al., 1997). Despite the use of different terminology, there is commonality among the description of elements. As Creer and Holroyd (1997) pointed out, apparent differences often result from the manner in which elements or processes are described, not from actual differences in conceptualization. Elements salient to the self-management of chronic illness include: (a) goal selection, (b) information collection, (c) information processing and evaluation, (d) decision making, (e) action, and (f) self-reaction. These elements, as well as the skills required to execute different aspects of self-management, serve as the framework for the discussion that follows.

Goal Selection

Goal selection only occurs after careful preparation. For example, it is necessary for health care providers and children/parents to have a basic understanding of and expectations for the role of self-management in the control of a chronic illness. Goal selection is the only activity where there is true collaboration between patients and their health care provider (Creer, 2000; Creer & Holroyd, 1997). Once children and their families have been taught about the treatment of a specific chronic disorder, health care providers can sit down with individual children and their parents to develop a treatment or action plan. Selecting an appropriate treatment goal, particularly one requiring medication compliance, is likely to involve the following steps:

1. *Discuss treatment options.* The physician or health care provider should describe treatment options available for control of a specific disorder. Specific strategies are needed to manage and control any chronic pediatric condition, such as monitoring blood sugar in juvenile diabetes.

2. *Select treatment option.* Physicians and other health care providers can discuss with patients and their parents the best option available for treating a particular disorder. In doing so, consideration should be given to the following issues (Creer, 1993): (a) decreasing the complexity of a regimen by prescribing as few medications as possible and introducing

longer lasting drugs; and (b) prescribing the simplest or easiest to administer medications first, followed by additional or more complex tasks that require additional instruction or shaping of behavior. A candid discussion of options, as well as the uncertainty surrounding what may happen when the selected choice is followed, can be helpful to health care providers, children, and their parents. It permits everyone to perceive potential outcomes within a probabilistic framework. Acquiring this perspective is critical to the decision making and action of children and their parents (Creer, 1990).

3. *Negotiate schedule and times of treatment.* Physicians or other health care providers often prescribe drugs to be taken *three times daily.* Rather than continue this common practice, Spector (1985) proposed that prescribing drugs to be taken *with each meal* prompts children to take their medicine each time they eat. Physiotherapy treatments for a patient with CF can be scheduled around the daily routine of a child and his or her family. Whatever treatment schedule is used should be negotiated by health care providers with children and their parents. The result should be a treatment regimen that fits the needs of individual children and their families with a minimum of lifestyle changes; the consequence should be improved compliance. Depending on the physical condition, there may be no room for negotiation on treatment options among health care providers, children, and their families. When this is the case, constraints imposed by a treatment or condition should be discussed in detail so that children and their families comprehend them. Such understanding is necessary if compliance to a regimen is to occur.

4. *Writing of contracts.* It is useful to negotiate contracts with older children and adolescents regarding medication use. They spell out, in as specific terms as possible, the exact duties of children and health care providers. The contract should contain input elicited from children or adolescents. Even if it is nothing more than how something is worded, it conveys to children and adolescents that their opinions are worthwhile. Once clauses of a contract have been debated and described in writing, the completed contract should be signed by both children and their health care providers. Such contracts generally enhance compliance in older children and adolescents (Creer, 1979).

5. *Introduce cues and reminders.* Two types of cues or reminders may be used. One type is designed solely for children and their families; it reminds them when to take medicines or perform other treatments. Examples might be daily calendars or pills set next to a plate at mealtime. A second type is diaries; these are used to not only categorize information for patients and their families, but as a way for health care providers to track the behavior of the families. When information from diaries is

shared by families and their health care provider, they allow adjustments to be made in treatment goals or strategies for achieving the goals.

After goals have been discussed, negotiated, and agreed on, they should be written up and described in some sort of treatment guidelines or illness action plan. These plans should, in an easy-to-read manner, provide a road map for treatment. By following them, children and their families know precisely what to do to treat a chronic condition, including exacerbations of the condition. It becomes the responsibility of individual patients to perform whatever self-management skills are needed to attain the goals as outlined in an action plan (Creer & Holroyd, 1997). In turn, it becomes the responsibility of health care providers to track and provide sustained follow-up services to the patient (Von Korff et al., 1997).

Several authors (Creer, 2000; Creer & Holroyd, 1997; Ford, 1987; Karoly, 1993) have described three positive consequences of goal selection: (a) it establishes preferences about desirable outcomes, (b) it increases the commitment of patients to perform goal-relevant self-management skills, and (c) it establishes expectancies on the part of patients that trigger their motivation and performance. In the case of chronic illness, goal selection can have an additional positive consequence: It sets an objective for managing an illness that can be attained only through the collaborative efforts of patients and health care providers (Creer, 2000). Ideally, patients begin to believe that, by developing and strengthening specific self-management competencies, they become partners with their physicians in controlling a chronic illness (Creer, 2000; Creer & Holroyd, 1997).

Information Collection

The mechanism of information collection is self-monitoring or the self-observation and self-recording of data. Self-monitoring is not only the foundation of self-management, but it is a necessary condition for determining if progress is made toward achieving goals (Creer, 2000). Self-monitoring is essential to the self-management of any physical problem; it is imperative if the child and family are to adhere to medical or medication instructions.

Creer and Bender (1993) offered three suggestions for improving the self-monitoring of behaviors related to chronic illness. First, children and their families should only observe and record data on phenomena that have been operationally defined as target behaviors by them and their health care providers. Anyone would be overwhelmed if asked to monitor too many categories of phenomena that constantly swirl about them. Second, whenever possible, an objective measure—such as use of reagent strip and computerized glucose meter to regulate insulin or peak flow meters to monitor airway obstruction—should be used in measuring selected target behaviors or responses. Such information can then serve as a benchmark to compare, for example, the taking of medications. Finally, it is imperative that individual children and their families observe and record information only during specified periods of time as agreed on with their physicians or health care personnel. It is virtually impossible— unless one is what Kirschenbaum and Tomarken (1982) referred to as an *obsessive–compulsive self-regulator*—to perform a task such as measuring blood pressure twice daily each day for the remainder of one's life.

Information Processing and Evaluation

Patients must process and evaluate the information they collect about themselves and their condition. Creer and Holroyd (1997) delineated five distinct steps involved in this process. First, children learn to detect physical changes in themselves that are related to their illness. In this manner, they can react quickly to adverse changes and initiate whatever steps are needed, such as taking medications, to deal with the problem. This may not be difficult when children and their families gather information with an objective measure, such as a blood glucose test. However, when children are asked to monitor and process information about subjective symptoms they experience, such as occurs with a headache or chronic pain, the task may be difficult. Here youngsters are asked to detect changes from some sort of personal baseline or adaptation level. There can be problems with children in that the benchmark is private information known only to a given child. Some youngsters are consistently accurate at detecting and interpreting changes in themselves, whereas others are unreliable. With the latter children, as well as with younger children, family members must pick up other observable cues, including changes in behavior, that may be correlated with a change in a youngster's physical condition.

Second, to make the assessment of changes consistent across children, standards must be established to permit youngsters to evaluate the data they collect and process about themselves. Such standards, in turn, can be used both by children/families and health care providers in establishing treatment goals. Public benchmarks have been developed for judging the severity of many chronic illnesses, including hypertension, diabetes, asthma, and HIV infections (Creer & Holroyd, 1997). There are no public standards for evaluating the severity of other disorders, including recurrent and chronic pain disorders. A number of attempts have been made to develop rating scales that can be used by patients. However, because information gathered and interpreted is available only to an individual patient, the severity of illness severity is often idiosyncratic to that patient (Creer, 2000).

Third, patients must make relevant judgments about the information they collect and process on themselves. Making judgments may be easy with objective data. For example, children and their families can match a child's breathing against an objective standard that denotes what is considered as a low peak flow rate. Matching to standard becomes difficult in the case of subjective symptoms. Children and their families must continually evaluate and refine their skills at matching their reaction to what, at the onset of their performance, may be ambiguous and fuzzy standards (Creer & Holroyd, 1997).

Fourth, children and their families must learn to evaluate changes that occur in a child vis-à-vis the antecedent conditions that may have led to the change, the behaviors performed to alter the changes, and the potential consequences of such action. An analysis of the ABCs—antecedents, behaviors, and consequences—of an event and the action taken to manage it provides feedback necessary for making the best decision about possible courses of action that can be taken in the future.

Finally, contextual factors must be considered in processing and evaluating information about the management of a chronic illness. Children with a chronic condition, for example, may not notice a change in that condition when they are doing something they enjoy with their peers. Their recognition of change may be considerably different, however, when they are alone or at home with their families.

Decision Making

Creer and Holroyd (1997) explained that decision making is a critical function in self-management: After patients collect, process, and evaluate the data they gather on themselves and their illness, they must make appropriate decisions based on the information. Despite a growing base of data regarding medical decision making, there is a paucity of information as to how individual patients make decisions about their condition and how they respond to it. This is ironic from two perspectives. First, particularly in the case of chronic illness, children and their families are asked not only to make accurate decisions about their condition and its treatment, but to make complex decisions. In asthma, for example, children and their families need to know how to adjust the preventive or maintenance drugs they take or when to take specified amounts of an as-needed medication. Second, evidence indicates that patient decision making is the epicenter of the successful self-management of chronic diseases (Caplin, 1998; Creer, 1990; Creer et al., 1988). If children and their families do not make the appropriate decision, they cannot initiate the action they and their health care providers have agreed should be taken.

Action

Action involves the performance of appropriate self-management skills to control a chronic illness (Creer & Holroyd, 1997). There are several steps involved in taking action.

Self-Instruction. Chronically ill children and their families should first contemplate the action they are going to need to take. They must consider the skills they have in their pooled behavioral repertoire and decide which are appropriate for managing whatever change has occurred. Self-instruction, including their prompting, directing, and maintaining performance, underlies whatever action individual children and their families decide to take. Creer and Bender (1993) explained that self-instruction is significant to self-management in two ways. First, control over a chronic illness requires that patients independently perform, often in a stepwise manner, the strategies they have worked out beforehand with their health care provider and outlined in their treatment action plan. Second, self-instruction may prompt the initiation of other strategies for coping with the illness. These could include relaxation, imagery, skill rehearsal, and self-desensitization (Creer, 1997; Creer & Bender, 1993).

Self-Statements. In taking action, children and their parents are guided by the self-statements they make to themselves. We all use such statements to guide our behavior from the time we awaken in the morning until we fall into bed at night. In perhaps the simplest case of self-statements, a child with asthma may tell himself, "The doc said I should use the inhaler when I get tight. I'm tight. I need to use my inhaler." Prompt use of an inhaler is apt to alleviate the tightness. However successful children and their families are in alleviating distress is, to a major extent, a function of the self-statements they provide to themselves to initiate and perform whatever actions they decide to take.

Self-Induced Response Change. A common trigger of childhood asthma is exercise. If a child's chest becomes tight while exercising, the youngster may say to herself, "I had better slow down and see if the tightness in my chest goes away." By using self-instructions to guide her behavior, the child engages in self-induced response change. The result, at least with exercise-induced asthma, should be an alleviation of the tightness in the chest and other symptoms of asthma.

Self-Induced Stimulus Change. Another common trigger of childhood asthma are allergens from cats and dogs. If a child is playing with a child and begins to feel tight, the child may say to himself, "Uh-oh. I'd better get away from the cat. It's causing my eyes to water and my chest to feel tight." By using self-statements to guide his behavior with respect to the cat, the child employs self-induced stimulus change. By escaping from the situation, the youngster should experience an improvement in his asthma, although, because the attack has commenced, inhaled medication may also be required.

Self-Reinforcement. Self-reinforcement is often difficult to pinpoint because it is private information available to an individual patient. Yet self-reinforcement seems to strengthen the action taken by children and their families. A youngster might tell herself after taking appropriate action that, "Hey, what I did worked! I'll have to tell my parents and my doc." Consequently, the child is apt to use the same actions in the future.

Children and their families may also use coping strategies to help manage an illness. These strategies include the following.

Relaxation. If chronically ill children relax when experiencing distress, they can make a major contribution to the control of their disorder. First, by relaxing, they can analyze the information they have about their condition, make correct decisions, and take appropriate actions. During an asthma attack, for example, a child may say, "Okay, I'm having an attack. I'll try and remain calm and remember what the doc and my family said I should do. Yeah, first I inhale from my inhaler." If children remain calm, they can use self-statements to guide themselves through the steps necessary for alleviating the episode. Second, children's behavior in managing the flare-up serves to prompt behaviors exhibited by others. If youngsters can remain calm and execute appropriate action, those around the youngsters will remain calm. If children panic, such behavior is likely to be contagious. As a result, those around them can also become upset and panicky (Creer, 1979).

Imagery. All of us use imagery—of one kind or another—to guide our everyday behavior. During an asthma attack, for example, a child may think, "Hey, I'm tight. If I inhale the medicine from my inhaler, I should be fine. I can then go back and finish the game I was playing." When chronically ill children can visualize all the steps of the treatment regime they agreed to follow, they can also imagine the outcome of their action: the control of the exacerbation they are experiencing or that they may experience in the future. These outcomes, in turn, build positive expectations as to the likely outcome of their action.

Skill Rehearsal. As treatments for chronic pediatric disorders become more complex, it is useful if children occasionally rehearse whatever skills are required to perform a particular action. For example, there are specific techniques to using a metered-dose inhaler (MDI) correctly in the management of an asthma attack (Creer & Levstek, 1996). Rather than wait until they have an attack to remember what to do, children may want to review the instructions they have received for the MDI and rehearse the steps required for correct use of the inhaler.

Self-Desensitization.   Older children and adolescents may use this technique to help them learn to relax when experiencing the distress that often accompanies the exacerbation of an illness. An adolescent girl once described her method to me:

> Attacks can be frightening, you know? So, I wrote down those things that scared me the most. Like you suggested, I put them in a hierarchy ranging from the thing that didn't scare me much up to the thing that frightened me the most. I put the hierarchy on a card I carried around with me. Whenever I had some free time, I'd relax and look over the list. By starting with the things that didn't scare me much, I worked my way up the list. By the time I got through it, I wasn't afraid of any of the things. Whenever I've had attacks since then, they haven't frightened me. I just go ahead and treat them.

Self-Reaction

Self-reaction refers to how individuals look at and evaluate their performance (Bandura, 1986). On the basis of their appraisal, they can establish realistic expectations about their future performance, as well as decide if they need more training and expertise. Children with a chronic illness and their families should also acquire realistic expectations about the limits of self-management in helping them control their condition. They should learn that self-management skills do not control every aspect of either their behavior or illness (Creer, 2000; Creer & Holroyd, 1997).

Self-efficacy influences the performance of self-management skills. Self-efficacy refers to the beliefs in one's capabilities to organize and perform the courses of action required to produce a given achievement (Bandura, 1977, 1997). With chronically ill children and their families, it means they have the belief that, either in the day-to-day management of the illness or in attempting to control an exacerbation, they can perform whatever skills are needed to manage the disorder. In contrast, if they lack self-efficacy, they are unlikely to perform these skills. Self-efficacy arises, in part, from patients' performance achievements; it guides and regulates the future action they will take with respect to their condition (Creer & Holroyd, 1997). Self-reaction, particularly self-efficacy, is not only an essential component in the performance of self-management skills, but is crucial to the maintenance of these skills over time and across settings (Creer, 2000).

SELF-MANAGEMENT AND CHRONIC ILLNESS

Application of Self-Management Techniques to Chronic Disorders

The characteristics of a chronic illness provide a compelling argument for teaching patients to perform self-management skills. As noted, recently there has been a rich and varied history of applying self-management techniques to help manage these disorders. Self-management programs have been developed and tested for arthritis, asthma, ataxia, chronic obstructive pulmonary disease (COPD), chronic pain, CF, epilepsy, fibromyalgia, glaucoma, headache, HIV infection, and multiple sclerosis (MS; Creer, 2000). Self-management procedures are especially useful with such chronic pediatric illnesses as diabetes, asthma, epilepsy, headache, JRA, and CF.

Outcome Variables Assessed in Chronic Illness

A range of outcome variables have been employed as outcome measures in studies of self-management and chronic illness (Center for the Advancement of Health, 1996). A list of these variables, as well as changes observed with the measures, are depicted in Table 5.2. As appropriate for a given measure, increases or decreases have been found in assessing these variables. Almost all of these outcome variables are relevant to the assessment of self-management and chronic pediatric illness. For example, a number of studies have reported that self-management increases knowledge of a disorder and its management, acquisition and performance of self-management skills, school and work attendance, quality of life, interactions with health care providers, and psychological well-being. At the same time, decreases in physical outcomes, hospital and emergency room use, symptom intensity and frequency of exacerbations, abnormal psychological reactions, and health care costs have been reported (e.g., Holroyd & Creer, 1986). Medication compliance, as well as correct use of prescribed medications and rapid initiation of treatment strategies, have also been found. Data gathered with these outcome measures suggest that chronically ill patients, including children, can become partners with their physicians and health care personnel in the management of the patients' illness (Creer, 2000).

Analysis of the Performance of Self-Management Procedures Over Time

Because duration is a prominent characteristic of chronic illness, most children with these conditions need to perform self-management skills for the remainder of their lives (Creer, 2000). Yet few studies have attempted

TABLE 5.2
Results Obtained in Self-Management Programs for Chronic Illness

Variable

Increases in following measures:
  Knowledge about chronic disorder and its management
  Physiological measures, including metabolic control and pulmonary functions
  School and work attendance
  Quality of life
  Psychological factors, including:
    Decision making
    Self-efficacy
    Positive attitudes toward illness and its management
    Mood
  Compliance to medication regimens:
    Correct use of prescribed medications
    Independent initiation of assessment and treatment strategies
  Acquisition and performance of self-management skills:
    Maintenance of self-management skills
  Interactions with health care providers
  Family involvement with illness and its management
Decreases in following measures:
  Physical outcomes, including smoking, weight, and blood pressure
  Hospital and hospital emergency room usage
    Home visits
  Medication use (e.g., less usage of more potent drugs)
  Symptoms, pain, insomnia, and dyspnea
    Decreases in symptom intensity and number of exacerbations of a chronic illness
  Psychological factors, including:
    Anxiety and distress
    Depression
  Activity restriction
  Costs of managing the disorder
  Relapse of behavioral skills

to answer this question: What happens to the performance of self-management for chronic illness over time and across settings? Three studies have attempted to collect such information for patients who received self-management training; these include a 4-year follow-up of adults with arthritis (Lorig & Holman, 1993), a 5-year follow-up of asthmatic children and their families (Creer et al., 1988), and an 8-year follow-up of adults with asthma (Caplin, 1998). There were common features among these studies: Self-management skills were taught over a period of time (6–8 weeks); and patients were treated by physicians or health care providers who enthusiastically referred patients to the program with the anticipation that, with the acquisition of self-management skills, the patients would become their partners. In addition, parents or siblings were invited to participate in the program for asthmatic children (Creer et al., 1988) while spouses, friends, or significant others were invited to join in the program for asthmatic adults (Kotses et al., 1995) followed up by Caplin (1998). Participants were taught in groups in the two studies (Creer et al., 1988; Kotses et al., 1995); the group format permitted adults, children, and adolescents to be exposed to materials specifically tailored to their needs while with their peers.

Highlights of the use of self-management procedures include the following.

Goal Selection. Once they completed the educational component of the programs, patients—especially children and their families—felt prepared to jointly establish goals with their physicians. Therefore, they continued, they had little difficulty in arriving at goals and treatment plans. Goals were incorporated into written treatment guidelines, which could be posted in a conspicuous place—usually on the door of a refrigerator. Parents explained that the written guidelines were invaluable given the variable and intermittent nature of asthma attacks.

Parents and children in the study by Creer and colleagues (1988) described several other factors related to goal selection. First, they noted that, once patients had proved themselves to be allies with their health care providers, the latter were readily amenable to making any changes in goals as necessitated by a child's condition. Often, children and their parents continued, they and their health care providers saw the need for a revision of goals at approximately the same time.

Second, informants reported that, by performing asthma self-management, the entire family became proactive in approaching health care providers. Children and their families not only gathered information on a youngster's asthma, but experienced no difficulty in asking questions about the data or other aspects of the child's condition. Physicians spontaneously described what a joy it was to have informed and inquiring patients (Creer, 1983). Finally, as also occurred in the study by Kotses et al. (1995), the number of interactions increased among patients and their health care providers. This took the form of scheduling more office visits or, as often occurred, telephoning their health care provider and staff more frequently to ask about a child's asthma.

The increase in activities was considered a positive outcome in the Creer et al. (1988) and Kotses et al. (1995) studies by both patients and health care providers. Patients and their families welcomed the increased interactions they had with their health care provider because it not only taught them more about their condition, but it reinforced their performance of self-management skills. Health care providers were ebullient about the increased number of interactions they had with their patients because it was accompanied by reductions in hospital admissions and emergency room visits for asthma (Kotses et al., 1995).

Information Collection. All asthma patients and their families recognized the necessity of self-monitoring—the observation and recording of information—throughout and after training. Children and their families reported they used the flow meter to obtain peak flow values; the values, in turn, could be compared against a child's predicted peak flow rate (Creer et al., 1988). They could then react to such information by following whatever steps were outlined in the treatment plan they had formulated with their health care provider. In addition, the parents of a few children suggested they used the peak flow data to predict future episodes. What they did was compare a given value against the baseline data they had collected and predict the likelihood of an attack sometime during the day. For example, if their data indicated that a child had experienced asthma two out of four times he blew a particular value, his parents assigned a 50% probability of an attack occurring in the next 12 hours. They could then prepare themselves in the event that the attack occurred. This rough type of prediction not only proved invaluable to several children and their families, but it stimulated research that resulted in a more refined and accurate approach to use of the peak flow meter to predict asthma attacks (e.g., Harm, Kotses, & Creer, 1985; Taplin & Creer, 1978).

Information Processing and Evaluation. Children and their families became sophisticated at processing and evaluating information they gathered on themselves (Creer, 1983; Creer et al., 1988). Several distinct trends were noted. First, children became skilled at detecting changes in their breathing. They began to notice changes earlier in attacks; they informed their parents of their condition or they quickly initiated treatment. Their parents became acutely aware of physical and behavioral signs that accompanied the onset of asthma episodes. Second, children and their families compared changes in a child's breathing to peak flow values. They were able to make refined judgments based on these comparisons. Third, they became keenly aware of the ABCs of asthma: the antecedents that occurred before an attack, the behaviors they performed, and the consequences of their action. Breaking down attacks in this manner not only helped them establish control over an episode, but it permitted children to avoid or escape potential triggers in the future. Finally, all family members became aware of contextual factors and how they influenced data collection. Children and their families, for example, became aware that the data they collected with a flow meter were dependent on the effort the children expended in collecting such information. They realized it was worthwhile to obtain accurate values and reduce any uncertainty with respect to future child and family activities.

Decision Making.   The least expected finding in the Creer et al. (1988) study concerned decision making. Creer (1990) found that children and their parents who were especially competent at asthma self-management used sophisticated decision-making rules to help control the disorder. In analyzing their responses, as described in reports of asthma episodes, it was found that the rules they used were identical to those obtained from a group of experienced physicians considered as a gold standard group by their peers. Both groups used judgment rules or heuristics described by Arkes (1981) as highly effective in the management of clinical problems. Members of both groups thought that using these skills had a major impact in how they controlled asthma. In addition, many children and their families noted that they used the decision-making skills they had been taught in all facets of their lives.

Action.   In the 5-year posttreatment interviews conducted by Creer et al. (1988), children and their families reported they had become skilled at taking appropriate actions to manage both their asthma and asthma attacks. They described how, in most cases, they followed a step-level method of managing attacks, such as those recommended by the guidelines for asthma (National Asthma Education and Prevention Program, 1997). However, many added two points regarding how they managed attacks. First, they developed short-hand procedures in that they often reduced treatment to only those steps that were absolutely necessary to abort an episode. This helped them establish control in a more rapid and efficient manner. A similar finding was also reported by Baum and Creer (1986) in their study of asthma self-management and medication compliance in children. Second, families described advanced forms of action where they tailored treatments according to such variables as severity of episode and context (Creer, 1983). Their initial action usually worked, although, as more children and families noted, they recognized the probabilistic nature of any potential outcome resulting from a given action.

Self-Reactions.   The mechanism for continuing to perform self-management skills appears to be self-efficacy. This was the case in the studies by Lorig and Holman (1993) on arthritis, by Kotses et al. (1995) and Caplin (1998) on adult asthma, and by Creer et al. (1998) on pediatric asthma. Three findings are especially relevant. First, participants in all the studies found that the development of self-confidence, especially self-efficacy, was the basic ingredient in their performance and maintenance in different contexts of these skills. In the study by Creer et al. (1988), for example, children and their parents reported that their confidence in performing self-management skills had increased over time. Second, participants said they developed positive outcome expectancies (i.e., they believed that if they reacted to their condition as they had been taught, they could make a difference in its control). However, their expectancies were tempered with reality: They recognized that if their initial treatment did not work with an exacerbation, they would have to take other steps to manage the condition. Finally, participants in the Creer et al. (1988) and Kotses et al. (1995) studies noted that they remained in contact with others they met during training. These interactions served not only to keep everyone up to date on the latest advances in asthma treatment, but as a source of support for performing self-management skills.

DISCUSSION

A revolution in two paradigms—providing health care services and shifting priorities of disease management—was discussed. Neither revolution is over; for that matter, it may be premature to speculate on the final outcome. Nevertheless, it is apparent that the march toward some type of managed health care system continues unabated. Economic pressures, spurred by an aging population and skyrocketing costs incurred in fighting biology at life's edge, push us toward a day of reckoning (Callahan, 1998). As a new paradigm for health care services has evolved, it has had an impact on the second revolution—shifting priorities in disease management. This consequence is inevitable given the inextricable linkage of the two paradigms. Indeed, the success of any paradigm of health care will ultimately be dependent on an a priori shift in priorities regarding the role of patients—a category that includes all of us—in managing our sickness and health.

Attempting to create a new paradigm with respect to priorities of disease management has not been easy. Part of the reason is that health care personnel, as well as the system within which they operate, are geared toward the management of acute illnesses. With acute diseases, the illness is central: health care personnel and the system do remarkably well in this situation in part because patients are often outside the realms of decision making and action. The problem arises in making a shift toward chronic illness where the person becomes central to management of the condition. Such a move has not been slow to develop in part because of the reluctance of most physicians to perceive patient care in a different light and, equally important, patients' grudging acceptance of their new role. The cautious attitudes of health care providers and patients are not necessarily bad: At this point in time, it is better that the momentum for change be carefully considered to arrive at a long-term solution involving patients and the emerging health care system.

Despite barriers, three factors were discussed that suggest progress is being made in generating a new treatment paradigm. First, there has been the inclusion of specific charges to patients in recently issued clinical treatment guidelines. These charges—ranging from inclusion in decision making to the performance of specific behavioral actions—are meant to empower patients to take a proactive position with respect to their own health. They go so far as to suggest that any treatment strategy be jointly developed by children, their families, and health care providers. Second, the pivotal role of self-management with respect to chronic pediatric illness, particularly chronic pediatric disorders, was discussed. Although in a nascent stage of development, self-management techniques have already shown their value to increase outcome variables such as medication compliance, school attendance, and quality of life, or decrease other outcome variables such as physical symptoms, hospital or emergency room use, and economic costs of the chronic illnesses. These changes would not have occurred without the whole-hearted cooperation of children and their families with their health care providers. Finally, buoyed by their own success, there is increasing evidence that, once acquired, children and their families continue to perform self-management skills. Because duration is a defining characteristic of a chronic illness, such endurance is required by children and their families.

It could be debated whether it is better to be in the first wave and create new ways to solve or manage persistent problems or follow the first wave and build on earlier findings. In the case of the self-management of chronic pediatric illnesses, it is better to be in the second wave. The reason is that most of the early self-management programs for chronic disorders relied on conceptual and research designs that failed to fit the nature of the phenomena being investigated. The approach entailed the use of a mechanistic model characterized by the assumption of a constant and additive effect of an independent variable onto a dependent variable (Ford & Urban, 1998). Such a reductionistic and linear model is considered outdated and totally inappropriate to what is studied by contemporary intervention theorists. These theorists, continued Ford and Urban, assume that we are complex, open systems that exist and develop only in transaction with contexts. We each construct our own developmental pathway and functional patterns within variable and changing conditions provided by our bodies and contexts. Chronically ill children and their families not only rely on specific self-management processes and behaviors, but must constantly use them to interact in the various contexts—generated by environmental, illness, health care, treatment, and developmental variables—within which they function. The result is a complex model of human behavior. However, it is one that closely approximates the day-to-day reality experienced by chronically ill children and their families.

REFERENCES

Abbey, F. B. (1997). Health care reform: The road lies with managed care. In P. R. Kongstvedt (Ed.), *Essentials of managed care* (2nd ed., pp. 17–35). Gaithersburg, MD: Aspen.

Arkes, H. R. (1981). Impediments to accurate clinical judgment and possible ways to minimize their impact. *Journal of Consulting and Clinical Psychology, 49*, 323–330.

Bandura, A. (1977). Self-efficacy: Toward a unifying theory of behavioral change. *Psychological Review, 84*, 191–215.

Bandura, A. (1986). *Social foundations of thoughts and action: A social cognitive theory.* Englewood Cliffs, NJ: Prentice-Hall.

Bandura, A. (1997). *Self-efficacy: The exercise of control.* New York: Freeman.

Baum, D., & Creer, T. L. (1986). Medication compliance in children with asthma. *Journal of Asthma, 23*, 49–59.

Callahan, D. (1998). *False hopes: Why America's quest for perfect health is a recipe for failure.* New York: Simon & Schuster.

Caplin, D. A. (1998). *Variables contributing to the long-term maintenance of self-management skills in patients with asthma.* Unpublished doctoral dissertation, Ohio University, Athens.

Cassell, E. J. (1997). *Doctoring. The nature of primary care medicine.* New York: Oxford University Press.

Center for the Advancement of Health. (1996). *An indexed bibliography on self-management for people with chronic disease.* Washington, DC: Author.

Creer, T. L. (1979). *Asthma therapy: A behavioral health care system for respiratory disorders.* New York: Springer.

Creer, T. L. (1983). *The self-management of a chronic physical disorder: Childhood asthma.* Unpublished manuscript, Ohio University, Athens.

Creer, T. L. (1990). Strategies for judgment and decision-making in the management of childhood asthma. *Pediatric Asthma, Allergy, & Immunology, 4*, 253–264.

Creer, T. L. (1997). *Psychology of adjustment: An applied approach.* Upper Saddle River, NJ: Prentice-Hall.

Creer, T. L. (1998). Editorial: The complexity of treating asthma. *Journal of Asthma, 35*, 451–454.

Creer, T. L. (2000). Self-management and chronic disease. In M. Boekaerts, P. R. Pintrich, & M. Zeidner (Eds.), *Self-regulation: Theory, research, applications* (pp. 601–629). Orlando, FL: Academic Press.

Creer, T. L., Backial, M., Burns, K. L., Leung, P., Marion, R. J., Miklich, D. R., Morrill, C., Taplin, P. S., & Ullman, S. (1988). Living with asthma: Part I. Genesis and development of a self-management program for childhood asthma. *Journal of Asthma, 25*, 335–362.

Creer, T. L., & Bender, B. G. (1993). Asthma. In R. J. Gatchel & E. B. Blanchard (Eds.), *Psychophysiological disorders* (pp. 151–208). Washington, DC: American Psychological Association.

Creer, T. L., & Holroyd, K. A. (1997). Self-management. In A. Baum, C. McManus, S. Newman, J. Weinman, & R. West (Eds.), *Cambridge handbook of psychology, health, and behavior* (pp. 255–258). Cambridge, England: Cambridge University Press.

Creer, T. L., & Levstek, D. A. (1996). Medication compliance and asthma: Overlooking the trees because of the forest. *Journal of Asthma, 33*, 203–211.

Creer, T. L., Levstek, D. A., & Reynolds, R. V. C. (1998). History and conclusions. In H. Kotses & A. Harver (Eds.), *Self-management of asthma* (pp. 379–405). New York: Marcel Dekker.

Creer, T. L., Tinkelman, D., & Winder, J. A. (1999). Guidelines for the diagnosis and management of asthma: Accepting the challenge. *Journal of Asthma, 36,* 391–407.

Creer, T. L., & Winder, J. A. (1986). Asthma. In K. A. Holroyd & T. L. Creer (Eds.), *Self-management of chronic disease. Handbook of clinical interventions and research* (pp. 269–303). Orlando, FL: Academic Press.

Ford, D. H. (1987). *Humans as self-constructing living systems: A developmental perspective on behavior and personality.* Hillsdale, NJ: Lawrence Erlbaum Associates.

Ford, D. H., & Urban, H. B. (1998). *Contemporary models of psychotherapy: A comparative analysis* (2nd ed.). New York: Wiley.

Fox, P. D. (1997). An overview of managed care. In P. R. Kongstvedt (Ed.), *Essentials of managed care* (2nd ed., pp. 3–16). Gaithersburg, MD: Aspen.

Gorovitz, S., & MacIntyre, A. (1975). Toward a theory of medical infallibility. *The Hastings Center Reports, 5,* 13–23.

Harm, D. L., Kotses, H., & Creer, T. L. (1985). Improving the ability of peak expiratory flow rates to predict asthma. *Journal of Allergy and Clinical Immunology, 76,* 688–694.

Herzlinger, R. E. (1997). *Market-driven health care: Who wins, who loses in the transformation of America's largest service industry.* Reading, MA: Addison-Wesley.

Hoffman, C., Rice, D., & Sung, H.-Y. (1996). Persons with chronic conditions: Their prevalence and costs. *Journal of the American Medical Association, 276,* 1473–1479.

Holroyd, K. A., & Creer, T. L. (1986). *Self-management of chronic disease: Handbook of clinical interventions and research.* Orlando, FL: Academic Press.

Kagan, J. (1998). *Three seductive ideas.* Cambridge, MA: Harvard University Press.

Karoly, P. (1993). Mechanisms of self-regulation: A systems view. *Annual Review of Psychology, 44,* 23–52.

Kazak, A. E., Segal-Andrews, A. M., & Johnson, K. (1995). Pediatric psychology research and practice: A family/systems approach. In M. C. Roberts (Ed.), *Handbook of pediatric psychology* (2nd ed., pp. 84–104). New York: Guilford.

Kirschenbaum, D. S., & Tomarken, A. J. (1982). On facing the generalization problem: The study of self-regulatory failure. In P. C. Kendall (Ed.), *Advances in cognitive-behavioral research and therapy* (Vol. 1, pp. 119–200). New York: Academic Press.

Kotses, H., Bernstein, I. L., Bernstein, D. I., Reynolds, R. V. C., Korbee, L., Wigal, J. K., Ganson, E., Stout, C., & Creer, T. L. (1995). A self-management program for adult asthma: Part I. Development and evaluation. *Journal of Allergy and Clinical Immunology, 95,* 529–540.

Kuhn, T. S. (1996). *The structure of scientific revolutions* (3rd ed.). Chicago: University of Chicago Press.

Lorig, K., & Holman, H. (1993). Arthritis self-management studies: A twelve year review. *Health Education Quarterly, 20,* 17–28.

Luntz Research Company. (1998, September 10). U.S. frustrated with managed care. *Reuters Ltd.* [Online].

MEDSTAT Group & J.D. Powers and Associates. (1998, September 15). Most U.S. physicians express opposition to managed care. *Reuters Ltd.* [Online].

Millenson, M. L. (1997). *Demanding medical excellence: Doctors and accountability in the information age.* Chicago: University of Chicago Press.

Moeller, K. A. (1998, January/February). In 16 years of providing consumer information, what have we learned? *Gratefully Yours From the National Library of Medicine,* pp. 1–3.

National Asthma Education and Prevention Program. (1997). *Highlights of the expert panel report: 2. Guidelines for the diagnosis and management of asthma* (Publication No. 97-4051A). Washington, DC: U.S. Department of Health and Human Services.

National Library of Medicine. (1998, March/April). From 7 million to 70 million . . . What a difference a year makes! *Gratefully Yours,* pp. 4–5.

Safran, D. G., Taira, D. A., Rogers, W. H., Kosinski, M., Ware, J. E., & Tarlov, A. R. (1998). Linking primary care performance to outcomes of care. *Journal of Family Practice, 47,* 213–220.

Smith, S., Freeland, M., Heffler, S., McKusick, D., & the Health Expenditures Projection Team. (1998). The next ten years of health spending: What does the future hold? *Health Affairs, 17,* 128–140.

Sontag, S. (1976). *Illness as metaphor.* New York: Farrar, Straus, & Giroux.

Spector, S. L. (1985). Is your asthmatic patient really complying? *Annals of Allergy, 55,* 552–556.

Stark, L. J., Jelalian, E., & Miller, D. L. (1995). Cystic fibrosis. In M.C. Roberts (Ed.), *Handbook of pediatric psychology* (2nd ed., pp. 242–262). New York: Guilford.

Taplin, P. S., & Creer, T. L. (1978). A procedure for using peak expiratory flow rate data to increase the predictability of asthma episodes. *Journal of Asthma Research, 16,* 15–19.

van Dulmen, A. M. (1998). Children's contributions to pediatric outpatient encounters. *Pediatrics, 102,* 563–568.

van Mier, H., Tempel, L. W., Perlmutter, J. S., Raichle, M. E., & Petersen, S. E. (1998). Changes in brain activity during motor learning measured with PET: Effects of hand on performance and practice. *Journal of Neurophysiology, 80,* 2177–2200.

Verbrugge, L. M., & Patrick, D. L. (1995). Seven chronic conditions: Their impact on U.S. adults' activity levels and use of medical services. *American Journal of Public Health, 85,* 173–182.

Von Korff, M., Gruman, J., Schaefer, J., Curry, S. J., & Wagner, E. H. (1997). Collaborative management of chronic illness. *Annals of Internal Medicine, 127,* 1097–1102.

Wandstrat, T. L., & Kaplan, B. (1997). Pharmacoeconomic impact of factors affecting compliance with antibiotic regimens in the treatment of acute otitis media. *Pediatric Infectious Disease Journal, 15,* S27–S29.

Wiesch, D. G., & Samet, J. M. (1998). Epidemiology and natural history of asthma. In E. Middleton, Jr., C. E. Reed, E. F. Ellis, N. F. Adkinson, Jr., J. W. Yunginger, & W. W. Busse (Eds.), *Allergy: Principles and practice* (5th ed., pp. 799–815). St. Louis: Mosby.

Wigal, J. K., Creer, T. L., Kotses, H., & Lewis, P. D. (1990). A critique of 19 self-management programs for childhood asthma: Part I. The development and evaluation of the programs. *Pediatric Asthma, Allergy, and Immunology, 4,* 17–39.

Wilson, S. R., Latini, D., Starr, N. J., Fish, L., Loes, L. M., Page, A., & Kubic, P. (1996). Education of parents of infants and very young children with asthma: A developmental evaluation of the Wee Wheezers program. *Journal of Asthma, 33,* 239–254.

Woolf, S. H., Grol, R., Hutchinson, A., Eccles, M., & Grimshaw, J. (1999). Potential benefits, limitations, and harms of clinical guidelines. *British Medical Journal, 318,* 527–530.

World Health Organization. (1998). *The World Health Report 1998: Life in the 21st century—A vision for all. Executive summary.* Geneva, Switzerland: Author.

PART IV

MEASUREMENT ISSUES

The contributions in this section deal with measurement issues in treatment adherence in childhood chronic illness, focusing on asthma and diabetes as key examples. In her comprehensive overview of treatment adherence in pediatric illness in chapter 6, Matsui underscores the need to identify the specific type of noncompliance, such as delayed or omitted doses, taking the wrong amount of medication, improper dosage intervals, taking the wrong medication, and premature discontinuation. Matsui points out that, although most studies of compliance are focused on whether patients consume medications that are available to them, it is important to determine whether patients actually fill their prescriptions because patients cannot take medications that they do not have.

Matsui also considers the advantages and disadvantages of available methods that can be used in the assessment of medication compliance such as self-report measures, pill counts, and direct measurement of drug levels and bodily fluids, such as blood or urine—microelectronic devices. Another important measurement issue noted by Matsui is the importance of assessing compliance in explaining treatment failure and targeting patients for more intensive interventions. One of Matsui's contributions is to consider the impact of noncompliance on measurement, clinical assessment, and decision making. For example, discovering the potential impact of poor compliance in a clinical trial of a new drug may result in a potentially beneficial medication being abandoned due to its apparent lack of efficacy. Another consequence is that medical decisions may be affected by noncompliance (e.g., children may be subjected to unnecessary medical tests). Medication doses may be increased due to perceived lack of clinical response with subsequent toxicity if compliance suddenly improves.

Matsui's recommendations for future research include determining the degree of compliance that is required for an adequate therapeutic outcome; developing tools to identify problematic adherence with treatment, including a practical, reliable method of assessing compliance with liquid medications; understanding parents' and children's reactions to having their treatment adherence monitored; evaluating intervention strategies to promote adherence; performing studies of cost-effectiveness of interventions; assessing prescription filling in children with chronic physical illness; and developing medications that are more palatable and hence easier for parents to administer to young children.

In chapter 7, Bender and his colleagues contribute a useful description of measurement issues in treatment nonadherence in children with asthma that has general implications. Researchers have identified a profile of high-risk children with asthma that includes pharmacotherapy in conjunction with severe disease, psychological dysfunction, African-American or Hispanic-American ethnicity, and residence in urban areas with a concentration of poverty. Bender and colleagues suggest that some of the morbidity experienced by these children may be linked to compliance-related issues, including excessive reliance on bronchodilators, along with insufficient use of inhaled corticosteroids and poor inhaler technique.

For Bender and colleagues, the assessment of adherence has potentially important clinical implications. For example, in the absence of a reliable and valid measure of behavior concerning treatment adherence, clinicians may rely unduly on their presumptions of what patients do between office visits and may not fully appreciate the degree and clinical consequences of noncompliance. Bender and his colleagues question the categorization of patients as adherent or nonadherent because it misses important variations in adherence behavior, including variability across time and across different components of the treatment regimen.

A range of measures has been used to assess adherence with pediatric asthma therapy, including clinical judgment, self-report, biochemical measurement, medication measurement, pharmacy database review, electronic measurement, and family interview. Factors that affect each of these measurement approaches and the strengths and weaknesses of these approaches are reviewed.

Bender and colleagues describe the challenges of assessing treatment nonadherence in clinical practice; they recommend ways to improve assessment of medication use, including conveying a nonjudgmental attitude, encouraging truthful answers, and avoiding asking for broad generalizations. For Bender and colleagues, clinical assessment is best accomplished by establishing a partnership between health caregivers and their patients that ensures a sufficient flow of information to facilitate a reasonable treatment plan.

Research recommendations include developing new, technology-based research (e.g., electronic devices) that can be used to assess the new dry powder inhalers for pediatric asthma, assessing the degree of concordance between electronic measures and indirect measures (e.g., pill counts, etc.), and documenting the circumstances in health caregiver behavior that elicit accurate self-report.

In chapter 8, Delamater identifies critical issues in the assessment of regimen adherence in children with diabetes. In a review of the medical management of diabetes in detail, Delamater notes that, based on data to support the impact of blood sugar control on health outcomes, many more children are now being prescribed more intensive regimens that require multiple insulin injections and blood glucose monitoring in the hopes of preventing or delaying the health-related complications of diabetes. Delamater recognizes that perfect or even near-perfect adherence to treatment is not necessarily associated with blood sugar control, which is influenced by a wide range of factors. Positive coping and emotional adjustment among children and families, family support, communication skills, and agreement about family responsibilities for diabetes management tasks all predict better regimen adherence. Although increased barriers to treatment adherence relate to lower compliance in adolescents, Delamater's analysis reveals that interventions that have targeted key areas of behavioral change (e.g., adherence to blood glucose testing as well as problem-solving interventions and parent training) have been associated with improvements in both treatment adherence and glycemic control.

Delamater's critical analysis considers the significant methodological issues that are involved in research on treatment adherence in diabetes and more generally concerning the management of childhood chronic illness. It also highlights the advantages and disadvantages of various adherence measures, including direct observations, self-reports, and health provider ratings. Recommendations for future research and clinical practice are that clinicians and researchers carefully document treatment prescriptions, utilize measures of self-care behavior, and rate and/or record specific behaviors over brief periods of time.

CHAPTER SIX

Children's Adherence to Medication Treatment

Doreen M. Matsui

Children's Hospital of Western Ontario, Canada

Modern research resulting in efficacious drug therapy has improved the outlook for many children with acute or chronic illness. However, for these children to benefit from the available treatments, they must actually take or be given their medication. In recent years, the extent of noncompliance has become increasingly recognized, and efforts have been undertaken to better measure compliance and develop strategies to improve it. Noncompliance, however, is not a new problem, as illustrated by Hippocrates' advice to physicians to "keep watch also on the fault of patients which often make them lie about the taking of things prescribed" (Tebbi, 1993).

Drug compliance is of particular concern with chronic medical conditions because therapy is often long term and, at times, lifelong. Asymptomatic patients may be required to take medication to prevent later complications without any immediate benefits noted. Both of these factors may make it more difficult for children to continually adhere to their treatment regimens. It is generally agreed that compliance with drug therapy for acute diseases is better than for chronic diseases (Rapoff & Barnard, 1991).

Evaluation of drug compliance in pediatrics is unique: Whether a younger child receives his or her prescribed medication is determined not only by the patient, but also by the parent—who is often responsible for giving the medication. There may be varying degrees of involvement of the parent in the case of the older child or adolescent. Administration of medication to a child is not always a simple matter because the child, often unaware of the purpose of the medication, may be reluctant to take

135

unpleasant tasting tablets and syrups, further compounding the problem of noncompliance (Dawson & Newell, 1994). Wherever possible, reference is made to pediatric studies.

DEFINITION OF COMPLIANCE

Compliance, a term often used interchangeably with *adherence*, is most commonly defined as the extent to which a person's behavior—in terms of medications, following diets, or executing lifestyle changes—coincides with medical and health advice (Sackett et al., 1991). Although, as this definition indicates, compliance may relate to a number of behaviors, the focus of this chapter is on medication compliance in pediatrics. The majority of information available regarding compliance with drug therapy pertains to adults; the literature dealing with children is more limited.

Uniform agreement as to the dividing line between compliance and noncompliance does not exist. Less than full adherence may be acceptable, provided the desired effect can still result (Tebbi, 1993). Often the designation of compliance is assigned if a minimum percentage or more of prescribed medication is taken (Thatcher Shope, 1981). However, this somewhat arbitrary distinction may have little meaning because it has not been shown for most pediatric regimens what degree of compliance is required for an adequate therapeutic outcome (Rapoff & Barnard, 1991).

FORMS OF MEDICATION NONCOMPLIANCE

Delayed or omitted doses are the most common errors made by patients in administering their medication (Urquhart, 1994). Other forms of noncompliance include incorrect dosage amount, improper dosage intervals, wrong medication, and premature discontinuation of the drug. Errors in timing were found to be common in a study of 75 mothers whose children (3½–10 years) had been prescribed antibiotics on at least one occasion during the previous 2 years. When timing of administration was considered, only seven parents were fully compliant with dosage instructions giving the medication within 2 hours of the optimal interval (Dawson & Newell, 1994). Such data suggest that regimens that require rigid timing of doses are perhaps best avoided if possible.

Premature discontinuation of medication is also common because compliance falls off dramatically soon after the patient has symptomatically improved (Jay, Litt, & Durant, 1984). In a study of oral penicillin prescribed as a 10-day course for either streptococcal pharyngitis or otitis media, 81% of children were taking penicillin as prescribed on the fifth day, whereas only 56% were taking it on the ninth day (Charney et al.,

1967). Similarly, in another study of penicillin compliance, 56% of children had stopped therapy by the third day, 71% by the sixth day, and 82% by the ninth day (Bergman & Werner, 1963). The possibility of illness relapse is a concern with this form of noncompliance.

The availability of electronic devices to monitor medication compliance has led to the description of additional drug dosing patterns. *Drug holidays*, defined as three or more drug-free days, occur more than twice a month in 20% of patients (Pullar, 1991) and are often associated with times of interruption of daily habits such as holidays and weekends (Kruse, 1992). These lapses in drug administration may be associated with breakthrough clinical events. An improvement in drug compliance, known as the *toothbrush effect* or *white coat compliance*, may occur during the several days prior to a scheduled medical appointment (Feinstein, 1990). This behavior may complicate the measurement of adherence when methods relying on recent compliance, such as drug levels, are conducted at the time of the medical visit.

Most studies on compliance have focused on whether patients take their medications. However, it is important to determine whether patients actually fill their prescriptions—because the first step in adherence with drug therapy is to actually obtain the medication. A small number of studies have examined the rate of prescription filling in the primary care or medical clinic setting and have found nonfilling rates from 5% to 20% (Beardon et al., 1993; Begg, 1984; Boyd et al., 1974; Krogh & Wallner, 1987; Rashid, 1982). With respect to patients with chronic diseases, it has been estimated that at least 30% of refillable prescriptions are not refilled (Levy, 1991). Although one study has suggested that age is an important factor, with a greater proportion of prescriptions being filled in the 15 years and younger age group (Beardon et al., 1993), information on failure to fill prescriptions in children is limited.

At the Children's Hospital of Western Ontario, our group determined the rate of compliance with filling of prescriptions written in a pediatric emergency department in 1,014 children ages 4.5 ± 4.2 years using a standardized telephone questionnaire. Compliance with prescription filling, defined as filling the same or next day, was 92.7% (Matsui et al., 1997a). The prescription nonfilling rate in children seen in our pediatric emergency room (7%) was lower than that for adults in a similar setting (Saunders, 1987; Thomas et al., 1996).

SCOPE OF MEDICATION NONCOMPLIANCE

Although the prevalence of compliance problems varies depending on the method of assessment, the criteria used for defining acceptable compliance, the regimen prescribed, and the setting in which compliance is assessed (Rapoff & Barnard, 1991), nonadherence with pediatric drug therapy appears to be a common and important problem. Studies in children suggest an overall drug noncompliance rate of approximately 50% (National Council on Patient Information and Education, 1989)—comparable with that reported in adults (Litt & Cuskey, 1980).

Chronic Diseases

In a comparison of three groups of male children with hemophilia, sickle cell disease, or asthma, differences in compliance patterns and attitudes toward treatment were noted, which may be attributed to adaptations and stresses uniquely associated with a particular disease and its treatment. Boys with hemophilia were rated as *somewhat compliant*, boys with sickle cell disease as between *somewhat compliant* and *consistently compliant*, and boys with asthma as *somewhat compliant* to *resistant* (Sciver et al., 1995). Although drug compliance rates may vary among different diseases, poor adherence has been demonstrated for a number of pediatric medical conditions.

In children with asthma followed in a specialist clinic, medication compliance of about 70% has been reported—similar to the rate in other groups of children taking long-term drugs for epilepsy, diabetes, and prevention of rheumatic fever recurrence (Phelan, 1984). In a study of 17 children with asthma, determination of canister weight and patient diaries showed that only 18% used their metaproterenol inhaler as prescribed (Zora, Lutz, & Tinkelman, 1989). Medications were forgotten some of the time by 45.2% of children who presented to an emergency department during an acute attack of asthma (Leickly et al., 1998). Poor compliance with inhaled asthma medication has been confirmed with the availability of an electronic inhaler timer device (Coutts, Gibson, & Patson 1992; Gibson, Ferguson, Aitchison, & Paton, 1995; Milgrom et al., 1996).

Estimates of pediatric patient adherence to anticonvulsant medication regimens for the treatment of seizure disorders range from 25% to 54% (Hazzard, Hutchinson, & Krawiecki, 1990). Less than half (47%) of patients with cystic fibrosis (CF) adhered to a recommended regimen of multivitamins (Borowitz, Wegman, & Harris, 1994). In a study of patients receiving growth hormone treatment, 50% failed to comply with all aspects of their treatment (Smith, Hindmarsh, & Brook, 1993). Difficulties associated with the administration of nightly subcutaneous deferoxamine for the treatment of iron overload in patients with ß-thalassemia has resulted in a significant decline in compliance between the ages of 10 and 20 years (McGee et al., 1989).

Lapses in adherence may be more common when treatment is prophylactic rather than therapeutic (Dajani, 1996). It may be particularly difficult for children who feel well to understand the necessity of taking medication for preventive purposes. Noncompliance with oral penicillin for rheumatic fever prophylaxis as assessed in children by urine assay was 32% (Gordis, Markowitz, & Lilienfeld, 1969). The penicillin prophylaxis compliance rate in adolescents and young adults previously treated for Hodgkin disease was low at 48% (Festa et al., 1992). Only 43.1% of sickle cell patients studied at the Children's Hospital of Buffalo were compliant with their penicillin prophylaxis (Teach, Lillis, & Grossi, 1998). In contrast, compliance with oral and intramuscular penicillin prophylaxis was good in 79% of splenectomized thalassemia children and adolescents, with only 7% constantly failing to take their medication (Borgna-Pignatti, DeStefano, Barone, & Concia, 1984).

Even children with life-threatening conditions are at risk of treatment failure due to nonadherence with their drug therapy. Despite the threat of cancer, several studies have confirmed less than optimal medication compliance in this population. The self-reported compliance rate of children and adolescents with cancer at 20 weeks after diagnosis was 60.5% (Tebbi, Cummings, & Zevon, 1986). Random urine assays for 17-ketogenic steroid in pediatric cancer patients suggested that 33% of children who were prescribed prednisone were not complying (Smith et al., 1979). In adolescents and young adults with acute lymphoblastic leukemia (ALL), 52% did not adhere with their prednisone therapy (Festa et al., 1992). Undetectable levels of 6-mercaptopurine were found in one third of children with ALL in remission (Snodgrass et al., 1984). Similarly, significant noncompliance has been reported in both pediatric renal and bone marrow transplant recipients (Blowey et al., 1997; Korsch, Fine, & Negrete, 1978; Meyers, Weiland, & Thomson, 1995; Phipps & DeCuir-Whalley, 1990).

Clinical Consequences

Although it may be argued that exact estimates of medication compliance have not been delineated for all chronic illnesses, there is irrefutable evidence that noncompliance is common and widespread in children. This would be of less concern if nonadherence with therapy were of little clinical significance. However, when present, it can compromise the efficacy of drug regimens resulting in failure to achieve the desired treatment goal. Disregarding poor compliance in a clinical trial of a new drug may result in a potentially beneficial medication being abandoned due to apparent lack of efficacy.

The treatment implications of noncompliance are numerous. Medical decisions may be adversely affected leading to inappropriate changes in treatment regimens. Children may be subjected to unnecessary medical tests, and medication doses may be increased due to perceived lack of clinical response, with subsequent toxicity if compliance suddenly improves. Thus, lack of adherence with drug therapy, as well as failure to appreciate noncompliance, may result in significant morbidity and costly wasting of resources. It has been suggested that 10% of all hospitalizations are due to a patient's inability to follow drug therapy (Berg et al., 1993). Researchers have estimated that prescription medication noncompliance costs the Canadian health care system between $7 and $9 billion per year (Coambs, Jensen, & Her, 1995).

As previously mentioned, it has not been determined for most pediatric regimens the degree of compliance that is necessary for an adequate therapeutic outcome (Rapoff & Barnard, 1991). However, the relationship between poor adherence with drug therapy and unfavorable disease outcome in children has been examined in a number of studies confirming the suspicion that clinical consequences of noncompliance are potentially enormous.

In a study of asthmatic children prescribed inhaled corticosteroids and ß-agonists, median compliance was 13.7% for those patients who experienced exacerbations and 68.2% for those who did not (Milgrom et al., 1996). Poor compliance with preventive treatment has been identified as a preventable factor in asthmatic children admitted to the hospital (Ordonez et al., 1998).

Children with recurrent urinary tract infections may be prescribed long-term antibiotic therapy to reduce the incidence of infection. When compliance was tested by urine assay in 93 children receiving antibiotics for this indication, the difference in infection rate between regular takers (3.9 infections per year) and nontakers (7.2 per year) and between irregular takers (4.8 per year) and nontakers was statistically significant (Daschner, & Marget, 1975). In a study of 123 patients with sickle cell disease prescribed penicillin prophylaxis, two episodes of pneumococcal bacteremia occurred, both in patients with measured noncompliance (Teach et al., 1998). Similarly, suboptimal compliance with prescribed penicillin was apparent in seven of eight cases of pneumococcal septicemia that occurred in 88 infants and young children with sickle cell anemia (Buchanan & Smith, 1986).

Although the outlook for childhood cancer has improved over the years, poor outcomes are still not uncommon. Less than optimal compliance with oral chemotherapy may be a contributing factor in relapse (Smith et al., 1981; Snodgrass et al., 1984). The evidence that poor compliance has an influence on disease-free survival is circumstantial but persuasive (Lilleyman & Lennard, 1996). In a study of adolescents with ALL or Hodgkin disease, 5 of 11 noncompliers with prednisone had relapses compared with 1 of 10 compliers (Festa et al., 1992).

Identification of children with renal transplants who do not adhere to their immunosuppressive drug regimen is important because they may be more at risk of graft failure. Noncompliant pediatric renal transplant recipients needed more grafts, had shorter graft survival, lost more grafts, and more died (Meyers et al., 1995). In 14 patients (13 adolescents) who interrupted their immunosuppressive medication at some time following transplantation, 8 experienced allograft failure requiring transplant nephrectomy and return to hemodialysis, whereas the other 6 suffered a reduction in allograft function (Korsch et al., 1978).

DETERMINANTS OF MEDICATION NONCOMPLIANCE

Although use of the term *noncompliance* implies fault of the parent or child (Hussar, 1987), in many instances this behavior is not a deliberate act, but rather a result of forgetfulness. Human error is the most probable cause of noncompliance in children and adolescents (Tebbi, 1993). Reasons given by parents as to why they were unable to administer medication as prescribed included forgetting, discontinuing medication because symptoms had resolved, misunderstanding of instructions, opposition from the child, apparent ineffectiveness or side effects of the medication (Thatcher Shope, 1981), and busy schedules (Tebbi, Cummings, & Zevon, 1986).

Unfortunately, although many different factors have been suggested as being associated with poor adherence, noncompliance is often difficult to anticipate due to a lack of accurate predictors. In addition, many of these factors may interact and work together in a complex way.

Regimen Factors

A number of characteristics of the drug regimen may influence adherence with therapy. In general, the more complex and demanding a regimen is, the lower the associated compliance (Rapoff & Barnard, 1991). Adherence with drug therapy is better when a smaller number of medications is prescribed (Thatcher Shope, 1981).

Drug schedules that are inconvenient and disrupt the child's or parent's normal routine or require lifestyle changes are less likely to be followed. For example, compliance tends to decrease the more frequently a medication must be taken. A review of the literature showed that once-a-day (73%) and twice-a-day (70%) regimens were associated with significantly better compliance than were three-times-daily (52%) and four-times-daily (42%) regimens (Greenberg, 1984). For children who attend school or parents who work during the day, any medication given more than twice daily will probably not be taken as often as prescribed (Dajani, 1996). In a study of 100 children who were prescribed antibiotics to be taken four times daily for the treatment of otitis media, 36 parents found that the day had elapsed by the time three doses had been given (Mattar & Yaffe, 1974). In asthmatic preschool children prescribed inhaled prophylactic therapy to be administered three or four times daily, it was generally the middle of the day doses that were missed (Gibson et al., 1995). It has also been suggested that drug compliance may be better in the evening than the morning (Lau et al., 1998; Moncica et al., 1995).

Several studies have shown that adherence to long-term regimens is poorer than with short-term ones (Fotheringham & Sawyer, 1995). Compliance tends to decay with time generally as the patient symptomatically improves.

Although financial cost of the medication may be a barrier to adequate drug therapy, a consistent relationship between compliance and socioeconomic status (SES) has not been demonstrated (Gordis et al., 1969). Similarly, not all studies have found a correlation between the occurrence of side effects and drug adherence in children and adolescent patients (Tebbi et al., 1986).

Palatability. It is reasonable to assume that when parents have difficulty giving a medication to a child drug compliance may suffer. This scenario is not uncommon in pediatrics. Variability in the acceptability of commonly prescribed antibiotic suspensions has been demonstrated (Dagan, Shvartzman, & Liss, 1994). In a study of 300 children with otitis media, parents reported difficulty in giving medication to 28% of children. Problems varied from outright refusal to take the medication to spitting out or vomiting the drug (Mattar, Markello, & Yaffe, 1975). One factor that may influence the ease with which parents are able to administer medication is the palatability of the preparation. Although tablets and capsules are usually more palatable than liquids or suspensions (Dajani, 1996), they are generally not practical for young children. Thus, palatability may be an important determinant of drug adherence, particularly in the younger age group. Considerations for drug selection should include palatability in addition to efficacy, safety, and cost.

Unfortunately, few studies of medication palatability have been carried out in pediatric subjects (Bagger-Sjoback & Bondesson, 1989; El-Chaar et al., 1996; Jahnsen & Thorn, 1987; Matsui, Barron, & Rieder, 1996; Matsui et al., 1997b; Powers, 1996; Sjoval et al., 1984). Although work has been done in adult volunteers (Demers et al., 1994; Ruff et al., 1991; Samulak, El-Chaar, & Rubin, 1996; Steele et al., 1997), it may not be appropriate to extrapolate the results of testing done in adults to children (Matsui et al., 1997b). It has also been shown that questioning children regarding flavors they do and do not like may not predict their antibiotic taste preferences (Matsui et al., 1996). Therefore, formal evaluation of taste is essential in the process of developing a new drug suspension. At the Children's Hospital of Western Ontario, our group conducted two studies of antibiotic taste in children 5 years of age and older—one testing various antistaphylococcal antibiotics (Matsui et al., 1996) and the other testing antibiotics effective against ß-lactamase-producing bacteria (Matsui et al., 1997b). Using a palatability assessment tool consisting of a visual analogue scale modified by the incorporation of a facial hedonic scale, significant differences in preference among different compounds were demonstrated (Matsui et al., 1996, 1997b).

Other Factors

Other factors that may influence compliance are only discussed briefly. For more information, the reader is referred to more detailed reviews of this topic (Matsui, 1997; Rapoff & Barnard, 1991).

Patient and Family Factors.   In general, demographic factors such as gender and SES have not been consistently related to compliance status (Rapoff & Barnard, 1991). The influence of age has been examined with several studies suggesting that adolescents are less adherent to medication regimens than young children (Fotheringham & Sawyer, 1995; Gordis et al., 1969; Liptak, 1996; Smith et al., 1979; Tebbi et al., 1986). Adolescents have been described as *abusers of nonprescribed drugs* on the one hand and as *nonusers of prescribed drugs* on the other (Litt & Cuskey, 1980). A supportive family environment is likely to be beneficial. A dysfunctional family situation may be a risk factor for poor compliance with therapy (Rapoff & Barnard, 1991; Thatcher Shope, 1981).

Disease Factors.   Although the type and duration of disease may have an effect on whether children take their medication, no disease process—even the more severe and life-threatening ones—is immune from poor adherence as previously described. Taking medication for asymptomatic conditions or prophylaxis against disease does, however, tend to be more difficult (Fotheringham & Sawyer, 1995). Knowledge of one's illness and its recommended treatment, although seemingly necessary, does not guarantee good compliance (Fotheringham & Sawyer, 1995). The health beliefs of the child (or parent), such as the perception of susceptibility to a particular illness, may be related to compliance with prescribed medical advice (Charney et al., 1967; Jay et al., 1984; Tebbi, 1993). However, in some studies, the assessment of disease severity by physicians has not been found to correlate with compliance (Rapoff & Barnard, 1991; Thatcher Shope, 1981).

In a study of prescription compliance conducted in the pediatric emergency department, parental reasons for not filling the prescription included medication not necessary (27%), financial (6.8%), and not enough time

(6.8%). Dissatisfaction with the explanation of the medical problem, instructions for treatment, and instructions for follow-up were also associated with noncompliance (Matsui et al., 1997a).

Physician Factors. The nature of the relationship between the patient and doctor may influence adherence with medical therapy. Better compliance is demonstrated by patients who are treated consistently by the same physician than by patients who are treated by different physicians on different occasions (Fotheringham & Sawyer, 1995; Litt & Cuskey, 1980). Higher rates of adherence are usually obtained by pediatricians in private practice than by pediatricians in a clinic setting (Litt & Cuskey, 1980).

ASSESSMENT OF MEDICATION COMPLIANCE

Given the potentially negative consequences of poor adherence with drug therapy, it is essential to identify noncompliance. Although there are several techniques that have been used to measure compliance, given the lack of a proved gold standard, drug compliance is best assessed using a combination of methods.

Available Methods

Unfortunately, although physicians think they know their patients, they tend to overestimate their drug compliance (Wang & Haynes, 1988). The physician's assessment of patient compliance has been found to be no more accurate than flipping a coin (Sackett et al., 1991). Patient self-report measures such as diaries, questionnaires, or interviews have been commonly used both in research settings and everyday practice. Relying on patient (or parental) reports of drug-taking behavior may be misleading because patients may be unwilling to admit to poor adherence. Self-reports of noncompliance are often more accurate than self-reports of compliance (Liptak, 1996). However, despite its limitations, this method may be of value, in particular if the information is gathered in a nonthreatening and nonjudgmental manner and is used as an adjunctive measure.

Noncompliance is often initially suspected as a reason for the failure to achieve a desired treatment target. However, because there is not always a predictable association between medication consumption and achievement of a treatment goal, this method of compliance assessment may be unreliable (Matsui et al., 1994). Not all patients respond to the same degree to a specific medical treatment, and indeed some patients may not respond at all although they take their medication.

Similarly the use of pill counts as a measure of drug therapy adherence may be misleading. This method involves determining the discrepancy between the number of pills remaining and the number of pills that should be missing if the recommended dosing regimen was followed. With liquid preparations, commonly used in children, the volume of remaining medication is measured. However, the assumption that any medication not returned has been ingested may not be justified. Patients may intentionally dispose of their medication to create the impression that they are taking their medication. Discarding unused drug, known as *pill dumping* (Rudd et al., 1989) or *the parking lot effect* (Urquhart, 1991), results in an overestimation of compliance. Medication may also be accidentally lost through spillage or misplacement of pills. This method may also not be feasible for practical reasons because patients often forget to bring their medication bottles to their visit. The reliability of this method also depends on the pharmacist dispensing the correct amount of medication with accurate dosing instructions, which may not always be the case (Johnson et al., 1996; Mattar et al., 1975).

A more direct estimation of medication compliance is provided by the measurement of drug levels in body fluids—most commonly blood or urine. The advantage of this method is that detection of drug confirms ingestion. However, the information obtained only reflects recent drug consumption (Matsui, 1997), which may be particularly relevant when the sample is collected at the time of a scheduled appointment because it has been shown that patients may alter their compliance during the several days prior to this visit (Feinstein, 1990). Other potential pitfalls include lack of available assay, cost, and variation in drug pharmacokinetics.

Most recently, various microelectronic devices have been introduced into the market for monitoring drug compliance. Although their use in the research setting has been a major advance, their feasibility for widespread use in clinical practice remains to be ascertained, although it may be helpful in differentiating between poor compliance and other reasons for suboptimal clinical effect in individual patients (Matsui et al., 1992). These automated devices have provided information on patterns of medication compliance over time, as well as evidence of the correlation of noncompliance with the occurrence of clinical events such as seizures (Cramer, Mattson, & Prevey, 1989).

The Medication Event Monitoring System (MEMS, Aprex Corporation) consists of a standard medication bottle with a microprocessor in the cap to record every container opening as a presumptive dose (Cramer, 1995). This tool has been used to measure drug compliance in several pediatric studies (Blowey et al., 1997; Lau et al., 1998; Moncica et al., 1995; Olivieri et al., 1991, 1995). An electronic inhaler timer device, the Nebulizer Chronolog (Forefront Technologies Incorporated), counts and times each actuation of a metered-dose inhaler (MDI) and has been used to measure adherence with medical therapy in children with asthma (Coutts et al., 1992; Gibson et al., 1995; Milgrom et al., 1996).

Although these microelectronic devices are considered by some investigators to be a breakthrough in the field of medication compliance, they are not without their drawbacks. In addition to being expensive and not readily available, they only confirm that the medication dispenser was used rather than guaranteeing ingestion. As well, patients must remember to bring the containers to their clinic visit and must use the device correctly to yield meaningful results (Matsui et al., 1994). How best to provide feedback to the child and parent to improve their compliance behavior using the information obtained remains to be determined.

Difficulties Encountered in Assessing Compliance in Clinical Practice

In clinical practice, the assessment of compliance may play an important role in explaining treatment failure and targeting certain patients for more intensive intervention. Physicians must have a high index of suspicion of noncompliance to provide the best possible care to their patients. However, the assessment of nonadherence with therapy is not always simple. In addition to the lack of a practical foolproof method, there are other difficulties associated with the process of evaluating the compliance behavior of patients in a nonresearch setting. Measurement of compliance on an isolated occasion or over a short period of time may not accurately reflect long-standing patterns of adherence with drug therapy (Friedman & Litt, 1986). Financial and time constraints may limit the physician's ability to thoroughly examine the area of drug compliance with each patient. In the case of chronic disease, other members of a multidisciplinary team may be in a better position to elicit evidence of poor adherence with treatment regimens. It has been suggested that if patients (or their parents) are aware that their compliance is being evaluated that they may alter their medication-taking behavior. Some physicians may fear that patients may react negatively to having their drug compliance monitored, thus discussions regarding adherence should be nonjudgmental in nature. Compliance assessment in everyday practice should also be unobtrusive and require minimal extra effort on the part of the parent and child.

Other Methodological Issues in Children

In addition to the difficulties associated with the assessment of medication compliance that pertain to all age groups, there are some unique issues specific to children. The evaluation of compliance in pediatrics is complicated by the need to assess the behavior of the parent in addition to that of the patient. The invasiveness of blood sampling to measure drug levels is particularly troublesome in children, making this method less desirable in this population.

The assessment of compliance with liquid medication poses special problems. Measuring the volume of remaining medication to estimate compliance may be misleading because error may be introduced when medication is spilled, spit out, or vomited (Rodewald & Pichichero, 1993). Variation may also exist in the measuring device used to administer the medication, which will also result in an unreliable estimate. The volumes of 130 teaspoons varied from 2.5 ml to 9 ml in a study of children with otitis media whose mothers often stated that they did not fill the spoon fearing the medication might be spilled (Mattar et al., 1975). As well, the microelectronic devices currently available for measuring medication compliance are not usable with liquid preparations, thus limiting their usefulness in young children who cannot take tablets or capsules (Berkovitch et al., 1998; Matsui, 1997).

RECOMMENDATIONS FOR FUTURE RESEARCH

Although knowledge in the area of pediatric adherence with medication regimens is increasing, much remains to be learned. With increasing appreciation of the scope of poor drug compliance, more research needs to be done in delineating the degree of compliance required for an adequate therapeutic outcome. Unfortunately, due to the lack of accurate predictors, noncompliance is difficult to anticipate. Therefore, there needs to be improvement in the tools for identifying poor adherence with drug therapy. In particular, in pediatrics, a practical and reliable method to assess compliance with liquid medications would be helpful. It would also be interesting to survey parents and children as to their reactions to having their adherence monitored. Although not addressed in this chapter, once noncompliance is demonstrated, better strategies for intervention need to be explored. The cost-effectiveness of these compliance-improving strategies also need to be examined.

Although prescription filling is a critical step in drug compliance, prescription filling in children with chronic disease has not been examined. The results of such a study may provide clues as to potentially helpful strategies to improve prescription redemption and thus enhance adherence with therapy. Finally, the role of pharmaceutical companies in developing medications that are more palatable, and hence easier for parents to administer to young children, requires consideration. Medications that are more forgiving in terms of still being effective in the face of less than perfect compliance would also be useful in practice.

REFERENCES

Bagger-Sjoback, D., & Bondesson, G. (1989). Taste evaluation and compliance of two pediatric formulations of phenoxymethylpenicillin in children. *Scandinavian Journal of Primary Health Care, 7,* 87–92.

Beardon, P. H., McGilchrist, M. M., McKendrick, A. D., McDevitt, D. G., & MacDonald, T. M. (1993). Primary non-compliance with prescribed medication in primary care. *British Medical Journal, 307,* 846–848.

Begg, D. (1984). Do patients cash prescriptions? An audit in one practice. *Journal of the Royal College of General Practitioners, 34,* 272–274.

Berg, J. S., Dischler, J., Wagner, D. J., Raia, J., & Palmer-Shelvin, N. (1993). Medication compliance: A health care problem. *Annals of Pharmacotherapy, 27* (Suppl.), S5–S24.

Bergman, A. B., & Werner R. J. (1963). Failure of children to receive penicillin by mouth. *New England Journal of Medicine, 268,* 1334–1338.

Berkovitch, M., Papadouris, D., Shaw, D., Onuaha, N., & Dias, C. (1998). Trying to improve compliance with prophylactic penicillin therapy in children with sickle cell disease. *British Journal of Clinical Pharmacology, 45,* 605–607.

Blowey, D. L., Hebert, D., Arbus, G. S., Pool, R., Korus, M., & Koren, G. (1997). Compliance with cyclosporine in adolescent renal transplant recipients. *Pediatric Nephrology, 11,* 547–551.

Borgna-Pignatti, C., DeStefano, P., Barone, F., & Concia, E. (1984). Penicillin compliance in splenectomized thalassemics. *European Journal of Pediatrics, 142,* 83–85.

Borowitz, D., Wegman, T., & Harris, M. (1994). Preventive care for patients with chronic illness—Multivitamin use in patients with cystic fibrosis. *Clincal Pediatrics, 33,* 720–725.

Boyd, J. R., Covington, T. R., Stanaszek, W. F., & Coussons, R. T. (1974). Drug defaulting: Part II. Analysis of noncompliance patterns. *American Journal of Hospital Pharmacy, 31,* 485–491.

Buchanan, G. R., & Smith, S. J. (1986). Pneumococcal septicemia despite pneumococcal vaccine and prescription of penicillin prophylaxis in children with sickle cell anemia. *American Journal of Diseases of Childhood, 140,* 428–432.

Charney, E., Bynum, R., Eldredge, D., Frank, D., MacWhinney, J. B., McNabb, N., Scheiner, A., Sumpter, E. A., & Iker, H. (1967). How well do patients take oral penicillin? A collaborative study in private practice. *Pediatrics, 40,* 188–195.

Coambs, R. B., Jensen, P., & Her, M. H. (Eds.). (1995). *Review of the scientific literature on the prevalence, consequences, and health costs of noncompliance and inappropriate use of prescription medication in Canada.* Ottawa, Ontario: Pharmaceutical Manufacturers Association of Canada.

Coutts, J. A. P., Gibson, N. A., & Patson, J. Y. (1992). Measuring compliance with inhaled medication in asthma. *Archives of Diseases in Childhood, 67,* 332–333.

Cramer, J. A. (1995). Microelectronic systems for monitoring and enhancing patient compliance with medication regimens. *Drugs, 49,* 321–327.

Cramer, J. A., Mattson, R. H., & Prevey, M. L. (1989). How often is medication taken as prescribed? *Journal of American Medical Association, 261,* 3273–3277.

Dagan, R., Shvartzman, P., & Liss, Z. (1994). Variation in acceptance of common oral antibiotic suspensions. *Pediatric Infectious Disease Journal, 13,* 686–690.

Dajani, A. S. (1996). Adherence to physicians' instructions as a factor in managing streptococcal pharyngitis. *Pediatrics, 97,* 976–980.

Daschner, F., & Marget, W. (1975). Treatment of recurrent urinary tract infection in children. *Acta Paediatrica Scandinavica, 64,* 105–108.

Dawson, D., & Newell, R. (1994). The extent of parental compliance with timing of administration of their children's antibiotics. *Journal of Advanced Nursing, 20,* 483–490.

Demers, D. M., Schotik Chan, D., & Bass, J. W. (1994). Antimicrobial drug suspensions: A blinded comparison of taste of twelve common pediatric drugs including cefixime, cefpodoxime, cefprozil and loracarbef. *Pediatric Infectious Disease Journal, 13*, 87–89.

El-Chaar, G. M., Mardy, G., Wehlou, K., & Rubin, L. G. (1996). Randomized, double blind comparison of brand and generic antibiotic suspensions: II. A study of taste and compliance in children. *Pediatric Infectious Disease Journal, 15*, 18–22.

Feinstein, A. R. (1990). On white-coat effects and the electronic monitoring of compliance. *Archives of Internal Medicine, 150*, 1377–1378.

Festa, R. S., Tamaroff, M. H., Chasalow, F., & Lanzkowsky R. S. (1992). Therapeutic adherence to oral medication regimens by adolescents with cancer: I. Laboratory assessment. *Journal of Pediatrics, 120*, 807–811.

Fotheringham, M. J., & Sawyer, M. G. (1995). Adherence to recommended medical regimens in childhood and adolescence. *Journal of Pediatrics and Child Health, 31*, 72–78.

Friedman, I. M., & Litt, I. F. (1986). Promoting adolescents' compliance with therapeutic regimens. *Pediatric Clinics of North America, 33*, 955–971.

Gibson, N. A., Ferguson, A. E., Aitchison, T. C., & Paton, J. Y. (1995). Compliance with inhaled asthma medication in preschool children. *Thorax, 50*, 1274–1279.

Gordis, L., Markowitz, M., & Lilienfeld, A. M. (1969). Why patients don't follow medical advice: A study of children on long-term antistreptococcal prophylaxis. *Journal of Pediatrics, 75*, 957–968.

Greenberg, R. N. (1984). Overview of patient compliance with medication dosing: A literature review. *Clinical Therapeutics, 6*, 592–599.

Hazzard, A., Hutchinson, S. J., & Krawiecki, N. (1990). Factors related to adherence to medication regimens in pediatric seizure patients. *Journal of Pediatric Psychology, 15*, 543–555.

Hussar, D. A. (1987). Importance of patient compliance in effective antimicrobial therapy. *Pediatric Infectious Disease Journal, 6*, 971–975.

Jahnsen, T., & Thorn, P. (1987). An acceptability study of two pivampicillin mixtures in children in general practice. *Scandinavian Journal of Primary Health Care, 5*, 241–243.

Jay, S., Litt, I. F., & Durant, R. H. (1984). Compliance with therapeutic regimens. *Journal of Adolescent Health Care, 5*, 124–136.

Johnson, K. B., Butta, J. K., Donohue, P. K., Glenn, D. J., & Holtzman, N. A. (1996). Discharging patients with prescriptions instead of medications: Sequelae in a teaching hospital. *Pediatrics, 97*, 481–485.

Korsch, B. M., Fine, R. N., & Negrete, V. F. (1978). Noncompliance in children with renal transplants. *Pediatrics, 61*, 872–876.

Krogh, C., & Wallner, L. (1987). Prescription-filling patterns of patients in a family practice. *Journal of Family Practice, 24*, 301–302.

Kruse, W. (1992). Patient compliance with drug treatment—new perspectives on an old problem. *Clinical Investigation, 70*, 163–166.

Lau, R. C. W., Matsui, D., Greenberg, M., & Koren, G. (1998). Electronic measurement of compliance with mercaptopurine in pediatric patients with acute lymphoblastic leukemia. *Medical and Pediatric Oncology, 30*, 85–90.

Leickly, F. E., Wade, S. L., Crain, E., Kruszon-Moran, D., Wright, E. C., & Evans, R. (1998). Self-reported adherence, management behavior, and barriers to care after an emergency department visit by inner city children with asthma. *Pediatrics, 101*, E8.

Levy, R. A. (1991). Failure to refill prescriptions. In J. A. Cramer & B. Spilker (Eds.), *Patient compliance in medical practice and clinical trials* (pp. 11–18). New York: Raven.

Lilleyman, J. S., & Lennard, L. (1996). Non-compliance with oral chemotherapy in childhood leukemia. *British Medical Journal, 313*, 1219–1220.

Liptak, G. S. (1996). Enhancing patient compliance in pediatrics. *Pediatrics in Review, 17*, 128–134.

Litt, I. F., & Cuskey, W. R. (1980). Compliance with medical regimens during adolescence. *Pediatric Clinics of North America, 27*, 3–15.

Matsui, D., Barron, A., & Rieder, M. (1996). Assessment of the palatability of antistaphylococcal antibiotics in pediatric volunteers. *Annals of Pharmacotherapy, 30*, 586–588.

Matsui, D., Hermann, C., Braudo, M., Ito, S., Olivieri, N., & Koren, G. (1992). Clinical use of the Medication Event Monitoring System: A new window into pediatric compliance. *Clinical Pharmacology and Therapeutics, 52*, 102–103.

Matsui, D., Hermann, C., Klein, J., Berkovitch, M., Olivieri, N., & Koren, G. (1994). Critical comparison of novel and existing methods of compliance assessment during a clinical trial of an oral iron chelator. *Journal of Clinical Pharmacology, 34*, 944–949.

Matsui, D., Joubert, G., Kim, S., & Rieder, M. J. (1997a). Compliance with prescription filling in the pediatric emergency department. *Clinical and Investigative Medicine, 20*, S12.

Matsui, D., Lim, R., Tschen, T., & Rieder, M. J. (1997b). Assessment of the palatability of ß-lactamase-resistant antibiotics in children. *Archives of Pediatric and Adolescent Medicine, 151*, 599–602.

Matsui, D. M. (1997). Drug compliance in pediatrics clinical and research issues. *Pediatric Clinics of North America, 44*, 1–14.

Mattar, M. E., Markello, J., & Yaffe S. J. (1975). Inadequacies in the pharmacologic management of ambulatory children. *Journal of Pediatrics, 87*, 137–141.

Mattar, M. E., & Yaffe, S. J. (1974). Compliance of pediatric patients with therapeutic regimens. *Postgraduate Medicine, 56*, 101–108.

McGee, A., Koren, G., Liu, P., Freedman, M., Rose, V., Benson, L., & Olivieri, N. F. (1989). Cardiac disease free survival in thalassemia major patients receiving deferoxamine: An update on the Toronto cohort. *Blood, 74*, 311a.

Meyers, K. E. C., Weiland, H., & Thomson, P. D. (1995). Pediatric renal transplantation noncompliance. *Pediatric Nephrology, 9*, 189–192.

Milgrom, H., Bender, B., Ackerson, L., Bowry, P., Smith, B., & Rand, C. (1996). Noncompliance and treatment failure in children with asthma. *Journal of Allergy and Clinical Immunology, 98*, 1051–1057.

Moncica, I., Oh, P. I., Qamar, I., Scolnik, D., Arbus, G. S., Hebert, D., Balfe, J. W., & Koren, G. (1995). A crossover comparison of extended release felodipine with prolonged action nifedipine in hypertension. *Archives of Diseases in Childhood, 73*, 154–156.

National Council on Patient Information and Education. (1989). *American Pharmacy, 29*, 436–437.

Olivieri, N. F., Brittenham, G. M., Matsui, D., Berkovitch, M., Blendis, L. M., Cameron, R. G., McClelland, R. A., Liu, P. P., Templeton, D. M., & Koren, G. (1995). Iron-chelation therapy with oral deferiprone in patients with thalassemia major. *New England Journal of Medicine, 332*, 918–922.

Olivieri, N. F., Matsui, D., Hermann, C., & Koren, G. (1991). Compliance assessed by the Medication Event Monitoring System. *Archives of Diseases in Childhood, 66*, 1399–1402.

Ordonez, G. A., Phelan, P. D., Olinsky, A., & Robertson, C. F. (1998). Preventable factors in hospital admissions for asthma. *Archives of Disease in Childhood, 78*, 143–147.

Phelan, P. D. (1984). Compliance with medication in children. *Australian Paediatric Journal, 20*, 5.

Phipps, S., & DeCuir-Whalley, S. (1990). Adherence issues in pediatric bone marrow transplantation. *Journal of Pediatric Psychology, 15*, 459–475.

Powers, J. L. (1996). Properties of azithromycin that enhance the potential for compliance in children with upper respiratory tract infections. *Pediatric Infectious Disease Journal, 15*, S30–S37.

Pullar, T. (1991). Compliance with drug therapy. *British Journal of Clinical Pharmacology, 32*, 535–539.

Rapoff, M. A., & Barnard, M. U. (1991). Compliance with pediatric medical regimens. In J. A. Cramer & B. Spilker (Eds.), *Patient compliance in medical practice and clinical trials* (pp. 73–98). New York: Raven.

Rashid, A. (1982). Do patients cash prescriptions? *British Medical Journal, 284*, 24–26.

Rodewald, L. E., & Pichichero, M. E. (1993). Compliance with antibiotic therapy: A comparison of deuterium oxide tracer, urine bioassay, bottle weights, and parental reports. *Journal of Pediatrics, 123*, 143–147.

Rudd, P., Byyny, R. L., Zachary, V., LoVerde, M. E., Titus, C., Mitchell, W. D., & Marshall, G. (1989). The natural history of medication compliance in a drug trial: Limitations of pill counts. *Clinical Pharmacology and Therapeutics, 46*, 169–176.

Ruff, M. E., Schotik, D. A., Bass, J. W., & Vincent, J. M. (1991). Antimicrobial drug suspensions: A blind comparison of taste of fourteen common pediatric drugs. *Pediatric Infectious Disease Journal, 10*, 30–33.

Sackett, D. L., Haynes, R. B., Guyatt, G. H., & Tugwell, P. (1991). Helping patients follow the treatments you prescribe. In *Clinical epidemiology: A basic science for clinical medicine* (pp. 249–281). Boston, MA: Little, Brown.

Samulak, K. M., El-Chaar, G. M., & Rubin, L. G. (1996). Randomized, double blind comparison of brand and generic antibiotic suspensions: I. A study of taste in adults. *Pediatric Infectious Disease Journal, 15*, 14–17.

Sauders, C. E. (1987). Patient compliance in filling prescriptions after discharge from the emergency department. *American Journal of Emergency Medicine, 5*, 283–286.

Sciver, M. M. V., D'Angelo, E. J., Rappaport, L., & Woolf, A. D. (1995). Pediatric compliance and the roles of distinct treatment characteristics, treatment attitudes, and family stress: A preliminary report. *Journal of Developmental and Behavioral Pediatrics, 16*, 350–358.

Sjoval, J., Fogh, A., Huitfeldt, B., Karlsson, G., & Nylen, O. (1984). Methods for evaluating the taste of pediatric formulations in children: A comparison between the facial hedonic method and the patients' own spontaneous verbal judgment. *European Journal of Pediatrics, 141*, 243–247.

Smith, S. D., Cairns, N. U., Sturgeon, J. K., & Lansky, S. B. (1981). Poor drug compliance in an adolescent with leukemia. *American Journal of Pediatric Hematology and Oncology, 3*, 297–300.

Smith, S. D., Rosen, D., Trueworthy, R., & Lowman, J. T. (1979). A reliable method for evaluating drug compliance in children with cancer. *Cancer, 43*, 169–173.

Smith, S. L., Hindmarsh, P. C., & Brook, C. G. D. (1993). Compliance with growth hormone treatment—are they getting it? *Archives of Diseases in Childhood, 68*, 91–93.

Snodgrass, W., Smith, S., Trueworthy, R., Vats, T. S., Klopovich, P., & Kisker, S. (1984). Pediatric clinical pharmacology of 6-mercaptopurine: Lack of compliance as a factor in leukemia relapse. *Proceedings of the Annual Meeting of the American Society of Clinical Oncology, 3*, 204.

Steele, R. W., Estrada, B., Begue, R. E., Mirza, A., Travillion, D. A., & Thomas, M. P. (1997). A double-blind taste comparison of pediatric antibiotic suspensions. *Clinical Pediatrics, 36*, 193–199.

Teach, S. J., Lillis, K. A., & Grossi, M. (1998). Compliance with penicillin prophylaxis in patients with sickle cell disease. *Archives of Pediatric and Adolescent Medicine, 152*, 274–278.

Tebbi, C. K. (1993). Treatment compliance in childhood and adolescence. *Cancer, 71*, 3441–3449.

Tebbi, C. K., Cummings, M., & Zevon, M. A. (1986). Compliance of pediatric and adolescent cancer patients. *Cancer, 58*, 1179–1184.

Thatcher Shope, J. (1981). Medication compliance. *Pediatric Clinics of North America, 28*, 5–21.

Thomas, E. J., Burstin, H. R., O'Neil, A. C., Orav, E. J., & Brennan, T. A. (1996). Patient non-compliance with medical advice after the emergency department visit. *Annals of Emergency Medicine, 27*, 49–55.

Urquhart, J. (1991). Real-time compliance data to help define optimal drug regimens. *Annals of the New York Academy of Sciences, 618*, 522–532.

Urquhart, J. (1994). Role of patient compliance in clinical pharmacokinetics. *Clinical Pharmacokinetics, 27*, 202–215.

Wang, E., & Haynes, R. B. (1988). Compliance with antimicrobial therapy in children. In G. Koren, C. G. Prober, & R. Gold (Eds.), *Antimicrobial therapy in infants and children* (pp. 105–114). New York: Marcel Dekker.

Zora, J. A., Lutz, C. N., & Tinkelman, D. (1989). Assessment of compliance in children using inhaled beta adrenergic agonists. *Annals of Allergy, 62*, 406–409.

CHAPTER SEVEN

Measurement of Treatment Nonadherence in Children With Asthma

Bruce G. Bender
Henry Milgrom
Frederick S. Wamboldt
National Jewish Medical Research Center, Denver, CO

Cynthia Rand
JHACC, Baltimore, MD

Nonadherence with an asthma treatment regimen contributes to treatment failure, human suffering, and unnecessary medical costs. Asthma can be treated effectively; significant improvements in pharmacotherapy have greatly enhanced our capacity to control this disease. Most notably, anti-inflammatory medications control chronic inflammation in the airways and dramatically reduce the need for hospitalization (Donahue et al., 1997). Despite the availability of effective treatments, many asthmatic patients do not adhere to their prescribed treatment and, consequently, are at increased risk for symptom exacerbation (Milgrom et al., 1996).

Although failure to adhere to the asthma regimen is widely recognized, the prevalence and impact of this problem are not fully recognized. Whether *medication adherence* is defined as proportion of appropriate use days or proportion of total prescribed medication taken, less than 50% adherence is typically reported. Creer found an average compliance rate of 48% in his review of 10 pediatric asthma adherence studies (Creer, 1993). Although a small proportion of nonadherence involves overuse of medication, most reflects underuse. The widespread underutilization of medication in the treatment of asthma has been reported in children (Gibson, Ferguson, Aitchison, & Paton, 1995) as well as adults (Bailey et al., 1990) regardless of whether the prescribed medication consists of tablets (Christiannse, Lavigne, & Lerner, 1989) or aerosolized medication (Milgrom et al., 1996).

The objective of this chapter is to examine the nature of treatment for pediatric asthma, the extent and circumstances of treatment nonadherence, and approaches to the measurement of treatment adherence in pediatric asthma and other childhood chronic illnesses. Finally, discussion of the implications of adherence include recommendations regarding both practice-based applications of this new knowledge and directions for future research concerning asthma treatment adherence.

TREATMENT OF CHILDHOOD ASTHMA

Children with asthma are frequently treated with more than one inhaled medication. This often includes beta agonists, which provide quick relief of asthma symptoms by acting directly on the bronchial muscles to open narrowed airways, and inhaled corticosteroids, which counteract inflammation in the lining of the airways. Inhaled corticosteroids serve an important preventive function, but do not provide the same immediate relief as beta agonists and hence are particularly susceptible to nonadherence.

RECENT TRENDS IN TREATMENT NONADHERENCE IN CHILDHOOD ASTHMA

Although a great deal of attention has been directed toward nonadherence to treatment of chronic illnesses such as asthma in recent years, there is no indication that the problem is resolving. Rates of adherence in recent reports (Bender, Milgrom, Rand, & Ackerson, 1998; Gibson et al., 1995) are no better than in the previous decade (Cluss et al., 1984; Christiannse, Lavinge, & Lerner, 1989).

In addition, reported prevalence rates and asthma death rates continue to increase nationally. A recent report from the Center for Disease Control and Prevention concluded that the increasing asthma morbidity and mortality would be entirely reversible with improvements in patient education and steps to increase treatment adherence (Mannino et al., 1998). In 1990, $3 billion of the $6.2 billion in asthma health care expenses were attributed to emergency room visits and hospitalization (Weiss, Gergen, & Hodgson, 1992). Much of this enormous cost is shared by a small group of patients who experience repeated emergency room visits and hospitalizations. That intensive adherence interventions resulted in dramatic reductions in emergency care use in this population suggests that nonadherence contributes significantly to urgent care use and its associated costs (Clark et al., 1986; Greineder, Loane, & Parks, 1995).

POTENTIAL CONSEQUENCES OF NONADHERENCE
TO TREATMENT IN ASTHMA

Despite the hope that parents should do all that is possible to manage a child's asthma, the incidence of nonadherence among asthmatic children is alarmingly high and the consequences often dire. In a 3-month pediatric asthma study, the median adherence rate of patients who suffered exacerbation was 13.7%, whereas those children whose disease remained under control demonstrated an adherence rate of 68.3% (Milgrom et al., 1996). Consistently low serum theophylline concentrations were found in children seeking emergency room care (Sublett, Pollard, Kadlec, & Karibo, 1979), as well as those being hospitalized for asthma (Cox, Webster, Ilett, & Walson, 1993). Adherence with anti-inflammatory medication prescribed for preschool-age children occurred on only 50% of days (Gibson et al., 1995). Use of inhaled bronchodilator medications was also low and sometimes unpredictable; parents often recorded their children's symptom exacerbations on study diaries but did not treat them (Ferguson, Gibson, Aitchison, & Paton, 1995).

A group of children with asthma who are at high risk for morbidity and mortality require particular concern. A high-risk profile for fatal or near-fatal asthma has emerged in the United Sates that includes suboptimal pharmacotherapy in conjunction with severe disease, psychological dysfunction, African-American race or Hispanic-American ethnicity, and residence in an urban area with a concentration of poverty (Gerbino, 1993). In contrast to a trend of declining hospitalization for other chronic diseases, the annual admission rate for asthma among persons 0 to 24 years old increased 28% from 1980 to 1993 (Lang, 1997). African Americans were 3.4 times more likely than Whites to require inpatient treatment. The death rate from asthma in the general population increased from .8 per 100,000 in 1977 to 2.0 in 1989 and has remained stable through 1994, the last year for which data are available (Centers for Disease Control and Prevention, 1996). In 1993, the asthma death rate of African Americans was six times higher than that of Whites in age groups 0 to 4 years and 15 to 24 years and four times higher among children ages 5 to 14 (Lang, 1997). In New York City, the mortality rate from asthma in patients under 35 years of age in the 1980s was 5.5 times higher for African Americans and 3 times higher for Hispanics than for Whites.

There is some evidence that adherence behavior may augment the risk of these groups. One worrisome finding among high-risk inner-city children with asthma is that excessive reliance on bronchodilators occurs frequently in association with insufficient use of inhaled corticosteroids and poor inhaler technique (Hartert, Windom, & Peebles, 1996). β-agonist overuse by children and adolescents is more common among males, minorities, and members of lower socioeconomic groups (Beausoleil, Weldon, & McGeady, 1997) and may signal the need for greater utilization of inhaled steroids (Donahue et al., 1997). Young children of racial minorities admitted for an asthma exacerbation are less likely to have received maximally effective anti-inflammatory therapy (Finkelstein et al., 1995)—a fact that points to likely links between poor patient adherence and inadequate medical attention. These aspects of management must be addressed to reduce asthma morbidity in the urban United States (Hartert et al., 1996). It is essential that the medical profession embrace the guidelines set down by the National Asthma Education and Prevention Program. Further, the guidelines must be linked to ongoing clinical and organizational processes to ensure their intended effect (Brooks et al., 1994; Greineder, 1996; Lang, Sherman, & Polanski, 1997). Education and training aimed at providing medical care consistent with the National Asthma Education and Prevention Program (NAEPP) guidelines and better self-care for minority children has resulted in marked improvement in illness management (Evans et al., 1997).

ADHERENCE MEASUREMENT

General Considerations

Limitations in adherence measurement have diminished full appreciation of the degree or consequence of treatment nonadherence. Without having a window to view actual patient behavior, clinicians have relied on presumptions of what patients actually do between office visits. Historically, these presumptions have been inaccurate, generally underestimating nonadherence and its consequences.

Another problem is that research has sometimes characterized adherence as a singular, homogeneous patient characteristic. Patients are frequently categorized as *adherent* or *nonadherent* (or as *compliant* or *noncompliant*). In other cases, patients' behavior may be assessed and rated by degree of adherence (e.g., patients are labeled as 50% adherent if they use one half of the medication that has been prescribed for them). This approach may miss important day-to-day variations in adherence behavior. Few patients are strictly adherent or nonadherent, and their medication use seldom falls into a consistent daily pattern of taking a particular percentage of drug.

Like most behavior, adherence behavior may follow certain patterns but is nonetheless variable over time. Variability in medication use reflects patients' views of their illness and belief in the advice of their physician, and it may be linked to periods of exacerbation or frequency of contact with the health caregiver. For this reason, more precise measures of actual patient behavior result in clearer understanding of the factors influencing treatment outcome, whereas less precise measures have provided only dim and partial insights. Less precise or ambiguous measures lead to inaccurate conclusions and may delay introduction of effective adherence interventions.

Types of Adherence Measures

The most common measures used to assess adherence with pediatric asthma therapy are clinical judgment, self-report, biochemical measurement, medication measurement, pharmacy database review, electronic measurement, and family interview (Dunbar, 1980; Rand & Wise, 1994; Sackett & Haynes, 1976).

Clinical Judgment.   Health care providers routinely form impressions of how well each of their patients is following the prescribed regimens. These clinical assessments of patient adherence shape the content of the patient–provider interaction, the selected therapy, and the follow-up plan. However, several classic studies have shown that physicians greatly overestimate the degree to which their patients comply with the formers' directives. Clinical judgment based on preconceived beliefs about the attributes of the typical compliant patient are destined to fail. Patient characteristics such as race, education, gender, socioeconomic status (SES), and personality have not been found to be reliable predictors of adherence. Physician interviewing skills and the qualities of the patient–provider interaction are more important in both measuring and facilitating adherence than stereotypical beliefs about adherence (Davis, 1966; DiMatteo, Sherbourne, Hays, & Ordway, 1993; Steele, Polard, Kadlec, & Karibo, 1979). Indeed, one recent study documented that quality of the relationship between children and parents with their health care providers is an important correlate of asthma treatment adherence to outcome in high-risk asthma (Gavin et al., 1999).

Self-Report.   Patient self-report of medication use is a standard measure of adherence in both clinical trials and behavioral intervention studies. Self-reports may be collected by interviews, diaries, and questionnaires. In the case of pediatric asthma, *self-report* refers to the combined reporting of parent and child. No validated adherence-specific questionnaire is currently in common use partly because most self-report questionnaires of adherence have been designed for specific studies. Self-report measures are common because they are simple, inexpensive, and generally brief. In addition, self-report (particularly in the clinical setting) is the best measure for collecting information about patient beliefs, attitudes, and experiences with medication regimens.

As a quantitative measure of medication use, self-report has been found to have a highly variable degree of accuracy. Studies have compared asthmatic patients' self-reports of inhaler usage with the objective adherence data collected by an electronic medication monitoring device and found that patient self-reports of adherence recorded in asthma diaries typically overestimate adherence often by a large margin (Coutts, Gibson, & Paton, 1992; Spector et al., 1986).

Self-reports of adherence are influenced by the setting in which the information is collected. The desire to please the physician or investigator can lead patients to exaggerate reports of medication use. Physicians' and investigators' skills and sensitivity in eliciting patients' self-reports influence the reliability and usefulness of the information they receive, particularly in research. When carefully collected, self-reported adherence information can provide critical information into the nature of the patients' problems with adherence. In addition, because there is no evidence to suggest that adhering patients misrepresent themselves as nonadherers, self-report measures identify the honest nonadherers (Coutts et al., 1992; Dolce, Crisp, Manzella, & Richards, 1991).

Biochemical Measurement. Inhaled medications are not easily detectable by biochemical assays because of the rapid and limited systemic absorption of these agents. For this reason, theophylline (via direct blood level assay) and oral corticosteroids (via indirect assessment of AM cortisol as a reflection of HPA-axis-suppression) are the only asthma medications for which adherence is commonly measured by biochemical assay. Because assays of theophylline are routinely measured as part of clinical care to determine whether a therapeutic level of theophylline has been achieved, the clinician or researcher can be provided with ongoing information about patient adherence levels.

Biochemical measurement is the only adherence measurement strategy that provides direct confirmation of drug use; however, these measures have several limitations. Biochemical measures can be confounded by diet and/or other drug use (e.g., the effect of smoking on theophylline), as well as by idiosyncratic pharmacokinetic abnormalities (e.g., delayed absorption or rapid metabolism). These measures cannot be used to measure day-to-day patterns of adherence with therapy. Finally, biochemical measures can be compromised if patients deliberately (or inadvertently) begin taking medications just before clinical samples are collected (Eney & Goldstein, 1976; Koysooko, Ellis, & Levy, 1974; Levy, Ellis, & Koysooko, 1974; Miller, 1982).

Medication Measurement. Counting pills, checking prescription refills, or weighing inhaler canisters or liquid medication are examples of medication measurement—an objective measure that allows researchers to infer the degree of medication adherence. This method requires recording the exact quantity of medication that is issued to a patient and returned by the patient at follow-up. Level of adherence is calculated by deriving average daily usage over the monitored period.

Although medication measurement data are both objective and reasonably simple to collect, they are limited by several factors. Medication measures can be influenced by a patient's efforts to deceive the investigator. Some patients may discard medication to appear adherent. Medications may be shared within households, particularly when family members are on the same medication. In addition, medication measures give no indication of the accuracy of dosages or the timing of the medication. However, in situations where patients are comfortable reporting nonadherence, the pattern of medication use is not critical; where the likelihood of medication sharing is low, medication measurement is a useful, objective, and valid means to assess adherence (Gordis, 1976; Haynes & Dantes, 1987).

Pharmacy Database Review. In some managed care settings, pharmacy databases can provide useful information on the exact regimen prescribed, the amount of medication dispensed, and the timing of refills. These data can be used to roughly calculate the average dose per day. In some health care data management systems, prescriptions written but never filled can also be monitored. Dispensing pharmacy data can also be matched with medical record and health care utilization databases to provide integrated analyses of the antecedents and consequences of patient adherence behaviors. Review of automated pharmacy records can also allow large-scale population studies of patient adherence with medication.

Pharmacy database review to identify nonadherence has several limitations. First, adherence estimates can only be calculated for patients who exclusively rely on the target pharmacy system for all prescriptions and refills. Second, pharmacy data can determine when a prescription was filled; however, it provides no confirmation of consumption or appropriate consumption patterns. Nevertheless, as more pharmacy data go online, this adherence measuring strategy has great potential to evaluate the compliance of both individuals and clinical populations (Kellaway & Brown, 1983; Spitzer et al., 1992; Steiner & Prochazka, 1997).

Electronic Medication Monitors. In the past 10 years, the increased availability of computer-based technology has introduced a new strategy for adherence monitoring. Electronic monitoring devices record and store the data (and, for some devices, time) from each medication use. Devices have been developed to monitor medication adherence behaviors including, but not restricted to, opening a pill bottle, releasing a blister-pak pill, discharging inhaled medications, and releasing eye drops. Electronic devices that have been used to investigate adherence in asthma treatment include the Nebulizer Chronolog and the MDILog (NC—Medtrac Technologies, Inc., Lakewood, CO), the Doser (NEWMED Corp. Newton, MA), the Smartmist (Aradigm Corporation, Hayward, CA), the Airwatch (Enart Health Management Systems, Inc., Nashville, TN), and the Asthma Monitor (Ferraris Medical, Inc., Holland, NY). All of these devices record the date and number of puffs taken. The MDILog and the Smartmist can detect the presence of vacuum at the point of discharge and thus can confirm that aerosolized medications have been consumed and not just dispensed into the air.

In recent years, the number of published studies that have used electronic adherence monitoring devices has dramatically increased. These devices provide a unique opportunity to investigate long-term patterns of presumptive adherence that were previously unavailable in such detail. The primary benefit of this type of monitoring is clear—electronic monitoring methods can provide a continuous record of timing of presumptive doses over period of months.

However, assessment of adherence provided by self-report, pill counts, or canister weights can be inaccurate because of recall, demand characteristics, deception, and provider biases. These methods are also insensitive to daily patterns of use over time. The phenomenon of medication *dumping*—a phenomenon found when patients discard medication to appear adherent in a clinical trial (Rand et al., 1992)—is nearly impossible to detect by traditional methods of adherence assessment. Inclusion of dumping data into a dose–response analysis can yield counterintuitive results because highly adherent subjects show poorer response than moderately adherent subjects. This phenomenon is likely to be present in any situation in which medication use is being monitored. Thus, it should be taken into consideration when making medication recommendations, although the risk of dumping may be greatest in clinical trial settings where the need to remain a good subject is enhanced by financial and social incentives.

Although electronic measures of adherence have a number of unique strengths, they also have a number of weaknesses. The cost for wide-scale use can be prohibitive for a small practice and may only be feasible in a clinical trial setting. Peer-reviewed data concerning the reliability and validity of these devices remain scant. Failure rate associated with the use of any type of electronic devices may be unacceptable (Wamboldt et al., 1997). The failure rate in electronic devices can be caused by patient misuse, device failure, or computer hardware/software problems. For these reasons, clinicians or researchers who use such devices must be careful to develop quality control procedures that ensure the ongoing monitoring of device performance and validity (Bender et al., 1998; Coutts et al., 1992; Mawhinney et al., 1991; Rand et al., 1992; Wamboldt et al., 1997).

The Interview. Although self-report of adherence, as provided by diary card or questionnaire procedures, often overstates adherence, the interviewing of patients and family members can provide more accurate information if properly conducted. Dew and colleagues (1996) developed an approach for assessing treatment adherence in patients who had undergone heart transplants. The interviews were conducted face to face and designed to emphasize the establishment of good rapport, nonjudgmental questioning, and encouragement of truthful and accurate answers. Information gathered through this method revealed dramatic nonadherence, including failure to take medications daily (22.1%) and smoking (24.4%).

An innovative approach to interview-based adherence assessment—the 24-hour interview—was developed by Johnson and colleagues (Johnson et al., 1986, 1992). Pediatric diabetic patients and their parents were interviewed by telephone regarding their illness-management behaviors during the previous day. Areas of illness management included injection regularity and timing, diet, exercise, and glucose testing. Correlations between parent and child reports were moderately high and increased with age. By limiting questioning to the previous 24-hour period, the investigators were able to avoid asking patients to provide broad generalizations about adherence and to focus instead on immediate behaviors, thus improving accuracy (Johnson et al., 1986). Interviews were conducted on nine occasions over 3 months to further increase accurate generalization about adherence (Johnson et al., 1992).

Behaviorally Focused Parent–Child Assessment. One methodology for assessing the family's ability to manage childhood asthma is the Family Asthma Management System Scale (FAMSS; Klinnert, McQuaid, & Gavin, 1997), a structured interview that includes both parent and child. The FAMSS includes interview guidelines for assessing strengths and weaknesses in the family asthma management system; it has 12 scales that describe the various behavioral domains and functional relationships that are key to effective asthma management for children. High functioning on a summary score encompassing all of the scales was related to fewer symptoms in a group of children with mild to moderate asthma from an outpatient setting (Klinnert et al., 1997). The interview and areas of functioning outlined by the FAMSS scales are particularly well suited for clinical assessments and treatment planning. The FAMSS was developed to assess adherence while beginning the process of changing behavior (Klinnert & Bender, in press).

SPECIAL CONCERNS ABOUT ADHERENCE MEASUREMENT

In addition to the unique strengths and weaknesses of each form of adherence measurement, there are also some cross-cutting issues that should be considered in selecting the most appropriate measurement strategy.

Social Desirability and Measurement Reactivity

Self-report adherence measures rely on the assumption that patients respond candidly when queried about their adherence with therapy. However, research suggests that, in an effort to present a positive or desirable appearance to health care providers, some patients may alter their self-report of adherence to appear more compliant (Rand, 1993). The extent to which this social desirability effect (Carnrike, McCracken, & Aikens, 1996) occurs may be influenced by many factors, including the setting where assessment occurs, the wording of the questions, and the relationship of the interviewer. If the consequences of candor are perceived as negative (e.g., being judged a neglectful parent), patients may be discouraged from admitting adherence problems.

Behavioral researchers have long recognized that the process of observing or measuring human behavior may alter the behavior under consideration (Gittelsohn, Shankar, Keith, & Gnywali, 1997). This measurement reactivity effect is most likely when the monitoring techniques are known by both the clinician and patient to be both accurate and revealing. For example, when medication counting is used as the monitoring strategy, patients may discard medications or take medications just prior to a clinic visit to appear adherent (Rand et al., 1992; Urquhart, 1991). Other studies using electronic monitoring have suggested that the actual levels of adherence may be improved when patients are aware that their behavior is being precisely monitored (Nides et al., 1993; Simmons et al., 1996). If the goals of the clinical interaction or study are to promote optimal adherence to the therapy, the reactivity inherent in known monitoring may be an asset to the study. However, when the focus is on the ability to generalize the study's conclusions (i.e., will most patients use enough bronchodilator to achieve therapeutic goals?), then the use of a specialized, highly reactive measurement methodology would be inappropriate. Therefore, it is important to clarify the goals of adherence assessment in each and every research or clinical application and then to select the most appropriate measurement strategies.

Predictors of Adherence

One of the questions most frequently asked by clinicians regarding adherence is: What patient characteristics predict adherence? Hundreds of studies have examined sociodemographic, psychosocial, and personality variables in an effort to characterize the type of patient who will experience adherence problems (Sackett & Haynes, 1976). Overall, efforts to identify a compliant personality type have not been successful, nor has the literature consistently found a relationship between patient characteristics and adherence behavior. Although some disruptive psychopathology, some addictive disorders, and chaotic family situations have been implicated as risks for nonadherence, personality, sociodemographic characteristics, and health beliefs have yielded inconsistent results (Sackett & Haynes, 1976). The literature on predictors of adherence makes it clear that stereotyping of patients' likely adherence by personal characteristics is an unsupported (and potentially misleading) strategy for assessing adherence (Dunbar, 1980).

One possible explanation for the often contradictory findings of adherence prediction studies may be attributable to the form of adherence measurement used. In a large-scale study monitoring adherence with an inhaled bronchodilator, Rand et al. (1995) found that women and more educated participants were more likely to have satisfactory self-reported inhaler adherence. However, when a validated objective measure of adherence was used in the analyses, both education level and gender dropped out of the model. This suggests that gender and education level were more strongly associated with reporting behavior than with actual medication use behavior. In this same study, no significant relationship was observed between race and self-reported adherence. However, analysis using objective adherence data found that non-Whites were less likely to have satisfactory adherence levels. This study raises the possibility that predictors of adherence behaviors may differ based on the adherence measure used. Those personal characteristics that may influence presenting oneself as adherent (i.e., self-reported adherence) may be different from those characteristics associated with actual adherence behavior.

Specific Challenges of Pediatric Adherence Measurement in Clinical Practice

Measuring children's adherence with therapy presents special challenges for the clinician and researcher. Pediatric adherence always occurs within the family context and may involve multiple members of the family. Responsibility for medication administration shifts as a child grows—from total parent management for a young child, to shared medication management for the school-age child, to complete self-management for the adolescent. As parents transfer responsibility for medication management, they generally become less accurate reporters of the child's medication adherence. Studies that have examined the concordance between parent–child reports of other health variables, such as symptoms, have found relatively poor agreement. Moreover, there can be great diversity between and within families in how medication management is implemented. Grandparents, siblings, and day-care providers may assume responsibility for regular medication delivery in some households. Because of the highly variable and often shifting family responsibility for a child's medication use, it is necessary for the health care provider to review medication use habits with both the parent and child to develop an adherence profile.

A Case Report

Addressing treatment nonadherence in clinical practice raises many challenges. It is not always apparent when nonadherence is a problem. Even when it is suspected, nonadherence can be difficult to detect. Further, the clinician's desire to reveal adherence behaviors may not be shared by the patient or family. The following case report provides an example of a patient who initially appeared to be fully adherent. However, his nonadherence was subsequently revealed to be contributing to treatment failure. The combined efforts of the medical caregivers and psychosocial team helped the patient eventually acknowledge his nonadherence, but resulted in only partial success in achieving improved illness control.

Jim, a 13-year-old with asthma, and his parents presented to the hospital staff as a normal, well-functioning family. Both his mother and stepfather held white-collar jobs, were invested in the patient's medical care, and were responsive to recommendations. Jim was a polite, eager-to-please young man who maintained good grades, had an active social life, and played on the high school football team. Jim's asthma was severe, and consequently his medication routine consisted of several asthma medications including theophylline, beta-agonists, and anti-inflammatory aerosols. He initially denied any significant difficulties adhering to his medical regimen. Later he admitted to occasionally overusing his inhaler and to exercising vigorously even while experiencing chest tightness. Serum theophylline concentrations measured in the office were in the range of 10 to 13 mcg/mL; however, concentrations measured during emergency room visits were below 5 mcg/mL.

Jim and his parents underwent an extensive psychosocial evaluation. Jim reported that, although he had been diligent with his therapy, his parents were overly critical about his medication compliance. They were all concerned about his problematic response to treatment. Over time, Jim and his mother began to talk about his anxiety during asthma attacks, his fear of dying, and family arguments about Jim's management of his illness. The stepfather was critical of Jim's technique with metered-dose inhalers (MDIs) and his lapses in taking medication. Jim began to complain about the difficulty of maintaining his regimen. The mother alternately defended Jim and sided with the stepfather in prompting Jim to take greater responsibility for his illness. Jim felt blamed for his illness and was angry with his parents for their inability to empathize with his plight. At the time of discharge from the hospital, after several meetings to work on these issues, individual and family therapy was recommended and arranged for in the home community.

Although Jim and his family did not follow through with psychotherapy, his symptoms were well controlled for approximately 6 months, at which point he began to experience increased nocturnal awakening. He continued to wheeze despite the reinstitution of methylprednisolone 20 mg every other day for 2 months. When a second inpatient stay was recommended, Jim became extremely upset and was especially sensitive to questions about his compliance. Jim indicated that he may have *slacked off* using the spacer on his inhaler, but, despite questions raised by his stepfather, he reported near-perfect compliance with all other aspects of his regimen. He was readmitted to the hospital 18 months after his initial hospitalization. A.M. cortisol level on admission was 8.6 mcg/dL. Three weeks later, following supervised administration of the same dose of methylprednisolone, it was 3.8 mcg/dL.

Although he appeared sincere, competent, and well motivated, Jim not only failed to comply with therapy, but he actively sought to mislead his parents and physicians. When he was gently confronted with the evidence of noncompliance, he continued to deny this to the medical team. Individual and family therapy addressed issues of body image, difficulty accepting his illness, the need to feel competent and in control, and anger and resentment toward the parents. As he began to explore these issues, Jim described periods of attempting to forget his illness and of being unsure of whether he took his medications. Later he denied these statements and reasserted angrily that he had been completely compliant. In the opinion of the psychosocial staff, Jim wanted to be perceived as someone who was cooperative, truthful, and working to control his illness. He had convinced himself, his physician, and his mother that he was taking his medications as prescribed. However, his anger about his illness, resentment toward his parents, and fear of steroid side effects hindered his ability to manage his disease.

CONCLUSIONS

On average, patients with asthma take only about half of their prescribed medications. Although the impact of partial medication adherence is difficult to assess, nonadherence clearly contributes to symptom exacerbation, human suffering, increased hospitalization, and unnecessary medical expense (Creer & Bender, 1993). More precise and insightful understanding of patient adherence behaviors will increase our understanding of why and how patients do not adhere to the treatment plan. This understanding will, in turn, lead to more effective adherence interventions. Introduction of adherence intervention based on incomplete or inaccurate assumptions about when and why patients do not take their medication will lead to failure. One example of this is the assumption that patient education alone can turn the tide of nonadherence. A meta-analysis of education intervention studies revealed little overall impact on treatment outcome (Bernard-Bonnin et al., 1995) and led one investigator to conclude that "to know is not to do" (Blessing-Moore, 1996).

CLINICAL APPLICATIONS

Physicians, physician assistants, nurses, and all other health care providers are concerned when their patients do not improve or get worse. Treatment nonadherence must also be given consideration as a potential cause of treatment failure. Even the most reasonable and intelligent patients may undermine illness control by failure to follow their treatment plan (Milgrom, Bender, Sarlin, & Leung, 1994). For this reason, clinical assessment of medication should begin with interviewing the patient and parents. Although patients frequently provide dramatic underestimates of medication use on a diary card, they may be more disclosing when talking to their doctor. The manner in which the health caregiver inquires about adherence greatly determines accuracy of the answers received. Conveying a nonjudgmental attitude, encouraging truthful answers, avoiding asking for broad generalizations, and asking about specific behaviors within specific time frames will gain a more accurate assessment. Conversely, the caregiver who appears in a hurry, who suggests by his behavior impatience or disinterest, and who is likely to shame or scold the patient who reveals that the treatment plan was not followed is unlikely to receive accurate information (Bender, Milgrom, & Rand, 1997).

The 1997 guidelines from the National Heart, Lung, and Blood Institute (NHLBI; 1997) Expert Panel emphasize the importance of establishing a partnership between health caregiver and patient within which a back-and-forth flow of information ensures that the patient and caregiver together will determine a reasonable treatment plan and assess its progress. Devices that measure medication-taking behavior can assist in developing this collaborative information flow. However, such measurement cannot be imposed on the patient and parents against their will. Rather, the introduction of any device into the health caregiver–patient relationship can only occur with the agreement of the patient and the understanding that the goal of this procedure is to facilitate better illness management. Because adherence-monitoring devices require the use of computer software and can malfunction, their use in clinical practice will succeed only if a staff member with sufficient time, interest, and skill assumes responsibility for their correct use.

Recommendations for Future Research

The science of adherence measurement in pediatric asthma is evolving, but is certainly not in an advanced state of development. Much remains to be learned about how to accurately measure patient health care behavior. The three areas of measurement have different capabilities. For example, direct measurement is composed of the electronic devices described earlier, which record on microchip the date and time of each use. The most significant recent improvement in this technology is the capacity to detect whether an inhalation has occurred when medication is dispensed from an MDI. These devices, which include the Smartmist and MDILog, avoid the problem of falsely recording medication dumping as adherence. However, they stop short of establishing ingestion of the medication. Because dry powder inhalers are increasingly replacing traditional 10CFC-driven inhalers, these devices may soon be unusable. No electronic devices are as yet marketed for use with dry powder inhalers. Furthermore, variation in size, shape, and delivery systems of these new inhalers obviates the development of a single universal adherence-monitoring device. Still the clear advantage of microchip-based recording of adherence events creates a compelling need for new technology-based research directed toward dry powder inhalers.

With respect to indirect measurements, pill counts, canister weights, and pharmacy databases all provide indirect adherence measurement. None can directly measure medication usage, nor can they provide time and date information essential to detecting patterns of medication use. Still such measures are effective as global indexes of patient adherence and can be widely applied to clinical trials and longitudinal studies of pediatric asthma. Computer-based pharmacy records are increasingly available as a source of information about refill frequency. Given the volume of evidence indicating that nonadherence is prevalent in all asthma studies, there seems little justification for failure to include such unobtrusive measures in all future pediatric asthma treatment studies.

Adherence assessments conducted via patient interviews show increasing promise as an accurate source of information about adherence behaviors. The interview approach holds the additional advantage of building strong patient–caregiver communication that can naturally lead to effective intervention. However, much research remains to be conducted to clarify the specific circumstances and health caregiver behavior that elicit accurate self-report. Johnson and colleagues (1986) determined that accurate interview assessment of adherence to a diabetes treatment regimen is enhanced when questions are specific and limited to behaviors occurring in the previous 24 hours. Future investigations of the effect of the 24-hour interviewing approach, telephone versus inperson interviewing, interviewer gender and behavior, and interview setting will help define those conditions that enhance the accuracy of interview assessments.

REFERENCES

Bailey, W. C., Richards, J. M., Brooks, C. M., Soong, S., Windsor, R. A., & Manzella, B. A. (1990). A randomized trial to improve self-management practices in adults with asthma. *Archives of Internal Medicine, 150,* 1664–1668.

Beausoleil, J., Weldon, D., & McGeady, S. (1997). β2-agonist metered dose inhaler overuse: Psychological and demographic profiles. *Pediatrics, 99,* 40–43.

Bender, B., Milgrom, H., & Rand, C. (1997). Nonadherence in asthmatic patients: Is there a solution to the problem? *Annals of Allergy and Asthma Immunology, 79,* 177–186.

Bender, B., Milgrom, H., Rand, C., & Ackerson, L. (1998). Psychological factors associated with medication nonadherence in asthmatic children. *Journal of Asthma, 35,* 347–353.

Bernard-Bonnin, A., Stachenko, S., Bonin, D., Charette, C., & Rousseau, E. (1995). Self-management teaching programs and morbidity of pediatric asthma: A meta-analysis. *Journal of Allergy and Clinical Immunology, 95,* 34–41.

Blessing-Moore, J. (1996). Does asthma education change behavior? To know is not to do. *Chest, 109,* 9–19.

Brooks, C. M., Richards, J. M., Kohler, C. L., Soong, S., Martin, B., Windsor, R. A., & Bailey, W. C. (1994). Integrating guidelines with continuous quality improvement: Doing the right thing the right way to achieve the right goals. *Journal of Quality Improvement, 20,* 181–191.

Carnrike, C. L. M. J., McCracken, L. J., & Aikens, J. E. (1996). Social desirability, perceived stress, and PACT ratings in lung transplant candidates: A preliminary investigation. *Journal of Clinical Psychology in Medical Settings, 3,* 57–67.

Center for Disease Control and Prevention. (1996). Asthma mortality and hospitalization among children and young adults, United States, 1990–1993. *Morbidity and Mortality Weekly Report, 45,* 350–353.

Christiannse, M. E., Lavigne, J. V., & Lerner, C. V. (1989). Psychosocial aspects of compliance in children and adolescents with asthma. *Journal of Developmental and Behavioral Pediatrics, 10,* 75–80.

Clark, N. M., Feldman, C. H., Evans, D., Levison, M. J., Wasilewski, Y., & Mellins, R. B. (1986). The impact of health education on frequency and cost of health care use by low income children with asthma. *Journal of Allergy and Clinical Immunology, 78,* 108–115.

Cluss, P. A., Epstein, L. H., Galvis, S. A., Fireman, P., & Friday, G. (1984). Effects of compliance for chronic asthmatic children. *Journal of Consulting and Clinical Psychology, 52,* 909–910.

Coutts, J. A. P., Gibson, N. A., & Paton, J. Y. (1992). Measuring compliance with inhaled medication in asthma. *Archives of Diseases of Childhood, 67,* 332–333.

Cox, S., Webster, M., Ilett, K., & Walson, P. D. (1993). Audit of theophylline plasma level monitoring in a pediatric hospital. *Therapeutic Drug Monitoring, 15,* 289–293.

Creer, T. L. (1993). Medication compliance and childhood asthma. In N. A. Krasneger, L. Epstein, S. B. Johnson, & S. J. Yaffe (Eds.), *Developmental aspects of health compliance behavior* (pp. 303–333). Hillsdale, NJ: Lawrence Erlbaum Associates.

Creer, T. L., & Bender, B. G. (1993). Asthma. In R. J. Gatchel & E. B. Blanchard (Eds.), *Psychophysiological disorders: Research and clinical applications* (pp. 151–203). Washington, DC: American Psychological Association.

Davis, M. S. (1966). Variations in patients' compliance with doctors' orders: Analysis of congruence between survey responses and results of empirical investigations. *Journal of Medical Education, 41,* 1037–1048.

Dew, M. A., Roth, L. H., Thompson, M. E., Kormos, R. L., & Griffith, B. P. (1996). Medical compliance and its predictors in the first year after heart transplantation. *Journal of Heart and Lung Transplantation, 15*, 631–645.

DiMatteo, M. R., Sherbourne, C. D., Hays, R. D., & Ordway, L. (1993). Physicians' characteristics influence patients' adherence to medical treatment: Results from the medical outcomes study. *Health Psychology, 12*, 93–102.

Dolce, J., Crisp, C., Manzella, B., & Richards, J. M. (1991). Medication adherence patterns in chronic obstructive pulmonary disease. *Chest, 99*, 837–841.

Donahue, J. G., Weiss, S. T., Livingston, J. M., Goetsch, M. A., Greineder, D. K., & Platt, R. (1997). Inhaled steroids and the risk of hospitalization for asthma. *Journal of the American Medical Association, 277*, 887–891.

Dunbar, J. M. (1980). Assessment of medication compliance: A review. In R. B. Haynes, M. E. Mattson, & T. O. Engebretson (Eds.), *Patient compliance to prescribed antihypertensive medication regimens: A report to the National Heart, Lung, and Blood Institute, NIH Publication No. 81-2102* (pp. 59–82). Washington, DC: Government Printing Office.

Eney, R. D., & Goldstein E. D. (1976). Compliance of chronic asthmatics with oral administration of theophylline as measured by serum and salivary levels. *Pediatrics, 57*, 513.

Evans, D., Mellins, R., Lobach, K., Ramos-Bonoan, C., Pinkett-Heller, M., Wiesemann, S., Klein, I., Donahur, C., Burke, D., Levison, M., J., Levin, B., Zimmerman, B., & Clark, N. (1997). Improving care for minority children with asthma: Professional education in public health clinics. *Pediatrics, 99*, 157–164.

Ferguson, A. E., Gibson, N. A., Aitchison, T. C., & Paton, J. Y. (1995). Measured bronchodilator use in preschool children with asthma. *British Medical Journal, 10*, 1161–1164.

Finkelstein, J. A., Brown, R. W., Schneider, L. C., Weiss, S. T., Quintana, J. M., Goldmann, D. A., & Homer, C. J. (1995). Quality of care for preschool children with asthma: The role of social factors and practice setting. *Pediatrics, 95*, 389–394.

Gavin, L. A., Wamboldt, M. Z., Sorokin, N., Levy, S. Y., & Wamboldt, F. S. (1999). Treatment alliance and its association with family functioning, adherence, and medical outcome in adolescents with severe, chronic asthma. *Journal of Pediatric Psychology, 24*(4), 355–365.

Gerbino, P. (1993). Forward. *Annals of Pharmacotherapy, 27*, S3–S4.

Gibson, N. A., Ferguson, A. E., Aitchison, T. C., & Paton, J. Y. (1995). Compliance with inhaled asthma medication in preschool children. *Thorax, 50*, 1274–1279.

Gittelsohn, J., Shankar, A., Keith, P. R. R., & Gnywali, T. (1997). Estimating reactivity in direct observation studies of health behavior. *Human Organ, 56*, 182–189.

Gordis, L. (1976). Methodologic issues in the measurement of patient compliance. In D. L. Sackett & R. B. Haynes (Eds.), *Compliance with therapeutic regimens* (pp. 51–66). Baltimore: Johns Hopkins University Press.

Greineder, D. K. (1996). The adaptation of asthma practice guidelines into clinical care: The Harvard Pilgrim Health Care experience. *Journal of Outcomes Management, 3*, 4–9.

Greineder, D. K., Loane, K. C., & Parks, P. (1995). Reduction in resource utilization by an asthma outreach program. *Archives of Pediatric and Adolescent Medicine, 149*, 415–420.

Hartert, T. V., Windom, H. H., & Peebles, R. S. (1996). Inadequate outpatient medical therapy for patients with asthma admitted to two urban hospital. *American Journal of Medicine, 100*, 386–394.

Haynes, R. B., & Dantes, R. (1987). Patient compliance and the conduct and interpretation of therapeutic trials. *Controlled Clinical Trials, 8*, 12–19.

Johnson, S. B., Kelly, M., Henretta, J. C., Cunningham, W. R., Tomer, A., & Silverstein, J. H. (1992). A longitudinal analysis of adherence and health status in childhood diabetes. *Journal of Pediatric Psychology, 17*, 537–553.

Johnson, S. B., Silverstein, J., & Rosenbloom, A. (1986). Assessing daily management in childhood diabetes. *Health Psychology, 5,* 545–564.

Kellaway, G. S. M., & Brown, S. A. (1983). Compliance failure and counseling in paediatric drug therapy. *New Zealand Medical Journal, 96,* 207–209.

Klinnert, M., & Bender, B. (in press). Psychological implications of pediatric asthma. In A. Kaptein & T. Creer (Eds.), *Behavioral sciences and respiratory disorders.* New York: Harwood.

Klinnert, M. D., McQuaid, E. L., & Gavin, L. A. (1997). Assessing the family asthma management system. *Journal of Asthma, 34,* 77–88.

Koysooko, R., Ellis, E. F., & Levy, G. (1974). Relationship between theophylline concentration in plasma and saliva in man. *Clinical Pharmacology Therapy, 15,* 454–460.

Lang, D., Sherman, M., & Polansky, M. (1997). Guidelines and realities of asthma management: The Philadelphia story. *Archives of Internal Medicine, 157,* 1193–1200.

Lang, D. (1997). Trends in U.S. asthma mortality: Good news and bad news. *Annals of Allergy and Asthma Immunology, 78,* 333–337.

Levy, G., Ellis, E. F., & Koysooko, R. (1974). Indirect plasma-theophylline monitoring in asthmatic children by determination of theophylline concentration in saliva. *Pediatrics, 53,* 873–876.

Mannino, D. M., Homa, D. M., Pertowski, C. A., Ashizawa, A., Nixon, L. L., Johnson, C. A., Ball, L. B., Jack, E., & Kang, D. S. (1998). Surveillance for asthma—United States, 1960–1995. *Mortality and Morbidity Weekly Report CDC Surveillance Summary, 47,* 1–27.

Mawhinney, H., Spector, S. L., Kinsman, R. A., Siegel, S. C., Rachelefsky, G. S., Katz, R. M., & Rohr, A. S. (1991). Compliance in clinical trials of two nonbronchodilator, antiasthma medications. *Annals of Allergy, 66,* 294–299.

Milgrom, H., Bender, B., Ackerson, L., Bowry, P., Smith, B., & Rand, C. (1996). Non-compliance and treatment failure in children with asthma. *Journal of Allergy and Clinical Immunology, 98,* 1051–1057.

Milgrom, H., Bender, B., Sarlin, N., & Leung, D. (1994). Difficult to control asthma: The challenge posed by non-compliance. *American Journal of Asthma and Allergy Pediatrics, 3,* 141–146.

Miller, K. A. (1982). Theophylline compliance in adolescent patients with chronic asthma. *Journal of Adolescent Health Care, 3,* 177–179.

National Heart, Lung, and Blood Institute. (1997, February). *Guidelines for the diagnosis and management of asthma: Highlights of the expert panel report II.* Washington, DC: Author.

Nides, M. A., Tashkin, D. P., Simmons, M. S., Wise, R. A., Li, V., & Rand, C. S. (1993). Improving inhaler adherence in a clinical trial through the use of the nebulizer chronolog. *Chest, 104,* 501–507.

Rand, C. S. (1993). Measuring adherence with therapy for chronic disease: Implications for the treatment of heterozygous familial hypercholesterolemia. *American Journal of Cardiology, 72,* 68D–74D.

Rand, C. S., Nides, M., Cowles, M. K., Wise, R. A., & Connett, J. (1995). Long-term metered-dose inhaler adherence in a clinical trial. The Lung Health Study Research Group. *American Journal of Respiratory and Critical Care Medicine, 152,* 580–588.

Rand, C. S., & Wise, R. A. (1994). Measuring adherence to asthma therapy. *American Journal of Respiratory and Critical Care Medicine, 149,* S69–S76.

Rand, C. S., Wise, R. A., Nides, M., Simmons, M. S., Bleecker, E. R., Kusek, J. W., Li, V., & Tashkin, D. P. (1992). Metered-dose inhaler adherence in a clinical trial. *American Review of Respiratory Diseases, 146,* 1559–1564.

Sackett, D. L., & Haynes, R. B. (1976). *Compliance with therapeutic regimens.* Baltimore: Johns Hopkins University Press.

Simmons, M. S., Nides, M. A., Rand, C. S., Wise, R. A., & Tashkin, D. P. (1996). Trends in compliance with bronchodilator inhaler use between follow-up visits in a clinical trial. *Chest, 109*, 963–968.

Spector, S. L., Kinsman, R., Mawhinney, H., Siegel, S. C., Rachelefsky, G. S., Katz, R. M., & Rohr, A. S. (1986). Compliance of patients with asthma with an experimental aerosolized medication: Implications for controlled clinical trials. *Journal of Allergy and Clinical Immunology, 77*, 65–70.

Spitzer, W. O., Suissa, S., Ernst, P., Horwitz, R. I., Habbick, B., Cockcroft, D., Boivin, J. F., McNutt, M., Buist, A. S., & Rebuck, A. S. (1992). The use of beta-agonists and the risk of death and near death from asthma. *New England Journal of Medicine, 326*, 501–506.

Steele, J. L., Pollard, S. J., Kadlec, G. J., & Karibo, J. M. (1979). Non-compliance in asthmatic children: A study of theophylline levels in pediatric emergency room population. *Annals of Allergy, 43*, 95.

Steiner, J. F., & Prochazka, A. V. (1997). The assessment of refill compliance using pharmacy records: Methods, validity, and applications. *Journal of Clinical Epidemiology, 50*, 105–116.

Sublett, J. L., Pollard, S. J., Kadlec, G., & Karibo, J. (1979). Non-compliance in asthmatic children: A study of theophylline levels in a pediatric emergency room population. *Annals of Allergy, 43*, 95–97.

Urquhart, J. (1991). Patient compliance as an explanatory variable in four selected cardiovascular studies. In J. A. Cramer & B. Spilker (Eds.), *Patient compliance in medical practice and clinical trials* (pp. 301–322). New York: Raven.

Wamboldt, F. S., Bender, B. G., O'Connor, S. L., McTaggart, S., Meltzer, L., Gavin, L. A., Wamboldt, M. Z., Milgrom, H., Szefler, S. J., Kamada, A., Kastner, W., Iklé, D., & Rand, C. (1997). Reliability of the Model MC-311 MDI chronolog. *American Journal of Respiratory and Critical Care Medicine, 155*, A259.

Weiss, K., Gergen, P., & Hodgson, T. (1992). An economic evaluation of asthma in the United States. *New England Journal of Medicine, 326*, 862–868.

CHAPTER EIGHT

Critical Issues in the Assessment of Regimen Adherence in Children With Diabetes

Alan M. Delamater
University of Miami School of Medicine

Research indicates that poor glycemic or blood glucose control in persons with diabetes is eventually associated with serious health complications, including kidney disease, retinopathy, and neuropathy (Clark & Lee, 1995). Attainment and maintenance of good glycemic control has therefore been considered a significant factor in diabetes management and prevention of complications (Diabetes Control and Complications Trial Research Group, 1993), with improved glycemic control shown to reduce the risk of health complications even among adolescents (Diabetes Control and Complications Trial Research Group, 1994). Therefore, although the goal of diabetes management is to achieve normal glycemic control, the process by which good glycemic control is achieved is through adherence to regimen prescriptions. Thus, it is important for health care professionals working with children and adolescents with diabetes to accurately determine whether they are adhering well to the prescribed medical regimen.

The issues involved in adherence with diabetic regimens can be considered as a model for other chronic illnesses affecting children. The regimen is complicated and essential for sustaining life and, in the absence of a cure, is chronic. The diabetic regimen impacts on virtually all areas of everyday life, including dietary intake and physical activity. Additionally, it requires the administration of specific types and amounts of insulin at certain times throughout the day (prior to eating), testing of blood for levels of glucose, and recording of blood glucose results in logbooks. Timing and amount of food intake, exercise, and insulin administration are all important relative to blood glucose levels and important to consider for avoiding hypoglycemia (low blood glucose) and hyperglycemia (high blood glucose). Without prompt treatment of hypoglycemia, the individual may lose consciousness, have a seizure, and even die. If hyperglycemia is sustained and progresses to ketoacidosis, without medical treatment the individual would likely die. Adherence to this regimen is therefore crucial to avoid serious symptoms as well as prevent long-term health complications. It involves the use of specialized medical equipment for monitoring health status and delivering medications, and everyday aspects of lifestyle such as eating and physical activity have significant impacts on blood glucose levels. Thus, this regimen is both complex and chronic—two characteristics of medical regimens associated with higher risk for adherence problems (Haynes, 1979).

The purpose of this chapter is to identify critical issues in the assessment of regimen adherence in children with diabetes. The medical management of diabetes is first discussed, followed by a review of studies addressing regimen adherence in children with diabetes. Methodological issues are then considered, including consideration of the definitions of compliance and adherence, the construct of regimen adherence, general approaches to its measurement, and specific tools for measurement that have been used in the literature. The chapter concludes with recommendations to improve the methodological quality of assessment of adherence in diabetes research and practice.

MEDICAL MANAGEMENT

Diabetes mellitus is the most common metabolic disease affecting children. Approximately 1 in 700 children have Type 1 diabetes (Arslanian, Becker, & Drash, 1994), with increasing rates of diagnosis among young children (Travis, Brouhard, & Schreiner, 1987).

Metabolic control is an integral aspect of disease management. A number of factors can potentially affect metabolic control. In the period after diagnosis, children go through a *honeymoon* period, during which their beta-cells produce some insulin (Madsbad, McNair, & Faber, 1980). This period generally lasts from 18 to 24 months, during which glycemic control is relatively easy to attain. However, after the residual pancreatic activity subsides, good glycemic control becomes more challenging.

Another critical time during which biological factors influence metabolic control is puberty. Studies indicate that the worsening of metabolic control typically seen during puberty is due in part to decreased insulin sensitivity (Amiel, Sherwin, Simonson, Lauritano, & Tamborlane, 1986; Bloch,

Clemons, & Sperling, 1987). Research has also shown a racial disparity in metabolic control, with African-American youths having greater metabolic control problems than White youths (Auslander, Anderson, Bubb, Jung, & Santiago, 1990; Auslander, Thompson, Dreitzer, White, & Santiago, 1997; Delamater, Albrecht, Postellon, & Gutai, 1991; Delamater et al., 1999).

Metabolic control is assessed in several ways. Patients can measure their own blood glucose with a drop of blood obtained by finger prick and then use a reflectance meter to accurately determine the current blood glucose within 2 minutes. In recent years, reflectance meters became equipped with memory so that several hundred values could be stored and downloaded to personal computers for statistical and graphical evaluation. Most families are asked to keep a written logbook of all blood glucose test results. Patients are usually prescribed two to four or more blood glucose tests each day. Urine tests for ketones may also be prescribed at certain times when there is high risk for diabetic ketoacidosis, such as during viral illness or after several days of hyperglycemia.

The gold standard of measurement of glycemic control for the past two decades has been the glycosylated hemoglobin A1 (or A1c) assay, which reflects the amount of glucose bound to hemoglobin in the blood (Gonen, Rachman, Rubenstein, Tanega, & Horwitz, 1977; Nathan, Singer, Hurxthal, & Goodson, 1984). Because the half-life of hemoglobin is about 2 months, this assay provides a measure of average blood glucose over that antecedent period. This blood test is usually conducted on a quarterly basis and has been increasingly used to evaluate the effectiveness of interventions. The glycohemoglobin (GHb) test typically requires a venous blood sample, but new technological advances have made it possible to attain via a finger stick sample of blood.

It is important to note that the GHb test does not reflect short-term changes and should not be used as a measure of regimen adherence (because glycemic control is affected by multiple biological, psychological, and behavioral factors). Furthermore, because it provides a measure of average blood glucose, the range of blood glucose values is not reflected in the test result. Norms for GHb vary across assays and laboratories. The range for most individuals without diabetes, across the various assays and laboratories, is 4% to 7%; the value for patients with diabetes in good control is less than 8%, whereas those in poor control would have values greater than 10%. Although GHb results are an important outcome measure, additional variables should be considered in evaluating control of diabetes, including the number of blood glucose values outside the target range both before and after meals, number of hypoglycemic episodes, and normal growth and development.

The goal of medical management is maintenance of normal or near normal blood glucose levels, with prevention of hypoglycemia (less than

70 mg/dl) and hyperglycemia (greater than 180 mg/dl). Education and involvement of the family is essential for good diabetes management. Besides daily glucose monitoring, the regimen requires adherence to a variety of medically prescribed behaviors, including daily insulin administration, planning and modification of diet and exercise, and timing of all these factors related to blood glucose levels. Children are typically prescribed two insulin injections each day (before breakfast and dinner), two to four blood glucose tests per day (generally before meals and at bedtime), and a balanced diet of meals and snacks with a daily caloric goal. Although most physicians encourage their patients to exercise, specific exercise prescriptions are not routinely made.

Insulin prescriptions usually involve the mixture of two types of insulin (short- and long-acting insulins) in specific amounts. The exact dosage may be fixed or may be on a sliding scale depending on the blood glucose level obtained prior to insulin administration. Patients are instructed to vary the sites where they inject insulin so as to avoid skin problems. Because short-acting insulin takes up to 30 minutes to be absorbed, children and families are instructed to wait a certain amount of time before eating. The amount of time depends on their blood glucose level before taking their insulin injection. For example, if a child were hyperglycemic, he or she would be instructed to wait 45 minutes to an hour before eating to give the insulin time to work. New insulin preparations that are fast acting have recently become available so that eating can occur immediately after taking the insulin.

With the results of the Diabetes Control and Complications Trial (DCCT) concluding that maintenance of normal GHb levels by intensive insulin therapy delays the onset and slows the progression of retinopathy, neuropathy, and nephropathy (Diabetes Control and Complications Trial Research Group, 1993, 1994), tight control of blood glucose has become the main goal of medical management of diabetes. Intensive therapy requires multiple insulin injections and blood glucose measures each day (up to six or more), with utilization of blood glucose data for adjustments in insulin dose, physical activity, and diet. Many more children are now being prescribed these more intensive regimens in the hopes of preventing or delaying the health complications of diabetes. Such intensive regimens may also consist of continuous subcutaneous insulin infusion using an insulin pump.

Dietary prescriptions have long been a cornerstone of diabetes management. In the past, this included a specific meal plan prescribed by a dietitian using the exchange method and a specific daily caloric goal. However, this method was difficult for most patients to successfully implement (Christensen, Terry, Wyatt, Pichert, & Lorenz, 1983; Delamater, Smith, Kurtz, & White, 1988; Lorenz, Christensen, & Pichert, 1985). More recently, carbohydrate counting has become popular. In most settings, dietitians work as part of the health care team caring for children with diabetes, and dietary goals and methods are individualized according to usual eating habits and lifestyle factors without prescription of any one diabetic diet (American Diabetes Association, 1999).

Perfect adherence is not necessarily associated with good glycemic control. This may be due to several factors, including regimen prescriptions that may be inappropriate or poorly communicated and endogenous factors (e.g., residual beta-cell activity, insulin resistance) that may exert independent effects on blood glucose. Conversely, poor adherence may still be associated with acceptable glycemic control in some cases. Thus, the interaction between biological and behavioral factors in diabetes management is complex. This complex interaction may help explain why some studies have found significant associations between regimen adherence and metabolic control (e.g., Brownlee-Duffick et al., 1987; Hanson, De Guire, Schinkel, Kolterman, Goodman, & Buckingham, 1996; Hanson, Henggeler, & Burghen, 1987; Johnson, Kelly, Henretta, Cunningham, Tomer, & Silverstein, 1992; Kuttner, Delamater, & Santiago, 1990; Schafer, Glasgow, McCaul, & Dreher, 1983), whereas others have not (Glasgow, McCaul, & Schafer, 1987; Johnson, Freund, Silverstein, Hansen, & Malone, 1990). When significant relationships between adherence and metabolic control are observed, the percentage of variance accounted for by adherence is generally less than 25%. Other factors may account for these findings, as discussed later in the chapter.

EMPIRICAL STUDIES OF REGIMEN ADHERENCE

Levels of Regimen Adherence

Studies have generally shown relatively low levels of adherence to various aspects of the regimen, especially among older children and adolescents (Johnson, Silverstein, Rosenbloom, Carter, & Cunningham, 1986). Insulin administration is of critical importance in preventing ketoacidosis and has been identified as a major adherence problem among the subgroup of patients hospitalized recurrently for poor metabolic control (White, Kolman, Wexler, Polin, & Winter, 1984). Studies indicate the vast majority of patients do take their insulin shots on a daily basis. However, many adolescent patients have been reported by their parents to have significant difficulty adhering with specific components of the insulin regimen, such as administering the correct dose (10%), administering it at the correct time (20%), and making appropriate adjustments in the insulin dose (19%; Delamater, Applegate, Eidson, & Nemery, 1998).

Although glucose testing is commonly prescribed two to four times per day, studies reveal adherence rates and utilization of blood glucose data are fairly low (Delamater et al., 1989; Wing et al., 1985). Furthermore, although some studies have indicated that blood glucose testing was not associated with improved metabolic control (Daneman et al., 1985; Mann, Noronha, & Johnston, 1984), recent studies suggest better metabolic control with more frequent blood glucose testing (Anderson, Ho, Brackett, Finkelstein, & Laffel, 1997). For example, a recent study of adolescents indicated the degree of significant adherence problems: By parent ratings, 31% did not adhere well with blood glucose testing prescriptions and 47% did not adhere well with recording their blood glucose test results (Delamater et al., 1998).

Dietary adherence is problematic for many young patients (Christensen et al., 1983; Delamater, Smith, Kurtz, & White, 1988; Lorenz et al., 1985), and poor dietary adherence has been associated with worse glycemic control (Delamater et al., 1988). The findings of a recent study of adolescents suggest that, by parent ratings, 48% did not eat the proper foods, 29% did not eat their meals on time, 32% did not eat regular snacks, and 28% did not carry a quick-acting sugar in case of hypoglycemia (Delamater et al., 1998). Exercise levels are generally low among diabetic youths (Johnson et al., 1986), but as noted earlier, exercise is not usually prescribed in a specific manner.

Psychosocial Factors

Research has shown a number of psychosocial factors are associated with regimen adherence (Johnson, 1995; Kurtz, 1990). For example, studies have shown good coping and adjustment of children (Jacobson et al., 1990) and healthier family functioning (Hauser et al., 1990) in the months just after diagnosis were predictive of better regimen adherence over the first 4 years of having diabetes. In studies with adolescents, higher levels of adherence have been associated with greater general and regimen-specific family support (Hanson, De Guire, Schinkel, Henggeler, & Burghen, 1992; La Greca et al., 1995; Schafer, Glasgow, McCaul, & Dreher, 1983) and more effective communication skills (Bobrow, AvRuskin, & Siller, 1985), whereas lower adherence has been associated with family conflict (Miller-Johnson et al., 1994).

It is important to assess children's abilities to assume responsibility for various components of the regimen, as well as who in the family is responsible for specific aspects of the regimen. Agreement about family responsibilities for diabetes management tasks has been associated with improved levels of metabolic control among youths (Anderson, Auslander, Jung, Miller, & Santiago, 1990). Studies have shown professionals often expect children to assume self-management responsibilities at relatively young ages (Wysocki, Meinhold, Cox, & Clarke, 1990), and that parents and professionals may differ in how they evaluate children's competence with regard to diabetes management tasks (Wysocki et al., 1992). This is particularly important in light of the finding that cognitive maturity among adolescents has been associated with more insulin self-adjustment and better glycemic control (Ingersoll, Orr, Herrold, & Golden, 1986). These findings call attention to the need for good communication between families and health care providers especially concerning the goals of treatment (Marteau, Johnson, Baum, & Bloch, 1987).

Personal factors such as health beliefs, appraisals, and psychopathology have also been studied in relation to regimen adherence. In accord with the Health Belief Model, studies by Brownlee-Duffeck et al. (1987) and Palardy, Greening, Ott, Holderby, and Atchison (1998) have shown that increased perceived costs of adherence are associated with lower levels of regimen adherence. Bond, Aiken, and Somerville (1992) found that perceptions of increased benefits relative to costs and more cues to action were related to better adherence; the best adherence was observed when perceived threat was low and perceived benefits to costs were high. Cognitive appraisals such as the perception of little internal control over health and the external attributional style for negative events have also been associated with lower levels of regimen adherence (Murphy, Thompson, & Morris, 1997). Additionally, major psychiatric disorder has been linked with poor regimen adherence (Kovacs, Goldston, Obrosky, & Iyengar, 1992).

Increased barriers to adherence have been related to lower regimen adherence in adolescent samples. Studies indicate a high number of barriers to the dietary and exercise components of the regimen (Glasgow, McCaul, & Scafer, 1986) and specific social barriers to dietary adherence (Delamater et al., 1988; Schlundt et al., 1994). Pressures to conform with peers in specific social situations have been shown to influence regimen adherence decisions (Thomas, Peterson, & Goldstein, 1997). Social demand has also been shown to influence reports of regimen adherence. In a study by Delamater, Kurtz, White, and Santiago (1988), adolescents under high social demand reported significantly lower blood glucose results than those under low social demand.

Knowledge About Diabetes Management

Diabetes knowledge and skills are of obvious importance in successful management, yet studies have shown substantial deficits (Johnson et al., 1982). Improving knowledge and skills has been assumed to lead to better adherence and metabolic control, but studies indicate this not to be the case (Bloomgarden et al., 1987). In fact, research findings indicate that children in poor metabolic control actually have high levels of diabetes knowledge (Weist, Finney, Barnard, Davis, & Ollendick, 1993), suggesting their poor control is not due to knowledge deficits.

Behavioral Intervention

Because knowledge and skills are necessary but not sufficient to improve good adherence and metabolic control, interventions that target behavioral change are necessary. A number of studies indicate that behavioral interventions can improve regimen adherence and metabolic control of children and adolescents with diabetes (Delamater, 1993). For example, blood glucose testing adherence has been improved through the use of individual clinic-based behavioral contracting (Wysocki, Green, & Huxtable, 1989), computer-assisted feedback (Marrero et al., 1989), and family-based behavioral contracting (Delamater et al., 1991), but without improvements in glycemic control. Other intervention programs, which have utilized peer groups for problem solving related to social situations associated with nonadherence (Kaplan, Chadwick, & Schimmel, 1985) and utilization of blood glucose data in combination with parent training (Anderson, Wolf, Burkhart, Cornell, & Bacon, 1989; Delamater et al., 1990), have led to improvements in both adherence and glycemic control. Peer group interventions targeting structured physical exercise have improved short-term glycemic control in children (Campaigne, Gilliam, Spencer, Lampman, & Schork, 1984) and adolescents (Stratton, Wilson, Endres, & Goldstein, 1987).

METHODOLOGICAL ISSUES

Definitions of Compliance and Adherence

It is helpful to consider the definitions of the two terms most often used when discussing patient behavior in relation to medical prescriptions—*compliance* and *adherence* (see Riekert & Drotar, chap. 1, this volume). *Compliance* has been defined as the degree to which a person's behavior is consistent with medical advice (Haynes, 1979); *noncompliance* thus implies disobedience, and the failure to comply can be viewed as the patient's fault. In this model, the patient has a passive role in relationship with the health care provider. In contrast, adherence "implies the active, voluntary, and collaborative involvement of the patient in a mutually acceptable course of behavior to produce a therapeutic result" (Meichenbaum & Turk, 1987, p. 20). In the adherence model, there is choice and mutuality in the treatment planning and implementation, as well as internalization of the health care provider's recommendations.

When planning to measure regimen-related health behavior, both of these models imply the comparison of some level of behavior relative to a specific goal or criterion (i.e., the prescription). Thus, measurement of compliance or adherence also implies measurement of regimen prescriptions, which may be problematic because precise regimen prescriptions may not be routinely recorded in medical charts (see Ievers-Landis & Drotar, chap. 11, this volume). Patients and parents may be asked what their regimen entails, but studies suggest that recall of regimen prescriptions is poor (Page, Verstraete, Robb, & Etzwiler, 1981). When planning interventions, the adherence model, because of its emphasis on patient involvement in goal setting, would appear to have advantages to the compliance model, although empirical tests of the relative effectiveness of the implementation of two different models of patient care on patient adherence have not yet been reported.

The Construct of Regimen Adherence

Regimen adherence is best considered a multivariate rather than a unitary construct (Johnson, Silverstein, Rosenbloom, Carter, & Cunningham, 1986). Four separate factors or components have been identified from empirical study utilizing factor analysis, including injection, diet type, eating/testing frequency, and exercise, with total calories and consumption of concentrated sweets considered separate, single-indicator constructs (Johnson, Tomer, Cunningham, & Henretta, 1990). However, many diabetes researchers have measured adherence as a unitary construct by creating composite scores based on the summation of individual items (e.g., Brownlee-Duffeck et al., 1987; Hanson et al., 1987, 1996). Although there can be some difficulties with the use of a single composite measure to reflect all the complex behaviors involved in the diabetes regimen, there is a precedent for this approach in controlled clinical trials (Henderson, Fisher, Cohen, Waltzman, & Weber, 1990).

General Measurement Approaches

Several approaches have been used to measure adherence, including self-report, collateral reports (parents), health care provider ratings, direct observations (of behavior or through the use of electronic devices), and treatment outcome. In all of these methods, data may be utilized in continuous or categorical ways. Self-reported and collateral-reported adherence has been measured by retrospective ratings, 24-hour recall interviews, or permanent products such as logbooks (written or electronic). Health care provider ratings have the disadvantage of being potentially biased by knowledge of metabolic control or other factors that may limit their reliability, validity, and clinical utility (Hays & DiMatteo, 1989). Direct observations may be useful in the clinic setting, but they yield data about skills rather than adherence in the natural environment. Direct observations in the natural environment would be too expensive and impractical for clinical work and have rarely been utilized in clinical research (Reynolds, Johnson, & Silverstein, 1990). Treatment outcome (e.g., GHb or blood glucose recordings) is flawed as a measure of regimen adherence given the imprecise relationship between health behaviors and health outcomes in diabetes.

To measure adherence, health care behaviors must be compared to some standard or criterion. Researchers have utilized both individually prescribed and group ideals for the entire population of diabetic children and adolescents. In the former case, it is obviously important to document the prescription for each regimen component. This can be determined by either asking the patient and/or parent what the regimen is or by going to the patient's medical record to record the regimen prescriptions. Unfortunately, as noted earlier, patients and parents often do not remember regimen prescriptions (Page et al., 1981), and medical records may not clearly indicate specific prescriptions. In addition, even if specific prescriptions can be accurately recalled or recorded, there is the possibility that the prescription is flawed or inappropriate so that even with perfect adherence glycemic goals may not be reached.

The alternative approach is to compare all patients to a universal ideal. An example of research using this approach is that of Johnson and colleagues (e.g., Johnson et al., 1986, 1990, 1992). In their work, these researchers have assumed a common ideal regimen for all children: It consists of a certain fixed number of injections, blood glucose tests, meals, and exercise periods per day; specific amounts of food consumed as protein, carbohydrates, and fat; and a specific amount of time elapsing between insulin injections and eating. This approach can be useful in large-group studies seeking to determine relationships between health behaviors and health outcomes, but becomes less meaningful in individual cases where the universal criterion may not apply.

This brings up the following issue: What is the optimal regimen prescription? This cannot be answered unequivocally because of the individual variation among patients and the fluid nature of managing this dynamic disease over time. Nevertheless, it can be asserted that intensive insulin regimens that approximate the way the pancreas naturally works, either by multiple injections per day or continuous subcutaneous insulin infusion (via the insulin pump), approach the ideal. Available data indicate that greater frequency of blood glucose monitoring is associated with better glycemic control (Anderson et al., 1997), particularly when data are utilized in an ongoing way for self-management. The research is not clear with regard to the precise type of diet or amount and type of exercise that is ideal. We can assume at this point that ideal regimen adherence would consist of appropriate modification of diet in light of preprandial blood glucose levels and insulin dose. Similarly, the ideal type and amount of exercise must depend on blood glucose levels because it is likely to be affected by insulin and food intake.

Another approach to assessment bypasses the problem of adherence relative to some criterion (whether individual or universal) and instead simply focuses on the frequencies of specific regimen-related or self-care health behaviors. For example, the measurement task is to quantify, over some specific time period, the number of blood glucose tests, the number of insulin injections, the amount of physical exercise, the type and amount of various foods consumed, and the time intervals between insulin injections and food intake. This absolute measurement method may have the advantage, in comparison with relative measurement approaches, of being better able to empirically determine the relationships between health behaviors and health outcomes.

Yet another approach utilizes these methods, whether relative or absolute, to categorize individual patients as being nonadherent or adherent with respect to various aspects of the regimen. This approach requires some decision to be made concerning the level at which various behaviors are judged to be suboptimal. However the decision to categorize is made (e.g., less than 80% of prescribed), in the absence of empirical data elucidating specific relationships between health behavior and health outcomes, it is to some degree arbitrary.

Another categorical method is to classify individual patients as nonadherent, as typified in the *DSM–IV* diagnosis, "Noncompliance With Medical Treatment." In this approach, patients are categorized when the problem of noncompliance is severe, but specific criteria for determining severity are not listed in the *DSM–IV* manual (other than requiring independent clinical attention). When this method was used by Kovacs et al. (1992), noncompliance was operationalized as a "behavior pattern whereby the patient showed serious and persistent negligence in at least two . . . diabetic management areas" (p. 1114; of insulin administration, glycemic monitoring, or dietary behavior). The diagnosis was made based on data obtained from interviews with parents and child and after consideration of history (i.e., duration of noncompliant behaviors).

Specific Measurement Tools

In this section, several specific measures of regimen adherence, as used in the pediatric diabetes literature, are reviewed. In general, four approaches have been used, including retrospective rating questionnaires or interviews, collection of record or logbooks, 24-hour recall interviews, and physician ratings. Another approach, based on categorizing patients as nonadherent using *DSM–IV* psychiatric criteria, has been used infrequently (e.g., Kovacs et al., 1992).

Retrospective Ratings.   Schafer et al. (1983) developed the Summary of Self-Care Activities (SSCA). This self-report measure asks respondents to rate the frequency of completing seven different regimen-related behaviors over the preceding 7-day period. Although some of the items are very specific (e.g., frequency of blood glucose testing), others are fairly global (e.g., extent following the diet). This measure has been significantly associated with both psychosocial factors and glycemic control as assessed by GHb (Schafer et al., 1983). The SSCA has been used by other investigators who have obtained significant relationships with health beliefs (Bond et al., 1992; Palardy et al., 1998). The instrument can be used as individual items or items combined to form a composite measure, which has been shown to be internally consistent (Bond et al., 1992).

Brownlee-Duffeck et al. (1987) developed a retrospective self-report questionnaire—the Diabetes Regimen Adherence Questionnaire (DRAQ). This measure consists of 15 items each rated on a 5-point scale, with 1 indicating *poor adherence* and 5 indicating *excellent adherence*; an overall adherence score ranging from 15 to 75 is computed, with higher scores reflecting better adherence. Internal consistency reliability was reported to be .79. Brownlee-Duffeck et al. (1987) found that the DRAQ total score was predicted on the basis of specific health beliefs (perceived costs of adherence). In addition, the DRAQ was significantly correlated with GHb, with eight items having significant correlations with GHb—seven of these pertained to diet and one to blood glucose testing. Other investigators have used the DRAQ and found it to be internally consistent (coefficient alpha = .78) and predicted by specific health beliefs (Bond et al., 1992). Similarly, Thomas, Peterson, and Goldstein (1997) found the DRAQ to have good internal consistency (coefficient alpha = .80) and to be associated with social problem-solving skills.

Another retrospective self-report questionnaire is the Self-Care Adherence Inventory (SCAI) developed by Hanson, Henggeler, and Burghen (1987). The SCAI consists of 15 items covering dietary behaviors, insulin adjustment, glucose testing, and hypoglycemia preparedness. Items are rated on a 4- to 5-point scale and are conducted during an interview. A total adherence score is computed by summing all items with acceptable internal consistency. The behaviors assessed by the SCAI appear to be relatively stable, with test–retest coefficients of .70 (Hanson et al., 1996). In addition, the overall adherence score as well as component scores relate significantly to GHb (−.20 to −.28; Hanson et al., 1992). Other investigators have similarly found the SCAI to have acceptable internal consistency and to be associated with GHb (Auslander et al., 1997). Higher levels of family support have been associated with better adherence as measured by the SCAI (La Greca et al., 1995).

La Greca and colleagues (1990) developed the Self-Care Inventory (SCI), another retrospective questionnaire approach to the measurement of regimen adherence. In this 14-item measure, respondents are asked to rate their adherence over the preceding 1-month period, on a 5-point scale, with higher scores indicating better adherence. Adequate internal consistency and test–retest reliability have been reported (Delamater et al., 1998; Greco et al., 1990). The SCI has also been significantly related with GHb, regimen barriers, family cohesion and stress (Delamater et al., 1998), and developmentally appropriate self-care autonomy (Wysocki et al., 1996).

Miller-Johnson et al. (1994) developed a method by which children, parents, and nurses rated each of 12 specific aspects of the regimen on a 0 to 100 scale reflecting percentage of adherence. The injection items were highly skewed and therefore deleted. The remaining items were summed to compute an average adherence score. Internal consistencies (i.e., coefficient alpha) for children, parents, and nurses were .76, .71, and .96, respectively (Miller-Johnson et al., 1994). Significant associations were obtained between overall adherence and GHb for all three informants.

Self-Monitored Records or Logbooks.   Miller-Johnson et al. (1994) also utilized a prospective method for measuring regimen adherence based on review of patient logbooks or self-monitored regimen-related behaviors. Patients and parents were instructed to complete postcards for each of 7 days following a clinic appointment. The postcards contained columns for recording relevant information concerning insulin injections, glucose tests, food intake, and exercise, including time of day for each regimen behavior. A nurse reviewed the records and computed adherence scores based on the expected frequencies of each regimen behavior. A timing variable was computed based on timing of food intake relative to insulin injection. Because the insulin injection variable was highly skewed (with almost all subjects reporting perfect adherence), this variable was eliminated. Exercise was not completed in enough detail to be useful. Therefore, only ratings of glucose testing, meals, snacks, and timing of injections relative to meals were utilized. This method is limited by the lack of reliability and the failure to find any relationships of this data with GHb. Delamater et al. (1988) evaluated patient records of blood glucose testing for a 1-week prospective period and found that reports of blood glucose were affected by social demand characteristics.

Rather than rely on patient records, which may be unreliable, some investigators have simply used electronic reports of specific regimen behavior. For example, one regimen behavior that can be electronically recorded is blood glucose monitoring (assuming patients have a blood glucose meter with a memory capability). Murphy et al. (1997) recorded the frequency of glucose monitoring over the past 7 days by inspecting the readings from the glucose meter. These investigators then grouped subjects into adherence groups: Three or more tests per day were considered good, one to two times per day were considered adequate, and those who averaged less than one per day were considered poor. Frequency of blood glucose monitoring was significantly correlated with GHb.

24-Hour Recall Interviews.   A different approach was taken by Johnson and colleagues in developing their 24-hour recall interview methodology for the assessment of regimen adherence (Johnson et al., 1986, 1990, 1992). In this method, children and parents are separately interviewed by telephone on three unannounced occasions over a 2-week period (one weekend day and two weekdays). The structured interview covers 13 specific aspects of regimen adherence over the preceding 24-hour period. Because young children may not be able to report on certain aspects of their self-care (e.g., those relating to time) and parents may not be able to observe their child performing all regimen-related behaviors (e.g., at school), data from children and parents are combined according to explicit coding rules.

This methodology has been extensively studied by Johnson and colleagues, and results have provided support for its reliability and validity (Johnson et al., 1986, 1990, 1992; Reynolds, Johnson, & Silverstein, 1990). Factor analytic research with this method has identified four regimen factors: exercise (type, duration, and frequency), injection (regularity, interval, and timing in relation to eating), diet type (carbohydrate and fat consumption), and frequency (eating and glucose testing). This method utilizes reference of regimen behaviors to ideal standards for the population of diabetic children. For example, all children's exercise is evaluated relative to a standard of three exercise periods per day; food intake is evaluated relative to a standard of three meals and three snacks per day, and consumption of calories based on tables for age and gender, with 60% of calories from carbohydrate and 25% from fat; and glucose testing is evaluated relative to an ideal of four tests per day.

Although this approach may limit the interpretation of adherence in individual cases, it does provide for tests of the relationship between adherence and metabolic control across individual patients. Studies have shown that data obtained from the 24-hour recall interview method have significant relationships with age (older less adherent than younger), health beliefs, and metabolic control (Bond et al., 1992; Johnson et al., 1990, 1992; Kuttner et al., 1990). Unfortunately, this method is labor-intensive in terms of both data collection and scoring, thus limiting its clinical utility.

Physician Ratings. Some investigators have utilized ratings by health care providers to quantify regimen adherence. Jacobson and colleagues (Hauser et al., 1990; Jacobson et al., 1990) had physicians and nurses make ratings of patient adherence on a 4-point scale ranging from *poor* to *excellent.* Acceptable reliability was obtained for ratings of adherence to diet, metabolic monitoring, and insulin use. A composite index was computed with internal consistency of .71. Psychological (Jacobson et al., 1990) and family (Hauser et al., 1990) factors were found to predict adherence. Anderson et al. (1997) modified this approach by having physicians rate patients' adherence in the preceding 3 to 4 months with respect to frequency of blood glucose monitoring. Parental involvement in blood glucose monitoring was significantly correlated with adherence to glucose monitoring, and frequency of glucose monitoring in turn was associated with GHb.

SUMMARY AND RECOMMENDATIONS

This chapter has shown that a number of approaches, including retrospective ratings, self-monitoring, 24-hour recall interviews, and physician ratings, have been used in the pediatric diabetes literature in studies of regimen adherence. In general, there is evidence for adequate levels of reliability and validity for the various measures. Findings indicate that adherence to insulin regimen prescriptions is generally good, but less than optimal adherence has been documented with respect to blood glucose monitoring and dietary prescriptions. Levels of physical exercise appear to be fairly low, but specific exercise prescriptions are not usually made. Better adherence has been associated with a number of demographic and psychosocial factors, such as younger age, better coping and psychological health, specific health beliefs, fewer barriers, and more effective family functioning, including support and clear responsibilities for the regimen.

Despite these conclusions, a number of problems have been identified in research on adherence in diabetes (Hays & DiMatteo, 1989; Johnson, 1995; Kurtz, 1990; La Greca & Schuman, 1995; McNabb, 1997). These have to do with the various conceptual and methodological approaches utilized by investigators. Adherence has been considered as absolute levels or frequencies of self-care behaviors or as behaviors occurring relative to some standard (as some percentage of the regimen goal). In the latter approach, the criterion has been either individually determined (relative to a specific regimen prescription) or considered in relation to a more universal standard that would apply to the entire population of patients. Measures have been obtained from various informants, including patients, their parents, or physicians and nurses who care for them. The resulting measures have been utilized as specific components reflecting a multidimensional construct or as a composite measure reflecting a global, unidimensional construct.

Although each of these approaches has some psychometric merit, there are problems specific to each. This is illustrated by the less than impressive relationships observed between adherence and metabolic control across the various measurement approaches. For example, unidimensional composite measures may utilize items such as foot care or wearing identification bracelets that would be expected to have no direct relationship with measures of metabolic control. Furthermore, composites may be weighted more toward some aspects of the regimen versus others, which, in the absence of any data demonstrating the validity of such weighting, cannot be justified.

Moreover, the time periods covered by the various specific assessment tools vary from three 24-hour recall interviews over 2 weeks, to 1-week retrospective ratings or self-monitored recording, to 1-month retrospective ratings. Given that the time period covered by the GHb assay is 2 to 3 months, it is not surprising that robust relationships have not been observed between adherence and metabolic control.

Regimen prescriptions may be inappropriate or ineffectively communicated so that even perfect adherence may not result in predictable relationships with glycemic control. In addition to these methodological concerns, it is clear that metabolic control is influenced by independent endogenous factors. Thus, even with acceptable reliability of measurement, relationships between health behaviors and health outcomes may not be expected to have large effect sizes and should therefore not be considered as the only validity criterion.

Recommendations for Clinical Practice

It is clear that regimen prescriptions vary considerably from patient to patient. In light of this fact, the use of universal regimen ideals may not have much utility in clinical practice. It is recommended that clinicians attend carefully to the documentation of regimen prescriptions and utilize relative measurement of self-care behaviors in relation to individually determined regimen goals, which may change over time. Care must be given to the communication of specific regimen prescriptions because studies have shown patients and families may not remember prescriptions or share the same treatment goals (Marteau, Johnson, Baum, & Bloch, 1987; Page et al., 1981; see also DiMatteo, chap. 10, this volume). Consequently, it is critical for clinicians to effectively and explicitly communicate regimen prescriptions and work collaboratively with the patient and family to determine whether treatment goals are reasonable and achievable for them at that time.

Inspection of blood glucose records and interviews or rating forms used to assess adherence should be conducted in an atmosphere of interest and trust, with information obtained from both parents and children and utilized as useful feedback rather than interpreted as evidence of treatment failure (see Drotar et al., chap. 20, this volume). It is also important to assess psychological and psychosocial factors that may serve as barriers to good regimen adherence, such as inappropriate health beliefs, lack of parental and peer involvement and support, as well as general levels of psychological adjustment difficulties and family dysfunction.

The precision and reliability of measurement can be maximized with the use of specific behaviors to be rated or recorded over fairly brief periods of time. The use of electronic monitoring devices such as memory reflectance meters have advantages for measurement of the glucose testing component. However, until technology advances to provide electronic measurement of other regimen components, patient self-reports remain the primary approach to assess regimen adherence. The use of multiple informants is preferable to reliance on one rater (whether child, parent, or health care provider). Specific measurement approaches depend on the precision of the regimen prescription: With specific recommendations, adherence should be operationalized relative to that standard; without specific recommendations, adherence should be operationalized in an absolute fashion as levels or frequencies of self-care behaviors over time.

Recommendations for Clinical Research

Continued refinement of existing measures for assessment of regimen adherence is needed. In particular, items and scoring must be modified to reflect advances in medical treatment and changes in prescribed regimens. For example, the use of the fast-acting new insulin preparations requires patients not to wait 30 minutes before eating, but rather to eat immediately after the injection. With more patients now using the insulin pump, new items related to the specifics of this specialized regimen need to be developed. The clinical utility of the various questionnaires for identification of patients having adherence problems needs to be demonstrated in clinical settings (see Drotar et al., chap. 20, this volume). Additionally, such instruments must be shown to be sensitive to the effects of intervention in treatment–outcome studies.

The major question of diabetes management remains: What behaviors matter most for attainment of good glycemic control? Although current research findings do not indicate strong associations between adherence and glycemic outcomes, methodological problems (such as varying time intervals between measurement of adherence and glycemic control) may have obscured significant relationships from being observed. Therefore, future research efforts should focus on measurement of health behaviors and health outcomes during consistent time periods. Because behavior is easier to measure reliably by self-report or ratings by others over shorter time intervals, these methods for assessing adherence should be compared with glycemic control data that are obtained over a similarly short period of time. More research is needed that can compare short-term adherence with blood glucose records or glycosylated proteins (such as fructosamine, measuring blood glucose over a 2- to 3-week antecedent period) over the same time period to increase the probability of finding significant relationships between adherence and glycemic control.

Another methodological problem is the relative lack of attention to measurement of the effects of various health behaviors that are contingent on blood glucose levels at the specific times these behaviors are measured. For example, the effects of physical activity on blood glucose would vary considerably depending on the blood glucose level at the time of exercise. The same amount and type of physical activity would have different effects on blood glucose if blood glucose were in the normal versus hypoglycemic or hyperglycemic range at the beginning of the exercise period. Similarly, the effects of the same amount and type of food intake would have different consequences on blood glucose depending on the initial premeal blood glucose as well as the amount of insulin in the system at the time the food is being absorbed.

Given the complexities of the relationships between regimen-related behaviors and blood glucose in diabetes, future research in this area would benefit from a more thorough consideration of assessment of specific health behaviors in their temporal context. Assessment approaches allowing computerized self-monitoring of various behaviors along with blood glucose would allow researchers to obtain the kind of data needed to sort out the complex relationships between health behaviors and health outcomes in this challenging area. With thousands of data points available for individual patients, statistical modeling techniques may be applied to identify which behaviors matter most.

Behavioral scientists have made substantial progress in the measurement of regimen adherence in children with diabetes. It can be concluded that there is no one method for assessing adherence that can or should be applied to all children with diabetes. Rather, individual differences or an idiographic approach utilizing one or more approaches is more likely to yield clinically useful information that can be utilized in both the clinical and research environments.

ACKNOWLEDGMENT

Preparation of this chapter was partially supported by grant #RO1 DK48031 from the National Institutes of Health.

REFERENCES

American Diabetes Association: Clinical Practice Recommendations. (1999). Nutrition recommendations and principles for people with diabetes mellitus. *Diabetes Care, 22*(Suppl. 1), S42–S45.

Amiel, S. A., Sherwin, R. S., Simonson, D. C., Lauritano, A. A., & Tamborlane, W. V. (1986). Impaired insulin action in puberty: A contributing factor to poor glycemic control in adolescents with diabetes. *New England Journal of Medicine, 315*, 215–219.

Anderson, B. J., Auslander, W. F., Jung, K. C., Miller, J. P., & Santiago, J. V. (1990). Assessing family sharing of diabetes responsibilities. *Journal of Pediatric Psychology, 15*, 477–492.

Anderson, B. J., Ho, J., Brackett, J., Finkelstein, D., & Laffel, L. (1997). Parental involvement in diabetes management tasks: Relationships to blood glucose monitoring adherence and metabolic control in young adolescents with insulin-dependent diabetes mellitus. *Journal of Pediatrics, 130*, 257–265.

Anderson, B. J., Wolf, R. M., Burkhart, M. T., Cornell, R. G., & Bacon, G. E. (1989). Effects of peergroup intervention on metabolic control of adolescents with IDDM: Randomized outpatient study. *Diabetes Care, 12*, 179–183.

Auslander, W. F., Anderson, B. J., Bubb, J., Jung, K. C., & Santiago, J. V. (1990). Risk factors to health in diabetic children: A prospective study from diagnosis. *Health and Social Work, 15*, 133–142.

Auslander, W. F., Thompson, S., Dreitzer, D., White, N. H., & Santiago, J. V. (1997). Disparity in glycemic control and adherence between African-American and Caucasian youths with diabetes. *Diabetes Care, 20*, 1569–1575.

Arslanian, S., Becker, D., & Drash, A. (1994). Diabetes mellitus in the child and adolescent. In D. Wilkens (Ed.), *The diagnosis and treatment of endocrine disorders in childhood and adolescence* (4th ed., pp. 969–971). Springfield, MA: Charles C. Thomas.

Bloch, C. A., Clemons, P. S., & Sperling, M. A. (1987). Puberty decreases insulin sensitivity. *Journal of Pediatrics, 110*, 481–487.

Bloomgarden, Z., Karmally, W., Metzger, M., Brothers, M., Nechemias, C., Bookman, J., Faierman, D., Ginsberg-Fellner, F., Rayfield, E., & Brown, W. (1987). Randomized controlled trial of diabetes patient education. *Diabetes Care, 10*, 263–272.

Bobrow, E. S., AvRuskin, T. W., & Siller, J. (1985). Mother–daughter interaction and adherence to diabetes regimens. *Diabetes Care, 8*, 146–151.

Bond, G., Aiken, L., & Somerville, S. (1992). The Health Belief Model and adolescents with insulin-dependent diabetes mellitus. *Health Psychology, 11*, 190–198.

Brownlee-Duffeck, M., Peterson, L., Simonds, J. F., Goldstein, D., Kilo, C., & Hoette, S. (1987). The role of health beliefs in the regimen adherence and metabolic control of adolescents and adults with diabetes mellitus. *Journal of Consulting and Clinical Psychology, 55*, 139–144.

Campaigne, B. N., Gilliam, T. B., Spencer, M. L., Lampman, R. M., & Schork, M. A. (1984). Effects of a physical activity program on metabolic control and cardiovascular fitness in children with IDDM. *Diabetes Care, 7*, 57–62.

Christensen, N. K., Terry, R. D., Wyatt, S., Pichert, J. W., & Lorenz, R. A. (1983). Quantitative assessment of dietary adherence in patients with insulin-dependent diabetes mellitus. *Diabetes Care, 6,* 245–250.

Clark, C. M., & Lee, D. A. (1995). Prevention and treatment of the complications of diabetes mellitus. *New England Journal of Medicine, 332,* 1210–1217.

Daneman, D., Siminerio, L., Transue, D., Betschart, J., Drash, A., & Becker, D. (1985). The role of self-monitoring of blood glucose in the routine management of children with insulin-dependent diabetes mellitus. *Diabetes Care, 5,* 472–478.

Delamater, A. M. (1993). Compliance interventions for children with diabetes and other chronic diseases. In N. Krasnegor, L. Epstein, S. Johnson, & S. Yaffe (Eds.), *Developmental aspects of health compliance behavior* (pp. 335–354). Hillsdale, NJ: Lawrence Erlbaum Associates.

Delamater, A. M., Albrecht, D., Postellon, D., & Gutai, J. (1991). Racial differences in metabolic control of children and adolescents with Type I diabetes mellitus. *Diabetes Care, 14,* 20–25.

Delamater, A. M., Applegate, B., Eidson, M., & Nemery, R. (1998). Increased risks for poor metabolic control in minority youths with Type 1 diabetes. *Diabetes, 47*(Suppl. 1), A326.

Delamater, A. M., Bubb, J., Davis, S., Smith, J. A., Schmidt, L., White, N. H., & Santiago, J. (1990). Randomized prospective study of self-management training with newly diagnosed diabetic children. *Diabetes Care, 13,* 492–498.

Delamater, A. M., Davis, S. G., Bubb, J., Smith, J. A., White, N. H., & Santiago, J.V. (1989). Self-monitoring of blood glucose by adolescents with diabetes: Technical skills and utilization of data. *The Diabetes Educator, 15,* 56–61.

Delamater, A. M., Kurtz, S. M., White, N. H., & Santiago, J. V. (1988). Effects of social demand on reports of self-monitored blood glucose testing in adolescents with Type I diabetes mellitus. *Journal of Applied Social Psychology, 18,* 491–502.

Delamater, A. M., Shaw, K., Applegate, B., Pratt, I., Eidson, M., Lancelotta, G., Gonzalez-Mendoza, L., & Richton, R. (1999). Risk for metabolic control problems in minority youth with diabetes. *Diabetes Care, 22,* 700–705.

Delamater, A. M., Smith, J. A., Bubb, J., Davis, S. G., Gamble, T., White, N. H., & Santiago, J. V. (1991). Familybased behavior therapy for diabetic adolescents. In J. H. Johnson & S. B. Johnson (Eds.), *Advances in child health psychology* (pp. 293–306). Gainesville, FL: University of Florida Press.

Delamater, A. M., Smith, J. A., Kurtz, S. M., & White, N. H. (1988). Dietary skills and adherence in children with insulin-dependent diabetes mellitus. *The Diabetes Educator, 14,* 33–36.

Diabetes Control and Complications Trial Research Group. (1993). The effect of intensive treatment of diabetes on the development and progression of long-term complications in insulin-dependent diabetes mellitus. *New England Journal of Medicine, 329,* 977–986.

Diabetes Control and Complications Trial Research Group. (1994). Effect of intensive diabetes treatment on the development and progression of long-term complications in adolescents with insulin-dependent diabetes mellitus. *Journal of Pediatrics, 125,* 177–188.

Glasgow, R. E., McCaul, K. D., & Schafer, L. C. (1986). Barriers to regimen adherence among persons with insulin-dependent diabetes. *Journal of Behavioral Medicine, 9,* 65–77.

Glasgow, R. E., McCaul, K. D., & Schafer, L. C. (1987). Self-care behaviors and glycemic control in Type I diabetes. *The Journal of Chronic Diseases, 40,* 399–412.

Gonen, B., Rachman, H., Rubenstein, A. H., Tanega, S. P., & Horwitz, D. L. (1977). Hemoglobin A1C as an indicator of the degree of glucose intolerance in diabetics. *Lancet, 2,* 734–737.

Greco, P., La Greca, A., Ireland, S., Wick, P., Freeman, C., Agramonte, R., Gutt, M., & Skyler, J. (1990). Assessing adherence in IDDM: A comparison of two methods [Abstract]. *Diabetes, 39*(Suppl. 1), 657.

Hanson, C. L., De Guire, M., Schinkel, S., Henggeler, S. W., & Burghen, G. A. (1992). Comparing social learning and family systems correlates of adaptation in youths with IDDM. *Journal of Pediatric Psychology, 17,* 555–572.

Hanson, C., De Guire, M., Schinkel, A., Kolterman, O., Goodman, J., & Buckingham, B. (1996). Self-care behaviors in insulin-dependent diabetes: Evaluative tools and their associations with glycemic control. *Journal of Pediatric Psychology, 21,* 467–482.

Hanson, C. L., Henggeler, S. W., & Burghen, G. A. (1987). Model of associations between psychosocial variables and health outcome measures of adolescents with IDDM. *Diabetes Care, 10,* 752–758.

Hauser, S. T., Jacobson, A. M., Lavori, P., Wolfsdorf, J. I., Herskowitz, R. D., Milley, J. E., Bliss, R., Wertlieb, D., & Stein, J. (1990). Adherence among children and adolescents with insulin dependent diabetes mellitus over a four-year longitudinal follow-up: II. Immediate and long-term linkages with the family milieu. *Journal of Pediatric Psychology, 15,* 527–542.

Haynes, R. B. (1979). Introduction. In R. B. Haynes, D. W. Taylor, & D. Sackett (Eds.), *Compliance in health care* (pp. 1–7). Baltimore: Johns Hopkins University Press.

Hays, R., & DiMatteo, M. (1989). Patient compliance assessment: Key issues and suggestions, sources of information, focus of measures, and nature of response options. *Diabetes Spectrum, 2,* 55–63.

Henderson, W. G., Fisher, S., Cohen, N., Waltzman, S., & Weber, L. (1990). Use of principal components analysis to develop a composite score as a primary outcome in a clinical trial: The VA Cooperative Study Group on Cochlear Implantation. *Controlled Clinical Trials, 11,* 199–214.

Huttunen, N. P., Lankelaa, S. L., Knip, M., Lautala, P., Kaar, M. L., Laasonen, K., & Puukka, R. (1989). Effect of onceaweek training program on physical fitness and metabolic control in children with IDDM. *Diabetes Care, 12,* 737–739.

Ingersoll, G., Orr, D., Herrold, A., & Golden M. (1986). Cognitive maturity and self-management among adolescents with insulin-dependent diabetes mellitus. *Journal of Pediatrics, 108,* 620–623.

Jacobson, A. M., Hauser, S. T., Lavori, P., Wolfsdorf, J., Herskowitz, R., Milley, J., Bliss, R., Gelfand, E., Wertlieb, D., & Stein, J. (1990). Adherence among children and adolescents with insulin-dependent diabetes mellitus over a four-year longitudinal follow-up: I. The influence of patient coping and adjustment. *Journal of Pediatric Psychology, 15,* 511–526.

Johnson, S. B. (1995). Diabetes mellitus in childhood. In M. Roberts (Ed.), *Handbook of pediatric psychology* (2nd ed., pp. 263–285). New York: Guilford.

Johnson, S. B., Freund, A., Silverstein, J., Hansen, C. A., & Malone, J. (1990). Adherence-health status relationships in childhood diabetes. *Health Psychology, 9,* 606–631.

Johnson, S. B., Kelly, M., Henretta, J. C., Cunningham, W., Tomer, A., & Silverstein, J. (1992). A longitudinal analysis of adherence and health status in childhood diabetes. *Journal of Pediatric Psychology, 17,* 537–553.

Johnson, S. B., Pollak, T., Silverstein, J. H., Rosenbloom, A., Spillar, R., McCallum, M., & Harkavy, J. (1982). Cognitive and behavioral knowledge about insulin-dependent diabetes among children and parents. *Pediatrics, 69,* 708–713.

Johnson, S. B., Silverstein, J., Rosenbloom, A., Carter, R., & Cunningham, W. (1986). Assessing daily management in childhood diabetes. *Health Psychology, 5,* 545–564.

Johnson, S. B., Tomer, A., Cunningham, W. R., & Henretta, J. C. (1990). Adherence in childhood diabetes. Results of a confirmatory factor analysis. *Health Psychology, 9,* 493–501.

Kaplan, R. M., Chadwick, M. W., & Schimmel, L. E. (1985). Social learning intervention to promote metabolic control in Type I diabetes mellitus: Pilot experimental results. *Diabetes Care, 8,* 152–155.

Kovacs, M., Goldston, D., Obrosky, D., & Iyengar, S. (1992). Prevalence and predictors of pervasive non-compliance with medical treatment among youths with insulin-dependent diabetes mellitus. *Journal of the American Academy Child Adolescent Psychiatry, 31,* 1112–1119.

Kurtz, S. (1990). Adherence to diabetes regimens: Empirical status and clinical applications. *Diabetes Educator, 16,* 50–56.

Kuttner, M. J., Delamater, A. M., & Santiago, J. V. (1990). Learned helplessness in diabetic youths. *Journal of Pediatric Psychology, 15,* 581–594.

La Greca, A., Auslander, W., Greco, P., Spetter, D., Fisher, E. B., & Santiago, J. V. (1995). I get by with a little help from my family and friends: Adolescents' support for diabetes care. *Journal of Pediatric Psychology, 20,* 449–476.

La Greca, A., Follansbee, D., & Skyler, J. (1990). Developmental and behavioral aspects of diabetes management in children and adolescents. *Children's Health Care, 19,* 132–139.

La Greca, A., & Schuman, W. B. (1995). Adherence to prescribed medical regimens. In M. Roberts (Ed.), *Handbook of pediatric psychology* (2nd ed., pp. 55–83). New York: Guilford.

Lorenz, R. A., Christensen, N. K., & Pichert, J. W. (1985). Diet-related knowledge, skill and adherence among children with insulin dependent diabetes mellitus. *Pediatrics, 75,* 872–876.

Madsbad, S., McNair, P., & Faber, O. K. (1980). Beta-cell function and metabolic control in insulin-treated diabetics. *Acta Endocrinology, 93,* 196–200.

Mann, N. P., Noronha, J. L., & Johnston, D. I. (1984). A prospective study to evaluate the benefits of long-term self-monitoring of blood glucose in diabetic children. *Diabetes Care, 7,* 323–326.

Marrero, D. G., Kronz, K. K., Golden, M. P., Wright, J. C., Orr, D. P., & Fineberg, N. S. (1989). Clinical evaluation of computer-assisted self-monitoring of blood glucose system. *Diabetes Care, 12,* 345–350.

Marteau, T. M., Johnson, M., Baum, J. D., & Bloch, S. (1987). Goals of treatment in diabetes: A comparison of doctors and parents of children with diabetes. *Journal of Behavioral Medicine, 10,* 33–48.

McNabb, W. (1997). Adherence in diabetes: Can we define it and can we measure it? *Diabetes Care, 20,* 215–218.

Meichenbaum, D., & Turk, D. (1987). *Facilitating treatment adherence: A practitioner's guidebook.* New York: Plenum.

Miller-Johnson, S., Emery, R., Marvin, R., Clarke, W., Lovinger, R., & Martin, M. (1994). Parent–child relationships and the management of insulin-dependent diabetes mellitus. *Journal of Consulting and Clinical Psychology, 62,* 603–610.

Murphy, L., Thompson, R., & Morris, M. A. (1997). Adherence behavior among adolescents with Type 1 insulin-dependent diabetes mellitus: The role of cognitive appraisal processes. *Journal of Pediatric Psychology, 22,* 811–826.

Nathan, D., Singer, D. E., Hurxthal, K., & Goodson, J. D. (1984). The clinical information value of the glycosylated hemoglobin assay. *New England Journal of Medicine, 310,* 341–346.

Page, P., Verstraete, D., Robb, J., & Etzwiler, D. (1981). Patient recall of self-care recommendations in diabetes. *Diabetes Care, 4,* 96–98.

Palardy, N., Greening, L., Ott, J., Holderby, A., & Atchison, J. (1998). Adolescents' health attitudes and adherence to treatment for insulin-dependent diabetes mellitus. *Developmental and Behavioral Pediatrics, 19,* 31–37.

Reynolds, L., Johnson, S. B., & Silverstein, J. (1990). Assessing daily diabetes management by 24-hour recall interview: The validity of children's report. *Journal of Pediatric Psychology, 15,* 493–510.

Schafer, L. C., Glasgow, R., McCaul, K., & Dreher, M. (1983). Adherence to IDDM regimens: Relationship to psychosocial variables and metabolic control. *Diabetes Care, 6,* 493–498.

Schlundt, D., Pichert, J., Rea, M., Puryear, W., Penha, M., & Kline, S. (1994). Situational obstacles to adherence for adolescents with diabetes. *The Diabetes Educator, 20,* 207–211.

Stratton, R., Wilson, D. P., Endres, R. K., & Goldstein, D. E. (1987). Improved glycemic control after supervised 8-week exercise program in insulin-dependent diabetic adolescents. *Diabetes Care, 10,* 589–593.

Thomas, A. M., Peterson, L., & Goldstein, D. (1997). Problem solving and diabetes regimen adherence by children and adolescents with IDDM in social pressure situations: A reflection of normal development. *Journal of Pediatric Psychology, 22,* 541–561.

Travis, L. B., Brouhard, B. H., & Schreiner, B. J. (Eds.). (1987). The child less than three years old. In *Diabetes mellitus in children and adolescents* (pp. 187–192). Philadelphia: W. B. Saunders.

Weist, M., Finney, J., Barnard, M., Davis, C., & Ollendick, T. (1993). Empirical selection of psychosocial treatment targets for children and adolescents with diabetes. *Journal of Pediatric Psychology, 18,* 11–28.

White, K., Kolman, M., Wexler, P., Polin, G., & Winter, R. J. (1984). Unstable diabetes and unstable families: A psychosocial evaluation of diabetic children with recurrent ketoacidosis. *Pediatrics, 73,* 749–755.

Wing, R. R., Lamparski, D. M., Zaslow, S., Betschart, J., Siminerio, L., & Becker, D. (1985). Frequency and accuracy of self-monitoring of blood glucose in children. Relationship to glycemic control. *Diabetes Care, 8,* 214–218.

Wysocki, T., Green, L., & Huxtable, K. (1989). Blood glucose monitoring by diabetic adolescents: Compliance and metabolic control. *Health Psychology, 8,* 267–284.

Wysocki, T., Meinhold, P. A., Abrams, K. C., Barnard, M. U., Clarke, W. L., Bellando, B. J., & Bourgeois, M. J. (1992). Parental and professional estimates of self-care independence of children and adolescents with IDDM. *Diabetes Care, 15,* 43–52.

Wysocki, T., Meinhold, P. A., Cox, D. J., & Clarke, W. L. (1990). Survey of diabetes professionals regarding developmental changes in diabetes self-care. *Diabetes Care, 13,* 65–68.

Wysocki, T., Taylor, A., Hough, B., Linscheid, T., Yeates, K., O., & Naglieri, J. (1996). Deviation from developmentally appropriate self-care autonomy: Association with diabetes outcomes. *Diabetes Care, 19,* 119–125.

PART V

INFLUENCES ON TREATMENT ADHERENCE IN CHILDHOOD CHRONIC ILLNESS

The wide-ranging influences on adherence to chronic illness treatment are considered in this section. These range from broad systemic factors, such as managed care and reimbursement for services to promote adherence, to more specific factors, such as the quality of patient–physician communication and patient and family knowledge of the treatment regimen.

Walders and colleagues' chapter (chap. 9) focuses on a description of the relationship among treatment adherence for chronic illness, child health policy, and managed care. Given the high rates of nonadherence and the potential health implications of children with chronic health conditions, understanding the effects of managed care on the ability of health care providers to promote treatment adherence is an important concern. Walders and colleagues review the potential impact of nonadherence to treatment in chronic illness on functional morbidity, health care costs, and evaluation of findings from clinical research.

Chapter 9 also considers the potential impact in changes in health care delivery on the care of children with chronic health conditions. The authors raise concerns about the potential for a mismatch between the principles of managed care arrangements and the needs of chronic health conditions. These include restrictions available in time for patient contacts and access to specialty care providers and mental health services, all of which may be needed to support optimal management of treatment adherence of chronic health conditions. Moreover, children with special health care needs are at risk for being denied coverage due to their financial risk and reimbursement arrangements that create physician disincentives to care for high-cost patients.

Walders and colleagues make several recommendations for advocacy to promote quality pediatric chronic illness care, including (a) ensuring access to specialty care for children with chronic health conditions in interdisciplinary clinics, (b) developing guidelines for the management of pediatric chronic illness, (c) designing tools for evaluation of the care of children with chronic illness, (d) supporting consumer advocacy efforts, and so on. In this regard, the efforts of the American Academy of Pediatrics to develop principles for managed care arrangements for health care of infants, children, and adolescents, as well as children with special health care needs, are seen as an important step. The authors review the results of innovative programs for management of asthma that have potential implications for the development of interventions to improve adherence and self-management in a range of chronic health conditions.

These authors advocate research to inform policy and practice concerning managed care for children with chronic health conditions. Specific recommendations include documentation of the effects of health care trends on treatment of chronic illness, impact of interdisciplinary care, and effectiveness of adherence promotion interventions.

In chapter 10, DiMatteo reviews the results of research concerning the relationship between treatment adherence and communication among providers, pediatric patients, and their families; and suggests clinical applications. DiMatteo's chapter suggests that patient adherence is heavily dependent on patient satisfaction with the psychosocial aspects of the physician–patient relationship, including the patient's trust in the physician and expectations for help. Research with pediatric populations indicates a discrepancy between pediatricians' and parents' expectations of their interaction. For example, parental comfort with disclosure of sensitive information may be affected by the pediatrician's interview style (i.e., parents disclose more specific concerns relevant to their child's mental health when pediatricians ask questions about psychosocial issues, make supportive statements, and listen attentively).

DiMatteo outlines the unique challenges of pediatric chronic disease care for patient–physician communication and treatment adherence. These include changes in beliefs, attitudes, social interaction patterns, and autonomy brought about by changes in the child's development; the importance of family conflict, especially during adolescence; and the complex nature of communication that is required for the management of pediatric chronic illness. For example, because information concerning the treatment regimen needs to reach several people, including the child or adolescent and at least one family member, opportunities for misunderstanding treatment-related expectations and procedures are increased.

Advocating a multidimensional approach, DiMatteo makes cogent rec-ommendations to improve clinical management of adherence, such as ensuring that patients fully understand what they are being asked to do to take care of themselves, encouraging patients and families to ask ques-tions, giving feedback and follow-up, and determining through sensitive questioning whether patients have any desire and/or intention to follow their treatment recommendations. Moreover, discussion of differences in perspectives, including disagreements between the physician and families concerning the treatment regimen and treatment-related barriers, may allow patients' and families' preferences to be incorporated into treat-ment-related decision making, thus enhancing compliance.

DiMatteo makes several important recommendations for research con-cerning adherence to treatment in chronic illness, such as formulation and validation of standardized methods for quantifying intensity of treatment, prospective research, meta-analytic reviews of pediatric adherence, concep-tualizing and operationalizing adherence measurement, and understanding the difference between adherence behaviors and treatment outcomes.

In chapter 11, Ievers-Landis and Drotar focus on the implication of parental and child knowledge of treatment regimens for treatment adher-ence. The authors note that various definitions of *knowledge* of treatment in various chronic illnesses have made it difficult to compare the results of different studies. Their proposal for a more precise operational definition of *knowledge* includes: (a) understanding the specifics of the treatment regimen (e.g., what are the prescribed treatments and how often should they be performed), (b) having the ability to accurately recall the pre-scribed treatments, and (c) knowing how to implement the prescribed treatment. The authors suggest that an accurate assessment of treatment knowledge should involve asking children with a chronic illness and the parents what they believe has been prescribed by their providers rather than asking them to report what they are currently doing in their treat-ment. Ievers-Landis and Drotar's review of research indicates that parents do not accurately recall what the providers have told them concerning their children's medical treatment, which may contribute to the problems of noncompliance with treatment for various chronic conditions.

Ievers-Landis and Drotar underscore the importance of tailoring clinical interventions to improve knowledge of medical treatment to the specific management demands of a chronic illness, and (b) developing strategies to increase children's and parents' recall of prescribed treatments (e.g., by giv-ing families written instructions for treatments at each clinic visit, reviewing the treatment plan with the child and/or parents at each visit, etc.).

Ievers-Landis and Drotar make several recommendations to improve the quality of research, such as distinguishing between what children and parents know to be the recommended treatments from their actual treatment-related behaviors, assessing medical recommendations obtained from medical charts and comparing these to the child or parents' understanding of the prescribed treatments, and evaluating the impact of educational interventions (e.g., alternative methods of presentation concerning medical treatments designed to enhance children's and parents' knowledge of treatment and treatment adherence).

CHAPTER NINE

Promoting Treatment Adherence in Childhood Chronic Illness: Challenges in a Managed Care Environment

Natalie Walders
Chantelle Nobile
Dennis Drotar
Case Western Reserve University

There is a critical need for pediatric professionals to serve as child advocates to enhance the physical, cognitive, emotional, and social potential of children and adolescents (American Academy of Pediatrics, 1998). One key area of advocacy focuses on promoting adherence to treatment regimens for children with chronic health conditions. The need for such advocacy efforts stems from the importance of treatment adherence as a public health concern and the difficulties in managing nonadherence complications within the current medical care system. The scope of nonadherence to prescribed medical regimens among pediatric populations has been well documented, with rates of nonadherence ranging from 17% to over 90% of pediatric patients (Lemanek, 1990). Nonadherence to medical treatment has been identified as a major public health problem implicated in potentially avoidable functional morbidity and economic consequences (Sclar, Tartaglione, & Fine, 1994).

Examining the effects of recent changes in health care on the capacity of pediatric health professionals to provide optimal care for children with chronic conditions, and on the ability of patients and families to adhere to medical regimens for chronic conditions, is an important advocacy concern (Kelly, 1995). In a relatively short time span, managed care has emerged as the dominant market force in health care, replacing the predominance of the traditional fee-for-service indemnity plan approach, in which enrollees have access to a largely unrestricted choice of health care professionals and provider discretion is primary in health care decision making. In contrast, the key features of managed care include a focus on cost-containment and reduction of health care utilization through restrictions on patient choice and provider autonomy (American Academy of Pediatrics, 1998). Although managed care may offer some advantages to pediatric populations, such as increased access to preventive, well-child care, several facets of managed care are potentially detrimental for the medical care of children with chronic health conditions. In particular, managed care could disrupt treatment adherence and self-management behaviors among families and children. The purpose of the present chapter is to describe the impact of managed care on the clinical management of childhood chronic illness with special reference to treatment adherence. Furthermore, recommendations are presented for improving health care delivery, advocacy efforts, and relevant research initiatives to enhance management.

RATES AND RISKS OF TREATMENT NONADHERENCE IN PEDIATRIC CHRONIC ILLNESSES

Nonadherence to pediatric treatment regimens for chronic conditions is prevalent across illnesses and has been associated with poor disease management and increased morbidity. Although precise cause-and-effect relationships have not been established (Johnson, 1994), nonadherence has been linked to higher levels of functional morbidity and health care costs in various chronic illness conditions. For example, in pediatric asthma patients, treatment nonadherence has been associated with increased symptoms, diminished pulmonary function, and lower asthma control (Bender, Milgrom, & Rand, 1997; Cluss, Epstein, Galvis, Fireman, & Friday, 1984). In pediatric renal transplants, treatment nonadherence has also been associated with complications such as shorter graft survival and increased graft rejection (Meyers, Weiland, & Thomson, 1995). In addition, within pediatric diabetes, noncompliance has been associated with poorer metabolic control and diminished outcomes (Kovacs, Goldston, Obrosky, & Iyengar, 1992).

In addition to complicating disease management, treatment nonadherence is associated with mortality among some children with chronic illnesses, such as those that require kidney transplantation (Rodriguez, Diaz, Colon, & Santiago-Delphin, 1991; Rovelli et al., 1989; Swanson, Hull, Bartus, & Schweizer, 1992). Evidence from other investigations also suggests that treatment nonadherence may be related to deaths in pediatric asthma patients (Strunk, 1987) and pediatric renal disease patients (Meyers, Weiland, & Thomson, 1995).

Financial Implications of Treatment Nonadherence

From the standpoint of health policy, the economic costs of treatment nonadherence are substantial and may lead to increased expenditures in health care (Hammond & Lambert, 1994). Increased hospital admissions and prolonged length of stay are both associated with nonadherence to medical regimens (Hammond & Lambert, 1994; Swanson et al., 1992). A study conducted with children diagnosed with insulin-dependent diabetes mellitus (IDDM) found an association between nonadherence with diabetes care and IDDM-related rehospitalizations (Kovacs et al., 1992). Furthermore, those children with a history of nonadherence were more likely to be rehospitalized (68% compared with only 39% for youths with no serious compliance problems) compared with those who adhered to the treatment plan.

Nonadherence to medical regimens that are necessary for organ transplants has been implicated as a substantial cost of such treatments for adults with chronic health conditions. Swanson and colleagues (1992) argued that nonadherent behavior decreases the effectiveness of adult kidney transplants by as much as 50% per patient per year. A difference in mean admission costs of almost $16,000 for nonadherent and adherent kidney transplant patients was detected. The mean admission cost for nonadherent patients was $28,541, whereas the mean admission cost for adherent patients only totaled $12,885. However, it should be noted that there may not be a consistent, direct causal link between nonadherence and higher health care expenditures. Rather, additional factors such as disease severity and poor efficacy of the treatment regimen may also play a role in this relationship.

Nonadherence and Clinical Research

Another important implication of treatment nonadherence is its impact on clinical trials (see Johnson, chap. 13, this volume; Matsui, chap. 6, this volume). Undetected nonadherence in a clinical trial can lead to the distortion of outcome data, overestimation of required dosage (Matsui, 1997), difficulties generalizing results (Bender, Ikle, DuHamel, & Tinkelman, 1997), and ultimately the future prescription of unnecessarily high doses of medications (Bender et al., 1997). One example of the impact of nonadherence on data from clinical trials is evident in a study that examined patient adherence to inhaled asthma medication (Mawhinney et al., 1991). Participants demonstrated underuse, overuse, and repeated activations of inhalers just prior to follow-up medical visits. Without efforts to track compliance behaviors, conclusions based on the complete patient sample, including those subjects evidencing erratic use of the experimental medications, would have been flawed (Mawhinney, 1991).

THE RELATIONSHIP BETWEEN NONADHERENCE
AS A POLICY ISSUE AND HEALTH CARE TRENDS

As evidenced earlier, nonadherence to medical treatment for pediatric chronic illness is a significant pediatric health policy and scientific concern. Consequently, it is important to critically examine the potential effects of shifting health care trends on adherence to chronic illness treatment and to define the role of pediatric professionals in promoting adherence within the current health care climate. The importance of an advocacy perspective in chronic illness management is underscored by recent health care trends that may jeopardize the ability of health care professionals to provide optimal care and pose new challenges for patients and families in the management of chronic illness.

CHANGES IN HEALTH CARE DELIVERY
AND POTENTIAL IMPACT ON THE CARE
OF CHILDREN WITH CHRONIC HEALTH CONDITIONS

Health care delivery in the United States has undergone a dramatic transformation in recent years, with the most widespread trend being the emergence of managed care. Between 1993 and 1995, the percentage of employees in the United States receiving health insurance coverage from a managed care plan increased from 51% to 73% (Jensen, Morrisey, Gaffney, & Liston, 1997). Currently, an estimated 85% of all employed families are receiving their health care through a managed care plan (Deal, Shiono, & Behrman, 1998). The prevalence of managed Medicaid plans is rising rapidly, and such plans predominantly serve women and children, with more than 13 million Medicaid recipients receiving care under managed care plans in 1996 (Deal et al., 1998). Overall, children are more likely than adults to receive health care coverage through a managed care plan, although the effect of managed care arrangements on child health outcomes remains largely unknown because managed care systems were developed for adult care models (Deal et al., 1998). Children with special health care needs are often covered by managed care and HMO plans. In 1994, over 40% of children with chronic conditions receiving private insurance were enrolled in an HMO (Newacheck, Hughes, Halfon, & Brindis, 1997).

The apparent mismatch between the major principles of managed care arrangements and the health and psychological needs of children with a chronic illness merits attention. Several specific concerns have been raised regarding the impact of health care changes on children with chronic health conditions and are addressed within the present chapter (see Table 9.1). First, access to health care, delays in initiation of health care coverage on employment, and implementation of lifetime benefit caps are of utmost concern for children with chronic health conditions. Second, the roles of pediatricians within the managed care setting have expanded. Providers may experience difficulties serving as gatekeeper, care coordinator, and patient advocate in addition to promoting cost-containment (Kelly, 1995). Third, access to specialty care providers is often restricted within managed care arrangements where gatekeeping systems are in place to limit patient access to providers (Deal et al., 1998). Pediatric patients with special health care needs often depend on subspecialty providers for medical care rather than primary care physicians, who may not be able to offer the highly specialized background and skills to manage certain chronic conditions (Legorreta et al., 1998; Sperber et al., 1995). Fourth, effective delivery of mental health services for children with chronic health conditions within the current health care environment may be compromised. Mental health services may be particularly important for children with chronic health conditions because of their elevated risk for mental health problems, which can necessitate behavioral intervention in conjunction with medical management of a chronic illness (Cadman, Boyle, Szatmari, & Offord, 1987; Creagan, 1993; Gortmaker, Walker, Weitzman, & Sobol, 1990). Finally, increased responsibility for family-based care and difficulties in navigating the new health care system are challenges that children with chronic health conditions and their families face.

Access to Health Care

The current health care climate may offer some potential advantages for patients—namely, an increased focus on certain aspects of preventive care. However, managed care structures limit access to other forms of health care, which carries implications for children with chronic health conditions that likely impact the ability to effectively adhere to treatment regimen. Horwitz and Stein's (1990) comparison of the benefits offered by HMOs versus indemnity plans for children with chronic health conditions outlines specific issues of concern. For example, HMOs were found to be more likely to have a longer waiting period between employment and initiation of health care coverage. Although such lag time typically would not pose a problem for children who require well-child coverage, delays in insurance coverage can potentially jeopardize the care of chil-

TABLE 9.1

Impact of Managed Care and Health Care Trends on Comprehensive Care of Children With Chronic Illness

Health Care Trend	Potential Threats to Comprehensive Care	Policy/Research Implications
Restricted access to health care services	• Restricted access to health care services interrupts the continuity of care • Delays in initiation of coverage may pose risks for children with special health care needs • Benefit caps restrict coverage for childhood chronic illness	• Managed care plans should recognize the need for continuous care for children with chronic illness • Design health care plans that are not tailored solely to children who require well-child care and that consider the needs of children with chronic health conditions • Study and document the impact of restricted access to health care on treatment outcomes and adherence rates
Restricted ability for physicians to provide children with chronic illness highest quality care that addresses and promotes adherence	• Less incentive to provide care for high-cost chronic illness under capitated model, which encourages limiting utilization and containing costs • Less time to assess adherence during physician–patient contact and less time to conduct adherence promotion intervention when indicated • Less physician autonomy in health-related decision making	• Study impact of capitated delivery systems on health status and adherence rates of children with chronic health conditions • Provide physicians the flexibility necessary for addressing the complex medical and behavioral factors involved in chronic illness • Incorporate adherence assessments into regular pediatric practice patterns
Decreased access to specialty providers	• Decrease in quality of care in addressing the needs of children with chronic health conditions	• Incorporate access to specialty care in managed care plans • Primary care providers should be given incentives to

	• Decreased focus on chronic illness management • Less time to identify adherence problems • Less time to devote to adherence promotion	• involve specialists • Study the impact of these innovations on quality and cost of care, including the incidence of adherence problems
Increased separation of health and mental health reimbursement and clinical care structure	• Decrease in access to mental health care for children with chronic illness • Decrease in access to providers who are experts on adherence promotion and the remediation of adherence problems in chronic illness • Less opportunity for coordinated health and mental health care for children with chronic illness	• Develop integrated/coordinated mental health and health services for children with chronic illness and their families • Provide reimbursement for integrated health and mental health care for children with chronic illness • Study the impact of these changes on children's mental health, adherence to treatment, costs of care
Transition from hospital-based, doctor-administered care to home-based, family-administered care	• Decrease in quality of care • Little to no checks on adherence behaviors • Decreased access to multidisciplinary team • Increased burden on families with decreased support from physicians and allied health specialists	• Assess family access to multidisciplinary teams • Assess families' thoughts regarding home-based care—specifically whether it's an improvement over hospital-based care and how they can be best supported for caring for their child with a chronic illness • Study the impact of this trend on quality (including consumers' opinions and adherence problems) and costs of care (including direct health care costs & indirect costs)

dren with special health needs who often require frequent medical attention and consistent prescription coverage. Based on their comparison of HMO and indemnity plan services for children with special health needs, Horwitz and Stein concluded that the feasibility of HMOs for providing more structured and coordinated care for children with chronic health conditions "may be more of a myth than a panacea" (p. 586).

In addition to restricted access to health care, families are also faced with the problem of lifetime benefit caps. The trend toward benefits caps that began in the 1970s is believed to have been an endeavor to ensure insurance holders that they would be covered regardless of the seriousness of their medical condition (Tighe & Hardy Havens, 1997). However, now more than two decades later, these caps have led to large numbers of children and adults exceeding their policy limits each year, and it is predicted that the number of individuals losing coverage because of lifetime cap policies will continue to rise (Price Waterhouse, 1995; Tighe & Hardy Havens, 1997). Children with chronic health conditions are among those who could be the most severely impacted by lifetime benefit caps. It is quite conceivable that children born with a chronic health condition or who develop one during childhood could reach their benefit cap limit before they reach adolescence. Not only would this result in the loss of coverage, but it could lead to delays in receiving services or, worse yet, the loss of services necessary to combat a chronic illness.

Changing Role of the Physician in Current Health Care System

Shifts in Payment Structure.   Under the traditional fee-for-service health care design, providers received financial incentives for patient contact, and greater financial returns were associated with more direct patient care. In contrast, under risk sharing through capitation, which is one increasingly prevalent type of managed care arrangement, financial incentives are offered to physicians for limiting care. Patient utilization rates and access to care have been lessened by changes in physician payment patterns. In comparison to fee-for-service arrangements, capitated reimbursement systems have been associated with fewer hospitalizations and outpatient medical visits (Hillman, Pauly, & Kerstein, 1989). Moreover, children with special health care needs are at risk of being denied coverage due to their high financial risk in capitated reimbursement arrangements that create physician disincentives to cover high-cost patients (American Academy of Pediatrics, 1998). As costs and health care utilization continue to be limited, it is possible that physicians' ability to assess the extent of patient nonadherence before problems arise and intervene to promote optimal care behaviors will be compromised.

Practice Constraints. One by-product of the cost-containment features of managed care has been reductions in the length of time available for direct patient contact. Shortened visits may ultimately result in communication problems between physician and patient (Emanuel & Dubler, 1995). Placing constraints on the amount of time that physicians can provide patients with direct care interferes with their ability to address adherence problems as well as conduct interventions to prevent such problems. Despite the critical importance of promoting optimal adherence within pediatric patients, research indicates that physicians are typically unable to devote the time to address adherence-related behaviors during contact with patients. Thompson et al. (1995) reviewed the medical charts of pediatric patients with juvenile rheumatoid arthritis and found that providers rarely discussed barriers to adherence faced by patients and seldom offered behavior modification strategies to improve treatment adherence. Furthermore, reductions in the amount of time available for direct patient care has been shown to reduce physician satisfaction and may contribute to deterioration in the quality of care offered to patients (Probst, Greenhouse, & Selassie, 1997). A recent survey of physicians indicated that, under managed care, physicians felt they had less time for their patients because of the increased drive for productivity (Feldman, Novack, & Gracely, 1998).

Effects on Patient–Provider Relationship. The quality of the patient–provider relationship, which has been shown to be important in promoting adherence to medical regimens, may be jeopardized within managed care (see DiMatteo, chap. 10, this volume; Friedman & DiMatteo, 1990; Hazzard, Hutchinson, & Krawiecki, 1990). Research has found that parents who had better interaction and communication with their children's provider were more likely to ensure that their children adhered to the prescribed regimen (Thatcher, 1981). Investigations with adults with chronic health conditions have found that physician characteristics (i.e., job satisfaction, specialty, style of practice) were related to adherence rates in patients with chronic diseases (i.e., hypertension, diabetes, heart disease, and depression; DiMatteo et al., 1993). Adults who trust their primary care physicians have been found to be more adherent to physician recommendations involving behaviors such as smoking, alcohol use, seatbelt use, exercise, and stress (Safran et al., 1998). Multiple studies have shown that being an active participant in the decision-making process during the medical visit is associated with increased treatment adherence in adult diabetic patients (Golin, DiMatteo, & Gelberg, 1996). Moreover, establishing a continuous patient–provider relationship has been associated with adherence to cancer screening in adults (Womeodu & Bailey, 1996).

The specific effects of current health care trends on the feasibility of maintaining strong patient–provider relationships that promote treatment adherence within pediatric contexts has not been studied. Nevertheless, one may speculate that the prospects for maintaining positive relationships between providers and children who have chronic health conditions and their families would be more difficult within managed care due to increased restrictions placed on physician time, autonomy, and hence ability to foster a strong, continuous relationship.

Access to Specialty Care Providers

The trend toward managed care has been accompanied by decreased access to specialty care providers through the system of primary care providers who serve as gatekeepers that regulate patient access to specialists. Research has demonstrated that restricted access to specialty care is a hallmark of managed care. For example, one recent investigation demonstrated that over half of a sample of 766 primary care physicians practicing in managed care structures experienced pressure from MCOs to limit referrals to specialty care services for their patients (Grumbach, Osmond, Vranizan, Jaffe, & Bindman, 1998). An additional survey of over 1,500 pediatricians compared referral patterns of pediatricians in managed care systems to those practicing in traditional fee-for-service arrangements; it found managed care to be more likely to restrict referrals to pediatric subspecialty and inpatient care (Cartland & Yudkowsky, 1992).

Fox et al. (1993) used data from the 1989 National Health Interview Survey to examine the level of benefits offered to children with special health needs receiving care from HMOs. Overall, HMOs were found to offer more extensive coverage than traditional fee-for-service plans for certain services, such as medical case management for children with special health needs. Despite the advantages, HMOs were also found to place restrictions on a number of aspects of care for chronic illness populations, particularly on specialty care access. Eighty-five percent of HMO plans surveyed restricted the referral base of primary care physicians to strictly inplan specialists. Depending on the range of skills and expertise of authorized providers within a specific plan, this practice may threaten the quality of care for children with special health care needs. Moreover, it is unlikely that pediatric providers who have the specialized training needed to manage relatively rare chronic health conditions (e.g., cystic fibrosis [CF], sickle cell anemia, cancer) and promote adherence to chronic illness treatment will be adequately represented within a single plan's provider panel.

For these reasons, restriction of access to specialists could potentially impact patient adherence to prescribed regimens. For example, asthma research has demonstrated that, compared with general pediatric providers, physicians who specialize in respiratory conditions are optimally qualified to manage asthma effectively (Legorreta et al., 1998; Sperber et al., 1995). Although the impact of restriction of access to specialty care providers on adherence rates remains unclear, it is possible that children with special health care needs are particularly vulnerable to problematic health care and less than optimal adherence to chronic illness treatment based on restricted access to specialty care.

Access to Mental Health Services

In some cases, mental health services become an important component of care for children with chronic health conditions because they experience stress and emotional strain related to their illness (Baum & Creer, 1986; La Greca & Schuman, 1995; Lavigne & Faier-Routman, 1992). Effectively managing comorbid behavioral and physical health concerns in an integrated manner has become increasingly difficult in the current health care system due to the trend of separating mental health services through independent managed behavioral health care organizations. The prevalence of mental health *carve-outs* escalated dramatically during the 1990s (Mihalik & Scherer, 1998; Sturm & McCulloch, 1998) and may pose a barrier to promoting adherence among children with chronic health conditions. In a carve-out fee structure, the delivery of mental health services is conducted separately from general health services (Frank, Huskamp, McGruire, & Newhouse, 1996). Such mental health carve-outs may run the risk of offering suboptimal and fragmented care for children with chronic health conditions and may potentially jeopardize adherence (Walders & Drotar, 1999). For example, mental health professionals involved in chronic illness management can be instrumental in detecting and addressing psychosocial factors that pose a threat to adherence to treatment as well as health outcomes (e.g., a comorbid eating disorder in IDDM). However, in a carve-out design, behavioral health care is handled as a separate entity, independent from medical management, which can limit integrated assessment and treatment of psychosocial concerns. The impact of mental health carve-outs on adherence rates for children with chronic health conditions has not been clearly documented. Nevertheless, it appears that this structure of care could pose a significant barrier to utilizing psychological services that could facilitate adherence.

Increased Demands on Patient and Family

The trend toward managed care has helped forge a health care system that presents increasing barriers for families who wish to obtain services for their children with chronic health conditions. Securing optimal care for a chronic illness is often a formidable challenge in any health care system. A chronic condition may require multiple office visits to a number of health care providers, prescriptions needing frequent refills, and other complicated tasks. In the current health care environment, a considerable amount of responsibility is placed on consumers to be informed and proactive to handle the tasks involved in accessing care. Fox et al. (1993) commented that the quality of care provided to children with special health needs within HMOs is largely dependent on the ability of families to advocate effectively and understand complex rules and technicalities associated with health care services. The necessity for such family advocacy creates an additional burden for families who are already juggling the demands of complex medical regimens; it may interfere with the amount of time and energy that can be devoted directly to promoting effective treatment adherence (Kelly, 1995).

Many families are also faced with the increasing responsibility of managing their children's chronic diseases independently at home. A recent trend in the care of children with chronic illness has been the transition from hospital-based, physician-directed care to home-based, self- or family-administered care (O'Brien & Hanley, 1992). Although home and family-administered care are viewed by some as helping patients and their families obtain increased control over their lives, the resources necessary to facilitate this type of care are often not in place (Anderson, 1990). For example, research has documented that families frequently lack access to multidisciplinary teams or reimbursement for services that can assist in administering home care (Smith, 1996). Consequently, when the role of home care is expanded, it is quite possible that families may have diminished control over their child's treatments and health-related outcomes. Although a great deal remains to be learned about the nature of adherence to home-based, family-administered care in childhood chronic illness, one may speculate that the added demands placed on families could potentially overtax families, making it difficult for them to adhere to all aspects of the medical regimen. Consequently, it may be important to individualize the source of care on the basis of patient need and family resources, rather than allowing system structures to independently determine the route of care. Some families may benefit from having more autonomous control over their child's health care, whereas other families may be burdened by home-based illness management and treatment adherence may be jeopardized.

INTERCHANGE AMONG RESEARCH, POLICY, AND PRACTICE

Thus far we have raised several key questions concerning the impact of managed care on the comprehensive care of children with chronic illness and their families. Empirical data are needed to address these critical questions concerning the impact of managed care and to provide an empirical foundation to inform and influence policy and advocacy for the needs of children with chronic health conditions (see Table 9.2). For this reason, it is instructive to consider empirical data that have been obtained from the management of exemplar chronic conditions that can inform policy and advocacy concerning comprehensive care (Vinicor, 1998). One such condition is asthma.

Asthma as a Model

As the most common childhood illness with rapidly increasing rates of prevalence, morbidity, and health care expenditures, asthma represents a model condition for empirical investigation (Centers for Disease Control, 1996; Newacheck, Budetti, & Halfon, 1986). Asthma is characterized by high rates of problematic nonadherence that interfere with functioning and outcome (Baum & Creer, 1986; Creer & Bender, 1995). To address this problem, as shown in Table 9.2, a number of studies have examined the effectiveness of interventions designed to promote self-management and treatment adherence in pediatric asthma; these interventions contain lessons for future policy and practice in relation to general issues in childhood chronic illness.

For example, Greineder, Loane, and Parks (1995, 1999) conducted two studies examining the effects of a pediatric asthma outreach program (AOP) conducted within a staff-model HMO serving a primarily African-American, inner-city population. The first implementation of the AOP involved a comparison of health care expenditures, emergency department visits, and hospitalization rates before and after participation in a program of asthma education, treatment planning, and long-term follow-up conducted by a nurse employed by the HMO. Significant reductions in emergency ward visits and hospital admissions were found following participation in the AOP, resulting in a cost savings estimated at $87,000 after accounting for the cost of implementing the intervention (part-time nurse salary of $11,115). The first phase of the study was expanded with a subsequent randomized, controlled trial that assigned patients to either a brief single-session educational program or a group that received asthma education combined with asthma outreach case management conducted by a nurse that involved consistent follow-up (Greineder et al., 1999). Both groups demonstrated significant reductions in emergency department visits, hospitalization, and outside of health plan expenditures. However, the asthma outreach group demonstrated significantly greater reductions in utilization rates and cost savings (Greineder et al., 1999). This series of studies demonstrates the feasibility and efficacy of implementing an adherence promotion intervention within a managed care setting. Sig-

TABLE 9.2

Review of Asthma Adherence Promotion Intervention Models for Potential Application in Managed Care Settings

Author(s)	Sample	Objective/Aim	Design	Outcome Measures	Results	Implications for Managed Care
Baum & Creer (1986)	• N = 20 children ages 6–12	• Implementation of educational sessions to achieve: -improved medication compliance -improved family-based management skills	• Longitudinal design	• Serum theophylline levels, parental pill counts • Self-monitoring (peak flow meters, reports of asthma attacks, symptom diary)	• Asthma management training showed no gains in compliance, self-concept, or health locus of control • Intervention group did show more responsibility taking for responding to attacks	• Providing education and asthma knowledge may not be sufficient, and more hands-on training tools may be indicated
Brazil et al. (1997)	• N = 50 families with children ages 6–12 • Compared inpatient treatment (n = 25) to outpatient asthma camp (n = 25)	• To compare illness outcomes and self-management skills between families who participated in an intensive 3-month inpatient program to families who participated in 3-week outpatient asthma camp	• Casual-comparative, pre- & posttest design of participants in either program over prior 2 years, matched for asthma severity	• Compared reports of asthma morbidity over 3-month period (medical records used as proxy for pretest measures) • Examined parental report of knowledge, child self-management, child adjustment, and impact of asthma and child report of asthma knowledge, self-management, and attitudes	• Parents of inpatient participants reported significantly fewer asthma attacks than parents of outpatient participants • No group differences were found in school absenteeism or medical utilization • No significant differences between outpatient and inpatient groups were found in parental report	• More abbreviated forms of asthma intervention used in a MCO setting may be insufficient for changing behavior • Two factors should be included in interventions: [a] opportunity for children to perform and practice asthma management tasks in controlled and supervised conditions, and [b] parental involvement in child asthma education and behavior

Clark et al. (1986)	• $N = 310$ children ages 4–17 • 290 low-income urban families randomized into either experimental ($n = 207$) or control ($n = 103$) group	• Determine efficacy of group education program on parents' and child's ability to manage asthma and reduce the use of health services	• Randomized control trial	• Hospitalizations, ER visits, cost savings	• No statistically significant differences between groups for # hospitalizations, ER visits, or cost savings • Children w/previous hospitalizations: Experimental group had fewer hospitalizations and greater reduction in # of ER visits than control group and $11.22 saved for every $1.00 spent	• Group intervention easily exported to managed care setting • Program development outlined for ease of use in managed care settings • Targeting children at risk for nonadherence and using group intervention may be useful in terms of reductions in future morbidity and cost savings
Colland (1993)	• $N = 112$ children ages 8–13 • Divided into experimental group ($n = 48$), minimal treatment control group ($n = 34$), and placebo control group ($n = 30$)	• Determine effects of an educational training program to improve asthma coping using ten 1-hour sessions of self-management and cognitive-behavioral group therapy	• Randomized controlled design that employed pretest selection and matching on age, asthma severity, and asthma coping ability	• Included an evaluation of coping, compliance, morbidity, and utilization at 3 weeks, 6 months, and 12 months posttreatment	• Significant improvements in coping, asthma knowledge, MDI technique, and in experimental group • Significant decrease in medical consumption was found in experimental group • Clinically and statistically significant effects of an asthma intervention program were found using a rigorous methodology and design, which employed multiple sites and practitioners	• Study demonstrates the feasibility of employing a standard program of asthma management across a number of sites • No attrition occurred and qualitative feedback from participants was very positive, demonstrating that patients were enthusiastic and motivated to learn how to better cope with asthma

(Continued)

TABLE 9.2 (Continued)

Author(s)	Sample	Objective/Aim	Design	Outcome Measures	Results	Implications for Managed Care
Dahl et al. (1990)	• N = 20 children with an average age of 12.2 years • randomized into medical tx (n = 10) or medical and behavioral tx (n = 10)	• Compare outcomes of standard medical treatment to medical treatment combined with short series of brief behavioral intervention sessions aimed at improving adherence, symptom management, and coping	• Randomized, controlled trial including baseline, intervention, and follow-up phases	• Use of PRN medication, school absences, asthma symptom days, and lung functioning	• Behavioral intervention resulted in significant reduced use of PRN medications and reductions in school absences • No significant differences in lung function were detected	• Demonstrates the applicability and feasibility of integrated programs that combine medical management and behavioral intervention • Brief behavioral protocol could be exported to other settings
Fitzpatrick et al. (1992)	• N = 84 children ages 5–10 • Predominantly African-American males from single-family homes	• Determine the efficacy of a 1-day asthma camp curriculum using an interdisciplinary approach to teach family-based asthma management strategies and improved medication adherence	• Longitudinal design	• Follow-up interviews were conducted to track medication usage and asthma management techniques	• High percentage of children engaged in new asthma management techniques (78% with aerosol techniques, 55% engaged in breathing warm up exercises) following participation in the program • Clinically significant improvements (36%–69% reduction in school absences, ER visits, and hospitalizations) found following participation in the program	• Asthma camp model could be exported to a managed care setting • Joint initiative between consumer advocacy group (American Lung Association), and managed care organization is a promising an innovative model that could be replicated

216

Gebert et al. (1998)	• $N = 81$ patients ages 7–14 • Group 1 ($n = 27$) family asthma training with follow-up; Group 2 ($n = 29$) received family asthma training w/out follow-up; Group 3 ($n = 25$) standard medical tx control	• Examined the long-term effects of family-based asthma training and investigated whether individual follow-up visits enhance training benefits	• Randomized controlled trial • All groups were matched according to age, sex, duration and asthma severity	• Compared groups on health locus of control, anxiety, self-management, medical utilization, and morbidity variables	• Intervention group with long-term follow-up demonstrated the most significant improvements in asthma self-management, including greater knowledge about preventive and emergency measures • Intervention group without follow-up showed some improvements • Control group demonstrated no effects • No sustainable differences in pulmonary function tests	• Results highlight the importance of utilizing interdisciplinary professionals (pulmonologists, psychologist, and physiologist were involved) and a variety of techniques (education, social activities, family methods) to improve asthma management • Significant improvements were found with a relatively brief intervention format (5-day workshop) • Study demonstrates the need for active follow-up contact with families to provide continuous and intensive care
Gillies et al. (1996)	• $N = 110$ children ages 3–11 years recruited from 12 different family practitioners in New Zealand	• Determine the effects of a written asthma attack intervention plan for patients with mild to moderate asthma who previously lacked any treatment plan	• Prospective, single-group pre-posttest comparison	• Examined morbidity, health care utilization, prescribed medications, and acceptability of the plan	• Statistically significant reductions were found in asthma symptoms, nocturnal awakening from asthma, and activity restriction • Statistically significant reductions were found in health care utilization	• Program demonstrates the feasibility and efficacy of implementing an asthma management intervention protocol via pediatric general practitioners

(Continued)

TABLE 9.2 (Continued)

Author(s)	Sample	Objective/Aim	Design	Outcome Measures	Results	Implications for Managed Care
					• Statistically significant reductions were found in the use of oral steroids and increases in use of preventive medications • A large majority of patients reported that they found the plan to be acceptable, manageable, and easy to implement	
Godding, Kruth, & Jamart (1997)	• N = 41 children (39 families); • Mean age = 11.4 ± 5.2 yr. old high-risk pediatric asthma patients in Belgium	• Determine efficacy of joint consultation between physician and child psychiatrist for high-risk asthmatic patients	• Longitudinal design (2 yrs. before & 2 yrs. after onset of treatment)	• Hospitalizations, days in hospital, symptom score, therapeutic score, theophylline level in blood, ICU admissions prior to intervention, cost savings	• Symptom and treatment scores, hospital admissions, and days in hospital were all statistically significantly reduced • Compliance and autonomy scores, and theophylline level all statistically significantly increased • Reduction in cost (presented in Belgian Francs)	• Asthma model developed for intervention easily exported to managed care setting • Highlights the efficacy of an interdisciplinary intervention program that increases adherence and reduces morbidity and financial costs.
Greineder, Loane, & Parks (1995)	• N = 53 children • 1- to 17-year-old	• Determine efficacy of asthma outreach nurse's educational intervention and	• Longitudinal design	• Emergency visits, hospital admissions, cost savings	• Emergency admissions were reduced by 79% and hospital admissions were reduced 86%	• Design was implemented and evaluated within an HMO setting

Study	Sample	Purpose	Design	Measures	Results	Comments
	low-income urban pediatric asthma patients in an HMO	coordination of care for improving morbidity and reducing service-related costs				• Simplicity of design makes implementation feasible at minimum cost and maximum gain for managed care company
Greineder, Loane, & Parks (1999)	• $N = 57$ patients ages 1–15 • all patients were enrolled in an HMO • randomized into standard care or asthma outreach program	• Compare the effectiveness of a single educational session to asthma education combined with follow-up management and asthma outreach	• Randomized, controlled design	• Emergency visits, hospital admissions, outside of health plan medical expenditures	• An estimated $87,000 in costs were saved in the follow-up year (compared with pre-treatment year) • Both groups demonstrated reductions in emergency department visits, hospitalizations, and external costs, with the asthma outreach intervention patients evidencing more significant reductions and direct cost savings	• Study underscores the benefits of providing patient education combined with outreach efforts to track the long-term functioning of patients and families • Results demonstrate the importance of continuous care that could be implemented through case management and interdisciplinary clinics
Mesters et al. (1995)	• $N = 46$ general practitioners of 85 pediatric patients • Intervention group: 28 GPs with 47 infants with asthma • Control group: 18 GPs with 38 patients	• Examined the effects of an asthma patient education protocol delivered by general pediatric practitioners to patients	• Randomized, controlled trial • Chart reviews were conducted for 1-year period	• Compared medical care consumption (ER, urgent care visits, referrals to specialists, home care, admissions, medication prescriptions) between intervention and control	• Intervention group showed more reductions in the number of physician contacts and urgent care visits	• Interesting model of delivering intervention directly from provider to patient • Could be implemented and further evaluated within a managed care setting by incorporating a standardized education protocol and packet delivered at primary care-patient contact

(Continued)

TABLE 9.2 (Continued)

Author(s)	Sample	Objective/Aim	Design	Outcome Measures	Results	Implications for Managed Care
Rakos et al. (1985)	• N = 43 children ages 7–12 years	• Evaluation of Superstuff program (a comprehensive self-help program for pediatric asthma)	• Randomized control trial comparing outcomes of children enrolled in the Superstuff program and the no contact control group	• Examined self-report, parental and physician report, and school data preintervention and at 2, 6 and 12 months post-program	• Children in Superstuff demonstrated increased asthma self-control skills, but no improvements in general self-control or self-esteem • Parents and physicians reported greater improvements in the Superstuff participants • No significant improvements in severity of asthma or intensity of average asthma episodes were found • No reduction in health care utilization among Superstuff participants	• Superstuff initiative is a low-cost, self-administered, easily adopted intervention that is based on a self-help model • Dissemination of the project via a MCO would likely be low cost and low burden to the organization
Tal et al. (1990)	• N = 28 children ages 8–12 and both parents (only two-parent households) • Sample divided into	• Developed curriculum for "Family Asthma Management School" for 6 weekly 2-hour sessions to improve asthma knowledge and family-based asthma manage-	• Two-group independent samples design with pre- and postmeasures conducted 3 months	• Collected data on morbidity, utilization, child initiated adherence, and family decision-making skills	• Children in intervention reported taking increased responsibility for daily care, increased independent medication usage, and reductions in asthma-related activity restriction	• Intervention model and results demonstrate the importance of family-based approaches to chronic illness management

Study	Sample	Intervention/Purpose	Design	Outcome Measures	Results	Implications
	18 intervention families and 10 control families	ment and prevention skills	prior to start and 12 months following completion		• Reductions in parental involvement in asthma management were found for intervention families	• Intervention design demonstrated application of adherence promotion in late adolescent age group
Tehan et al. (1989)	• N = 22 late adolescents (college age) with asthma	• Implemented the "Breathe Free" program in a college health service setting that focused on medical management, psychosocial issues, behavior modification, and attack response strategies	• Pre- and posttest design	• Tracked asthma morbidity, health care utilization, and level of asthma knowledge • Combined objective measures and self-report	• Participants reported improvements in self-care, illness knowledge, perceived control of asthma symptoms, and illness attitudes • Objective measures demonstrated improvements in pulmonary functioning	
Volsko (1998)	• N = 27 pediatric asthma clinic patients	• Determine efficacy of self-management education for improving asthma patient outcomes	• Pre/posttest design	• Examined ED visits, hospitalizations, and health care costs as outcome variables comparing patient's pre-clinic data (3 months prior to participation) to postintervention (7-month period)	• Reduction in ED visits, hospitalizations, and costs associated w/ED and inpatient hospital care • Improvement in patient/family compliance in keeping appointments • Estimated cost savings per patient = $1,544	• Demonstrates cost savings associated with accomplishing improved family-based self-management

(Continued)

TABLE 9.2 (Continued)

Author(s)	Sample	Objective/Aim	Design	Outcome Measures	Results	Implications for Managed Care
Wein- stein et al. (1992)	• N = 44 chil- dren • 6 mos–17- yr-old severe asth- matic patients	• Determine efficacy of multidisciplinary approach using short-term hospi- talization and psy- choeducational self-management program for severely asthmatic patients	• Longitudinal design	• Hospital days, emergency care visits, pul- monary mor- bidity, and cor- ticosteroid bursts • Psychological fx (CBCl, FGAS, CGAS)	• Statistically significant reductions in hospital stays, ER visits, and corticosteroid bursts 1 year following inter- vention compared to 1 year prior • Dysfunctional families had children with sig- nificantly more steroid bursts/year and more hospitalizations	• Specific inclusionary criteria clearly stated and thus easily import- ed to managed care • Program development outlined for ease of use in managed care settings
Whitman et al. (1985)	• Preschool study: n = 21 children	• Evaluated the application of the Self-Care Rehabili-	• Randomized control design	• Examined morbidity and knowledge 3	• Decrease in asthma episodes but not sever- ity was found in both	• The decreases in mor- bidity found among both groups indicates

	randomly assigned to study or control • School-age study: n = 38 children who served as their own controls	tation in Pediatric Asthma Project for preschoolers and school-age patients	• Pre- and posttest design • Family-focused intervention protocol to improve asthma management skills	months prior to a following training	control and intervention groups • Increases in knowledge and skills were found for the school-age study group	that family monitoring of symptoms may be beneficial and could be implemented into a comprehensive care program for asthma
Wilson et al. (1996)	• N = 76 children ages 1–7	• Evaluation of the Wee Wheezers program • Aimed to reduce asthma morbidity and improve parental asthma management knowledge and skills	• Randomized control trial	• Tracked outcomes in both groups at 3-month follow-up	• Subjects enrolled in the Wee Wheezers groups demonstrated significant reductions in symptom days, nocturnal symptoms, and asthma sick days	• Intervention is a manualized program to reduce asthma complications that could be implemented by a managed care organization

223

nificant reductions in health care utilization and sizable cost benefits were found within both phases of the study, which was conducted in an inner-city setting with patients at an elevated risk for asthma complications, underscoring the effectiveness of the adherence promotion efforts. The results demonstrate the benefits of extending clinical services to incorporate family-based education and providing long-term follow-up contact with patients, both of which are jeopardized within a managed care framework. The work of Greineder et al. (1995, 1999), which was conducted within an HMO, suggests that other managed care settings might also benefit from offering extended clinical services and case management to pediatric patients.

Weinstein et al. (1992, 1996, 1997) developed a potentially cost-effective model of interdisciplinary inpatient asthma treatment that promotes effective family-based asthma management. The program combined educational and behavioral techniques to increase the quality of self-management, symptom monitoring, and medication usage during a short-term inpatient hospitalization using family-centered behavioral and educational techniques. The clinical strategies implemented during the program were specifically targeted toward improving adherence to asthma management regimens by maximizing the role of patients and family members in active self-management. Implementation of the intervention model, which emphasizes the relevance of behavioral principles for treatment adherence, has resulted in significant reductions in hospitalizations, emergency care, and reliance on certain medications. Furthermore, the program has demonstrated significant improvements in family management skills and reductions in medical costs sustained over an extensive 4-year follow-up period (Weinstein & Faust, 1997; Weinstein, McKee, Stapleford, & Faust, 1996). The experience of Weinstein and colleagues (1992, 1996, 1997) demonstrates the effectiveness of incorporating mental health professionals who have specific training in behavioral strategies and family management techniques in adherence promotion programs. Managed care could offer the structure needed to include mental health professionals within medical settings in such a systematic manner.

The randomized, controlled trial conducted by Dahl, Gustafsson, and Melin (1990) is an additional source of evidence that integration of mental health and medical services is a potentially valuable tool for improving the management of pediatric asthma within a managed care context. In their study, children with severe asthma were randomly assigned to either standard medical care or medical care combined with behavioral intervention. The behavioral intervention protocol included a series of brief sessions covering adherence promotion, symptom discrimination, relaxation training, and contingency management. The researchers compared the outcomes of the traditional medical group to patients who received the behavioral intervention in addition to medical treatment. The integration of behavioral intervention was associated with decreased reliance on certain medications and a decrease in school absences—a major problem for children with severe asthma (Dahl, Gustafsoon, & Melin, 1990). The study demonstrated both the feasibility and effectiveness of merging medical and behavioral efforts in the treatment of pediatric asthma. From a managed care perspective, the study underscored the potential benefits of integrating mental health services within standard treatment plans for children and families who need to manage chronic illness.

Another potentially valuable model of comprehensive chronic illness management includes Volsko's (1998) examination of an interdisciplinary approach to care that incorporates the expertise of pediatricians, allied health professionals, and mental health professionals in the management of severe asthma. The interdisciplinary clinic examined in the study was based on a three-session protocol including: (a) education regarding pathophysiology of asthma and the need for family-based adherence to a treatment plan, (b) identification of asthma triggers and training for symptom control through environmental modifications, and (c) integration of education and self-management behaviors. The program was associated with reductions in emergency department visits and hospitalizations, as well as an estimated cost savings of $1,544 per patient. The interdisciplinary clinic developed and tested by Volsko (1998) could be adopted by managed care companies as a cost-effective treatment protocol for managing severe asthma.

Based on available data from these and other exemplar programs (see Table 9.2) the following key principles of comprehensive care for children with chronic health conditions are suggested; they may have broad applicability toward enhancing the management of childhood chronic illness and related adherence rates: (a) developing collaborative care partnerships that merge the efforts of several pediatric professionals (e.g., physicians, psychologists, allied health professionals), (b) using long-term intervention in cases of difficult to manage illnesses, and (c) developing targeted interventions that address behavioral and medical factors in illness management. Such principles may have broad applicability to enhance the management of chronic illness in children.

FUTURE DIRECTIONS AND "ACTION STRATEGIES" FOR ADVOCACY, RESEARCH, AND CLINICAL ENDEAVORS

Our analysis and review suggests several recommendations to develop clinical care, research, and policy (see Table 9.3). These efforts are aimed at assisting patients and families to effectively adhere to treatment regi-

TABLE 9.3
Unmet Needs and Future Directions for Research and Advocacy

Unmet Research Needs in Childhood Chronic Illness	Potential Advocacy Applications of New Data
• From the patient/family perspective, what health care system factors *promote* adherence to treatment regimen?	• Collecting data on which features of health care delivery promote adherence (e.g., quality of relationship with provider, access to comprehensive services) will enable the identification of advocacy priorities
• From the patient/family perspective, what health care system factors are *barriers* to adherence?	• Identifying aspects of health care delivery that are risk factors for nonadherence will help to develop advocacy strategies
• From the provider perspective, what aspects of health care *facilitate* versus *prevent* the delivery of high-quality care?	• Providers can serve as powerful advocates on behalf of patient and professional interests, and empirical as well as anecdotal data are necessary to communicate their experiences of working in new health care settings
• What elements of clinical interventions are directly linked to improvements in adherence?	• Reviewing a range of interventions across sites and conditions to abstract the clinical features that lead to improved adherence would inform and influence managed care practices. Results from single isolated interventions are unlikely to make a widespread impact.

mens for chronic health conditions. Further, the recommendations are targeted toward facilitating the delivery of optimal pediatric health care to patients with special health care needs.

Development of Guidelines for Treatment of Pediatric Chronic Illness in a Managed Care Environment

The development of comprehensive practice guidelines outlining optimal care pathways for pediatric chronic illness (Coleman, 1992) is a cornerstone of effective clinical management and comprehensive care of chronic illness and is necessary for several reasons: (a) objective clarification of treatment goals for chronic illness, (b) communication of these goals and details of treatment to children and families, and (c) evaluation of the impact of treatment guidelines. The American Academy of Pediatrics developed two relevant policy documents entitled "Guiding Principles for Managed Care Arrangements for Health Care of Infants, Children, Adolescents and Young Adults" (1995) and "Managed Care and Children with

Special Health Care Needs: A Subject Review" (1998). These articles outlined several key recommendations for designing and implementing pediatric managed care and define the potential role of managed care in serving children and adolescents in primary and specialty care settings. Guiding principles include the following: (a) access to primary care and pediatric specialty care, (b) appropriate treatment authorization, (c) quality assurance, and (d) acceptable reimbursement procedures (American Academy of Pediatrics, 1995, 1998).

Unfortunately, practice guidelines for the treatment of chronic illness do not consider the optimal ways to integrate behavioral and medical management approaches to promote adherence to treatment and high-quality comprehensive care. Such treatment recommendations could serve as standards from which to evaluate the services provided by managed care organizations. Currently, guidelines for clinical management of pediatric chronic conditions to address nonadherence are absent, and such practice parameters may be potentially useful as leverage to ensure that patients receive optimal care (Kovach, 1996). Concrete recommendations could be established for reimbursement to enhance the management of pediatric chronic conditions (i.e., discontinue lifetime caps, provide access to mental health providers, etc.) and provide the services necessary to promote treatment adherence (e.g., integration of mental health services, interdisciplinary clinics, etc.). Moreover, managed care companies are not yet held to standards of practice related to the care of children with chronic illness, including adherence concerns. Consequently, patient/families and providers do not have a platform from which to advocate for more extended coverage of necessary medical and/or behavioral services.

Document the Effects of Health Care Trends on Treatment Adherence in Childhood Chronic Illness

We have raised a number of significant concerns about the impact of health care trends on treatment adherence in childhood chronic illness. Data are needed to document the specific implications of managed care changes. To effectively advocate on behalf of children and adolescents with chronic health conditions who are at some level of risk for diminished quality of care under current and future managed care arrangements, the following questions need to be addressed in future studies: How has managed care impacted the economic burden placed on families caring for a child with a chronic health condition? Have managed care system requirements (e.g., primary care provider as gatekeeper) placed barriers to accessing care for children with chronic health conditions? If so, what are the most significant barriers and what is their impact? How has managed care altered the psychological and physical challenges of achieving successful treatment adherence for children with chronic health conditions? Gathering further empirical evidence concerning the answers to these questions would extend beyond clinical anecdotes and vignettes to assist policymakers and advocates in efforts to promote treatment adherence and healthy functioning. This information may also be used to influence policy within managed care agencies.

Developing Tools to Evaluate the Care of Children With Chronic Illness

The development of research concerning the impact of patterns of health care on treatment adherence should be enhanced by the development of tools to evaluate the quality of care provided by managed care plans (such as the Health Plan Employer Data and Information Set [HEDIS] developed by the National Committee for Quality Assurance [NCQA]). Recommendations have also been made to improve the applicability of HEDIS indicators to adequately monitor the quality of care provided to children with chronic health conditions (Kuhlthau et al., 1998). These recommendations include increasing accurate identification of the number of children with chronic health conditions covered by health plans and add structure, process, and outcome indicators specifically focused on children with special health care needs.

Developing Tracking Systems to Monitor the Prevalence and Impact of Nonadherence to Pediatric Chronic Illness Treatment

Another recommendation is to develop tracking systems to identify and monitor the rates and impact of nonadherence for different illnesses for children covered by managed care organizations. Incorporating adherence rates in services delivered by health plans may encourage managed care companies to expend resources to maximize the ability of providers to promote adherence and optimize the ability of patients and families to successfully implement complex treatment regimen.

Initiating Interdisciplinary Clinics to Promote Comprehensive Care

The complex nature of many chronic health conditions may necessitate the involvement of an interdisciplinary team of health professionals (i.e., psychologists, social workers, allied health professionals) for optimal care, including adherence promotion (Creer, Levstek, & Reynolds, 1998). For example, within diabetes, the involvement of an interdisciplinary team, including the expertise of a pediatric endocrinologist, dietitian, psychologist, and pediatrician, may be indicated (Walders & Drotar, 1999). As further research documents the applicability and effectiveness of interdisciplinary care for children with chronic health conditions, it is recommended that access to interdisciplinary clinics become standard practice. Pediatric patients with chronic health conditions may need access to care that merges the expertise of primary and specialty care pediatrics along with behavioral providers, such as pediatric psychologists, who are trained to promote adherence to treatment regimen.

Research has shown that the quality of the patient–provider relationship has a role in adherence behavior (see DiMatteo, chap. 10, this volume), and interdisciplinary clinics may be able to provide patients and families with the individualized and specialized attention necessary to translate into an increased capacity for treatment adherence. Consequently, such clinics may have the potential to improve the quality of health care and potentially decrease the problems associated with nonadherence. The specific structures and financial strategies that are necessary to implement this care should be documented and described. The Children's Multidisciplinary Specialty Service, a program funded by the Michigan State Department of Public Health and implemented by Siegel (1995), serves as an example of this interdisciplinary, comprehensive care approach. In this program, pediatric health care for chronic conditions is delivered by a team of providers, including pediatric specialists, psychologists, and social workers. Families enrolled in the program receive a comprehensive evaluation and are provided with access to the type and extent of services necessary to handle their medical and behavioral health care needs (Seigel et al., 1995). Program evaluation on this initiative is currently underway, and it is expected that the service will be related to improved adherence and outcomes.

Studying the Impact of Interdisciplinary, Comprehensive Care on Adherence to Pediatric Chronic Illness Treatment and Health Care Outcomes

Although preliminary evidence exists that supports an integrated health and mental health service package for children with special pediatric health care needs, it is necessary to collect further evidence concerning the effectiveness of such programs on children's mental health, adherence to chronic illness treatment, and costs of care. Evaluations are recommended for existing interdisciplinary programs. Moreover, program evaluation plans should be included in the development of new interventions to increase the available data concerning the impact of comprehensive approaches to health care management. At a minimum, such program evaluations should include morbidity (e.g., frequency and intensity of symptoms), impact of chronic illness on child and family (e.g., school and work days missed), and health care utilization and expenditure (e.g., frequency and intensity of medical visits, visits to other professionals, emergency department visits, hospitalization) outcomes. Tracking these care delivery and outcome variables will enable mental health researchers and clinicians to better understand the specific improvements in health status associated with interdisciplinary comprehensive care.

Conducting Research on Adherence Promotion Interventions Conducted in Practice Settings

An additional research need is for the continued evaluation of adherence promotion interventions designed to maximize the healthy functioning of children and adolescents with chronic health conditions (see Anderson et al., chap. 15; Rapoff, chap. 14; Stark, chap. 18; Quittner et al., chap. 17; Wysocki et al., chap. 16, this volume). Randomized, controlled intervention trials that employ methodologically rigorous techniques and examine a range of outcome variables, including adherence behaviors and health care utilization rates and costs, are valuable and necessary. The structure of managed care organizations offers opportunities to conduct both controlled clinical trials to study adherence behaviors and clinical interventions to promote adherence and adaptation to a chronic illness. England and Cole (1995) noted that public or private managed care settings can be viewed as clinical laboratories to implement and examine the efficacy of behavioral interventions to promote adherence to a medical regimen.

Supporting Consumer Advocacy Efforts

Our review of current clinical care, research, and policy activities related to the management of treatment adherence in childhood chronic illness has suggested a number of action strategies. An important next step in meeting the needs of children with chronic health conditions includes facilitating the role of patient and family advocacy organizations in monitoring the quality of care provided within managed care settings. Consumer-based coalitions have mobilized influential advocacy movements in other areas, such as the effort to gain parity for mental health services and developing managed care *report cards* that evaluate services provided by insurers to special populations (i.e., persons with mental illness; National Alliance for the Mentally Ill [NAMI]). A parallel effort examining the effects of health care system factors on the ability of patients and families to adhere to complex medical regimens would be an extremely valuable contribution.

The organization *Family Voices®*, a consumer group working on behalf of children with special health care needs and their families, has initiated such an effort and advocates through several important avenues. For example, the Family Partners project collects and disseminates data on the experiences of children with special health care needs. It does so to document the effects of different health care systems and trends on the quality of care provided to these children. In addition to the organization's efforts to appraise the performance of different health care plans in serving children with special health care needs, *Family Voices®* has produced a variety of informational and advocacy resources to assist families, including documents that define managed care terms, lists of questions for families to ask when considering entering a managed care arrangement, and a set of standards and criteria for managed care. These valuable tools are available by contacting the agency at 1-888-835-5669 or via the Internet at http://www.familyvoices.org. It is recommended that the efforts of this agency, and the results of the Family Survey in particular, are widely disseminated to patients, families, providers, and payors in an effort to advocate on behalf of children with special health care needs within the managed care marketplace. As well, it is important that providers encourage families with children with chronic illness to become involved in such organizations because their input is extremely valuable.

Facilitating Professional Advocacy Efforts

Professional advocacy is another powerful tool for influencing health care policy to ensure that patients receive access to high-quality care and limit barriers that prevent professionals from delivering such care. In particular, the American Academy of Pediatrics (AAP) has been particularly invested in advocacy for children with chronic health conditions. One of the AAP's significant efforts in patient advocacy has been through the Ad Hoc Task Force on Definition of the Medical Home (American Academy of Pediatrics, 1992) and the Medical Home Program for Children with Special Needs (MHPCSN; American Academy of Pediatrics, 1999). The medical home concept supported by the AAP articulates the need for "accessible, continuous, comprehensive, family-centered, coordinated, and compassionate" pediatric care (American Academy of Pediatrics, 1992, p. 774) and lists the specific services necessary for accomplishing comprehensive pediatric health care. The MHPCSN provides a similar platform regarding the medical home concept tailored for children with special health care needs. The academy has produced a checklist of the necessary elements of the *medical home* for children with special needs that incorporates 38 specific items divided into elements of access to primary care pediatricians, specialty services, quality assurance, and outcome evaluation.

Although not specifically geared toward adherence promotion, the checklist serves as a valuable and broad advocacy tool for improving health care for children with chronic health conditions. It also serves as a model for future policy statements that relate more directly to adherence to chronic illness treatment.

CONCLUSIONS

The present chapter has demonstrated the importance of considering adherence as a pediatric advocacy concern and has proposed several next steps in the areas of clinical care, research, and policy development. The relevance of viewing adherence from an advocacy perspective and responding with appropriate clinical, research, and policy efforts is underscored by the current health care climate, which poses a number of threats to the quality of care for childhood chronic illness as evidenced by the present chapter. Patients, families, providers, and professional organizations each have a role in trying to shape the care provided to children with chronic health conditions within the rapidly expanding managed care environment.

REFERENCES

American Academy of Pediatrics. (1992). Ad hoc task force on definition of the medical home. *Pediatrics, 90,* 774.

American Academy of Pediatrics. (1995). Guiding principles for managed care arrangements for the health care of infants, children, adolescents, and young adults. *Pediatrics, 95,* 613–615.

American Academy of Pediatrics. (1998). Managed care and children with special health care needs: A subject review. *Pediatrics, 102,* 657–660.

American Academy of Pediatrics. (1999). *Medical home program for children with special needs* [Brochure]. Elk Grove Village, IL: Author.

Anderson, J. M. (1990). Home care management in chronic illness and the self-care movement: An analysis of ideologies and economic processes influencing decisions. *Advances in Nursing Science, 12,* 71–83.

Baum, D., & Creer, T. L. (1986). Medication compliance in children with asthma. *Journal of Asthma, 23,* 49–59.

Bender, B., Ikle, D., DuHamel, T., & Tinkelman, D. (1997). Retention of asthmatic patients in a longitudinal clinical trial. *Journal of Allergy & Clinical Immunology, 99,* 197–203.

Bender, B., Milgrom, H., & Rand, C. (1997). Nonadherence in asthmatic patients: Is there a solution to the problem? *Annals of Allergy, Asthma, & Immunology, 79,* 177–185.

Brazil, K., McLean, L., Abbey, D., & Musselman C. (1997). The influence of health education on family management of childhood asthma. *Patient Education and Counseling, 30,* 107–118.

Cadman, D., Boyle, M., Szatmari, P., & Offord, D. R. (1987). Chronic illness, disability, and mental and social well-being: Findings of the Ontario Child Health Study. *Pediatrics, 79,* 805–813.

Cartland, J. D. C., & Yudkowsky, B. K. (1992). Barriers to pediatric referral in managed care systems. *Pediatrics, 89,* 183–189.

Centers for Disease Control. (1996). Asthma mortality and hospitalization among children and young adults—United States, 1980–1993. *Morbidity and Mortality Weekly Report, 45*, 350–353.

Clark, N. M., Feldman, C. H., Evans, D., Duzey, O., Levison, M. J., Wasilewski, Y., Kaplan, D., Rips, J., & Mellins, R. B. (1986). Managing better: Children, parents, and asthma. *Patient Education and Counseling, 8*, 27–38.

Cluss, P. A., Epstein, L. H., Galvis, S. A., Fireman, P., & Friday, G. (1984). Effects of compliance for chronic asthmatic children. *Journal of Consulting and Clinical Psychology, 52*, 909–910.

Coleman, R. L. (1992). Promoting quality through managed care. *American Journal of Medical Quality, 7*, 100–105.

Colland, V. T. (1993). Learning to cope with asthma: A behavioural self-management program for children. *Patient Education and Counseling, 22*, 141–152.

Creagan, E. T. (1993). Psychosocial issues in oncologic practice. *Mayo Clinic Proceedings, 68*, 161–167.

Creer, T. L., & Bender, B. G. (1995). Pediatric asthma. In M. C. Roberts (Ed.), *Handbook of pediatric psychology* (2nd ed., pp. 219–240). New York: Guilford.

Creer, T. L., Levstek, D. A., & Reynolds, R. V. (1998). History and evaluation. In H. Kotses & A. Harver (Eds.), *Self-management of asthma* (pp. 379–405). New York: Marcel Dekker.

Dahl, J., Gustafsson, D., & Melin, L. (1990). Effects of a behavioral treatment program on children with asthma. *Journal of Asthma, 27*, 41–46.

Deal, L. W., Shiono, P. H., & Behrman, R. E. (1998). Children and managed health care: Analysis and recommendations. *The Future of Children, 8*, 4–24.

DiMatteo, M. R., Sherbourne, C. D., Hays, R. D., Ordway, L., Kravitz, R. L., McGlynn, E. A., Kaplan, S., & Rogers, W. H. (1993). Physicians' characteristics influence patients' adherence to medical treatment: Results from the medical outcomes study. *Health Psychology, 12*, 93–102.

Emanuel, E. J., & Dubler, N. N. (1995). Preserving the physician–patient relationship in the era of managed care. *Journal of the American Medical Association, 273*, 323–329.

England, M. J., & Cole, R. F. (1995). Children and mental health: How can the system be improved? *Health Affairs, 14*, 131–138.

Feldman, D. S., Novack, D. H., & Gracely, E. (1998). Effects of managed care on the physician-patient relationships, quality of care, and the ethical practice of medicine. *Archives of Internal Medicine, 158*, 1626–1632.

Fitzpatrick, S. B., Coughlin, S. S., & Chamberlin, J. (1992). A novel asthma camp intervention for childhood asthma among urban blacks. The Pediatric Lung Committee of the American Lung Association of the District of Columbia (ALADC) Washington, DC. *Journal of the National Medical Association, 84*, 233–237.

Fox, H. B., Wicks, L. B., & Newacheck, P. W. (1993). Health maintenance organizations and children with special health needs: A suitable match? *American Journal of Diseases in Childhood, 147*, 546–552.

Frank, R. G., Huskamp, H. A., McGuire, A. G., & Newhouse, J. P. (1996). Some economics of mental health "carve-outs." *Archives of General Psychiatry, 53*, 933–937.

Friedman, H. S., & DiMatteo, M. R. (1990). Patient–physician interactions. In S. A. Shumaker, E. B. Schron, & J. K. Ockene (Senior Eds.) & C. T. Parker, J. L. Probstfield, & J. M. Wolle (Co-Eds.), *The handbook of health behavior change* (pp. 84–101). New York: Springer.

Gebert, N., Hummelink, R., Konning, J. Staab, D., Schmidt, S., Szczepanski, R., Runde, B., & Wahn, U. (1998). Efficacy of a self-management program for childhood asthma—a prospective controlled study. *Patient Education and Counseling, 35*, 213–220.

Gillies, J., Barry, D., Crane, J., Jones, D., MacLennan, L., Pearce, N., Reid, J., Toop, L., & Wilson, B. (1996). A community trial of a written self management plan for children with asthma. *New Zealand Medical Journal, 109*, 30–33.

Golin, C. E., DiMatteo, M. R., & Gelberg, L. (1996). The role of patient participation in the doctor visit. *Diabetes Care, 19,* 1153–1163.

Godding, V., Kruth, M., & Jamart, J. (1997). Joint consultation for high-risk asthmatic children and their families, with pediatrician and child psychiatrist as co-therapists: Model and evaluation. *Family Process, 36,* 265–280.

Gortmaker, S. L., Walker, D. K., Weitzman, M., & Sobol, A. M. (1990). Chronic conditions, socioeconomic risks, and behavioral problems in children and adolescents. *Pediatrics, 85,* 267–276.

Greineder, D. K., Loane, K. C., & Parks, P. (1995). Reduction in resource utilization by an asthma outreach program. *Archives of Pediatric Adolescent Medicine, 149,* 415–420.

Greineder, D. K., Loane, K. C., & Parks, P. (1999). A randomized controlled trial of a pediatric asthma outreach program. *Journal of Allergy and Clinical Immunology, 103,* 436–440.

Grumbach, K., Osmond, D., Vranizan, K., Jaffe, D., & Bindman, A. B. (1998). Primary care physicians' experience of financial incentives in managed-care systems. *New England Journal of Medicine, 339,* 1516–1521.

Hammond, S. L., & Lambert, B. L. (1994). Communicating about medications: Directions for future research. *Health Communication, 6,* 247–251.

Hazzard, A., Hutchinson, S. J., & Krawiecki, N. (1990). Factors related to adherence to medication regimens in pediatric seizure patients. *Journal of Pediatric Psychology, 15,* 543–555.

Hillman, A. L., Pauly, M. V., & Kerstein, J. J. (1989). How do financial incentives affect physicians' clinical decisions and the financial performance of health maintenance organizations? *New England Journal of Medicine, 321,* 86–92.

Horwitz, S. M., & Stein, R. E. K. (1990). Health maintenance organizations vs. indemnity insurance for children with chronic illness. Trading gaps in coverage. *American Journal of Diseases of Children, 144,* 581–586.

Jensen, G. A., Morrisey, M. A., Gaffney, S., & Liston, D. K. (1997). The new dominance of managed care: Insurance trends in the 1990s. *Health Affairs, 16,* 125–136.

Johnson, S. B. (1994). Health behavior and health status: Concepts, methods, and applications. *Journal of Pediatric Psychology, 19,* 129–141.

Kelly, A. (1995). The primary care provider's role in caring for young people with chronic illness. *Journal of Adolescent Health, 17,* 32–36.

Kovach, J. S. (1996). Need for standardization of cancer practice via nationally accepted treatment guidelines. *Oncology, 10,* 41–43.

Kovacs, M., Goldston, D., Obrosky, D. S., & Iyengar, S. (1992). Prevalence and predictors of pervasive noncompliance with medical treatment among youths with insulin-dependent diabetes mellitus. *Journal of the American Academy of Child and Adolescent Psychiatry, 31,* 1112–1119.

Kuhlthau, K., Walker, D. K., Perrin, J. M., Bauman, I., Gortmaker, S. L., Newacheck, P. W., & Stein, R. E. K. (1998). Assessing managed care for children with chronic conditions. *Health Affairs, 17,* 42–52.

La Greca, A. M., & Schuman, W. B. (1995). Adherence to prescribed medical regimens. In M. C. Roberts (Ed.), *Handbook of pediatric psychology* (2nd ed., pp. 55–83). New York: Guilford.

Lavigne, J. V., & Faier-Routman, J. (1992). Psychological adjustment to pediatric physical disorders: A meta-analytic review. *Journal of Pediatric Psychology, 17,* 133–157.

Legorreta, A. P., Christian-Herman, J., O'Connor, R. D., Hasan, M.M., Evans, R., & Leung, K. M. (1998). Compliance with national asthma management guidelines and specialty care: A health maintenance organization experience. *Archives of Internal Medicine, 158,* 457–464.

Lemanek, K. (1990). Adherence issues in the medical management of asthma. *Journal of Pediatric Psychology, 15,* 437–458.

Matsui, D. M. (1997). Drug compliance in pediatrics. *Pediatric Clinics of North America, 44,* 1–14.

Mawhinney, H., Spector, S. L., Kinsman, R. A., Siegel, S. C., Rachelefsky, G. S., Katz, R. M., & Rohr, A. S. (1991). Compliance in clinical trials of two nonbronchodilator, anti-asthma medications. *Annals of Allergy, 66,* 294–299.

Mesters, I., van Nunen, M., Crebolder, H., & Meertens, R., (1995). Education of parents about pediatric asthma: Effects of a protocol on medical consumption. *Patient Education and Counseling, 25,* 131–136.

Meyers, K. E., Weiland, H., & Thomson, P. D. (1995). Pediatric renal transplantation non-compliance. *Pediatric Nephrology, 9,* 189–192.

Mihalik, G., & Scherer, M. (1998). Fundamental mechanisms of managed behavioral health care. *Journal of Health Care Financing, 24,* 1–15.

Newacheck, P. W., Budetti, P. P., & Halfon, N. (1986). Trends in activity-limiting chronic conditions among children. *American Journal of Public Health, 76,* 178–184.

Newacheck, P. W., Hughes, D. C., Halfon, N., & Brindis, C. (1997). Social HMOs and other capitated arrangements for children with special health care needs. *Maternal and Child Health Journal, 1,* 111–119.

O'Brien, P., & Hanley, F. L. (1992). New directions in pediatric heart transplantation. *Critical Care Nursing Clinics of North America, 4,* 193–203.

Price Waterhouse, LLP. (1995, November 8). *Estimating the financial impact of removing health insurance lifetime coverage caps.* Report to Genzyme Corporation.

Probst, J. C., Greenhouse, D. L., & Selassie, A. W. (1997). Patient and physician satisfaction with an outpatient care visit. *Journal of Family Practice, 45,* 418–425.

Rakos, R. F., Grodek, M. V., & Mack, K. K. (1985). The impact of a self-administered behavioral intervention program on pediatric asthma. *Journal of Psychosomatic Research, 29,* 101–108.

Rodriguez, A., Diaz, M., Colon, A., & Santiago-Delphin, E.A. (1991). Psychosocial profile of noncompliant transplant patients. *Transplantation Proceedings, 23,* 1807–1809.

Rovelli, M., Palmeri, D., Vossler, E., Bartus, S., Hull, D., & Scweizer, R. (1989). Noncompliance in renal transplant recipients. *Transplantation Proceedings, 21,* 833–834.

Safran, D. G., Taira, D. A., Rogers, W. H., Kosinski, M., Ware, J. E., & Tarlov, A. R. (1998). Linking primary care performance to outcomes of care. *Journal of Family Practice, 47,* 213–220.

Sclar, D. A., Tartaglione, T. A., & Fine, M. J. (1994). Overview of issues related to medical compliance with implications for the outpatient management of infectious diseases. *Infectious Agents and Disease, 3,* 266–273.

Shope, T. J. (1981). Medication compliance. *Pediatric Clinics of North America, 28,* 5–21.

Siegel, P. T. (1995). A description of Michigan's multidisciplinary specialty services program for chronically ill children and families. *Child, Youth, and Family Services Quarterly, 18,* 4–5.

Smith, C. E. (1996). Quality of life and caregiving in technological home care. *Annual Review of Nursing Research, 14,* 95–118.

Sperber, K., Ibrahim, H., Hoffman, B., Eisenmesser, B., Hsu, H., & Corn, B. (1995). Effectiveness of a specialized asthma clinic in reducing asthma morbidity in an inner-city minority population. *Journal of Asthma, 32,* 335–343.

Strunk, R. C. (1987). Asthma deaths in childhood: Identification of patients at risk and intervention. *Journal of Allergy & Clinical Immunology, 80,* 472–477.

Sturm, R., & McCulloch, J. (1998). Mental health and substance abuse benefits in carve-out plans and the Mental Health Parity Act of 1996. *Journal of Health Care Finance, 24,* 82–92.

Swanson, M., Hull, D., Bartus, S., & Schweizer, R. (1992). Economic impact of noncompliance in kidney transplant recipients. *Transplantation Proceedings, 24,* 2722.

Tal, D., Gil-Spielberg, R., Antonovsky, H., Tal, A., & Moaz, B. (1990). Teaching families to cope with childhood asthma. *Family Systems Medicine, 8,* 135–144.

Tehan, N., Sloane, B. C., Walsh-Robart, N., & Chamberlain, M. D. (1989). Impact of asthma self-management education on the health behavior of young adults. A pilot study of the Dartmouth College "Breathe Free" program. *Journal of Adolescent Health Care, 10,* 513–519.

Thompson, S., Dahlquist, L. M., Koenning, G. M., & Barholomew, L. K. (1995). Brief report: Adherence-facilitating behaviors of a multidisciplinary pediatric rheumatology staff. *Journal of Pediatric Psychology, 20,* 291–297.

Tighe, P., & Hardy Havens, D. (1997). Lifetime benefit caps: It could happen to you. *Journal of Pediatric Health Care, 11,* 243–246.

Vinicor, F. (1998). Diabetes mellitus and asthma: "Twin" challenges for public health and managed care systems. *American Journal of Preventative Medicine, 14,* 87–92.

Volsko, T. A. (1998). A pediatric asthma clinic pilot program reduces emergency department visits, hospitalizations, and costs of care. *Respiratory Care, 43,* 107–110.

Walders, N., & Drotar, D. (1999). Integrating health and mental health services in the care of children and adolescents with chronic health conditions: Assumptions, challenges, and opportunities. *Children's Services: Social Policy, Research, and Practice, 2,* 117–138.

Weinstein, A. G., & Faust, D. (1997). Maintaining theophylline compliance/adherence in severely asthmatic children: The role of psychologic functioning of the child and family. *Annals of Allergy, Asthma, and Immunology, 79,* 311–318.

Weinstein, A. G., Faust, D. S., McKee, L., & Padman, R. (1992). Outcome of short-term hospitalization for children with severe asthma. *Journal of Allergy and Clinical Immunology, 90,* 66–75.

Weinstein, A. G., McKee, L., Stapleford, J., & Faust, D. J. (1996). An economic evaluation of short-term inpatient rehabilitation for children with severe asthma. *Journal of Allergy and Clinical Immunology, 98,* 264–273.

Whitman, N., West, D., Brough, F. K., & Welch, M. (1985). A study of a self-care rehabilitation program in pediatric asthma. *Health Education Quarterly, 12,* 333–342.

Wilson, S. R., Latini, D., Starr, N. J., Fish, L., Loes, L. M., Page, A., & Kubic, P. (1996). Education of parents of infants and very young children with asthma: A developmental evaluation of the Wee Wheezers program. *Journal of Asthma, 33,* 239–254.

Womeodu, R. J., & Bailey, J. E. (1996). Barriers to cancer screening. *Medical Clinics of North America, 80,* 115–133.

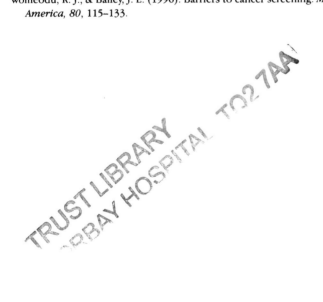

CHAPTER TEN

Practitioner–Family–Patient Communication in Pediatric Adherence: Implications for Research and Clinical Practice

M. Robin DiMatteo
University of California, Riverside, CA

Failure to adhere to medical treatment regimens is a complex and often frustrating phenomenon that appears to be influenced by a vast array of social and psychological factors. In the case of adult chronic illness, the influences of the physician–patient relationship and patients' beliefs, feelings, habits, social norms, and social support on patients' choices to follow or avoid medical advice are well established. When the adherence of a child or adolescent to chronic illness treatment is at stake, there is the potential for even greater complexity in determining adherence if only because more people, each with their unique perspectives, opinions, developmental stages, and relationships, are involved.

The conceptual work and empirical research on the role of communication in adherence is relatively well established in research on adults with chronic illness. Issues of communication have received less attention, however, in the study of interactions in the pediatric realm (Glasgow & Anderson, 1995). Consequently, there is much to be learned about relationships among patients, pediatricians, and families, as well as about issues of active patient involvement, trust, and negotiation—particularly about how these factors foster or inhibit adherence to prescribed treatments.

To address this need, the goals of this chapter are several. The first is to delineate the relationship between adherence and communication among providers, pediatric patients, and their families and to review this relatively new area of empirical research for pediatric populations. Another goal is to suggest some possible clinical applications of what is currently known, guided by the extensive research on adult chronic illness. Further, necessary research directions and methodological considerations are delineated. It is hoped that this analysis ultimately contributes to health psychology research and practice on pediatric chronic disease management.

THE ISSUE OF PATIENT ADHERENCE

Despite recent impressive advances in the medical management of chronic diseases and the enhanced potential for improvement in quality of life, the behavioral phenomenon of noncompliance (also called *nonadherence*) continues to plague medical care delivery and threaten the outcomes of health care (Trostle, 1997). Noncompliance may be a major cause of the proliferation of drug-resistant diseases, serious drug reactions and interactions, and the waste of billions of health care dollars (Fox, 1983).

The broadest definition of *noncompliance* is that the patient fails to manifest behaviorally the health professional's (usually physician's) intended treatment regimen. Because medical care is delivered through the interpersonal interaction between health professional and patient, any intended regimen must be communicated to the patient. Once communicated, it must be fully understood, believed in, committed to, and acted on. Decades of research on (primarily) adult and pediatric populations suggest that this chain of events should not be taken for granted. Nearly half of adult patients with chronic diseases fail to adhere to their regimens—many because they do not understand them or do not want to carry them out, or simply cannot succeed in doing so (DiMatteo & DiNicola, 1982; Epstein & Cluss, 1982; Meichenbaum & Turk, 1987). The extent of the problem appears to be similar in the care of pediatric chronic illness. For example, in the treatment of pediatric insulin-dependent diabetes mellitus (IDDM), one study found that 25% of patients regularly missed their insulin injections, 81% ate an improper diet, and 29% did not conduct all of their required blood glucose monitoring (sometimes reporting false results to their health professionals; Johnson et al., 1992).

THE CENTRAL ELEMENTS OF PEDIATRIC HEALTH PROFESSIONAL–PATIENT COMMUNICATION

Effective communication is not an easy thing to accomplish in any medical care delivery setting. Technological advances in the treatment of the chronically ill, including children and adolescents, have in some ways limited communication more than ever. There are now so many occasions to do things to patients that often there is little time to talk with patients and their families and learn how a given chronic illness affects their present lives and threatens their hopes for the future (Kleinman, 1988). Health professionals, particularly physicians, are often quite separated from patients and their families by the *competence gap* (Parsons, 1951), which grows wider as the science of medicine progresses. In this competence gap, health professionals typically have far more technical information about patients' cases than do patients and their families. As Kleinman (1988) noted, such differences can cause patients/families and their physicians to have quite different perspectives on the illness. Specifically, physicians tend to view illness in terms of altered biology, whereas patients and their families view illness in terms of its effects on functioning and quality of life. Further, unless they examine these issues explicitly, physicians may know little about the beliefs, commitment, supports, difficulties, and outcome preferences of the patient and family members and about the dynamics of family members' relationships to each other and to the regimen.

As Kleinman (1988) noted, such issues must be addressed in order to provide effective care for patients. In the pediatric realm, where several family members in addition to the patient may be involved, careful attention to communication may be essential to bring patient, family, and physician expectations and goals into alignment. The following sections examine the role of communication in helping patients and their families make effective choices about following their recommended care.

THE COMPLEXITIES OF COMMUNICATION

In the treatment of childhood chronic diseases (examples being IDDM and childhood asthma), effective communication is required not only about the medical regimen, but also about a multitude of factors. These include: (a) what patients and their families know and believe about the disease and its treatment, (b) how the regimen fits with their family life and habits, (c) what supports are available to the patient and family, and (d) how the patient and family relate to their health professionals. The existing research on such aspects of communication is far more extensive in the realm of adult care than in that of pediatrics. The research on adults has clearly demonstrated that communication regarding adherence is indeed multifaceted, and that the issues of concern are both task-oriented and socioemotional in nature (DiMatteo & Lepper, 1998). In the following sections, the findings of research with pediatric populations are reviewed, work with adult populations is applied to the communciation between pediatricians and patients/families, and an approach to research and clinical application is suggested.

Information About the Regimen

It seems obvious that patients (and, in the case of pediatric care, families) need to understand what they are being asked to do by health professionals before they have any hope of doing it. Yet at least in the medical care of adults, communication of the therapeutic regimen is often so unclear that about half of adult patients leave their physicians' offices and do not know what they have been asked to do in order to take care of themselves (Ley, 1979). Studies suggest that the information actually provided to patients is often surprisingly inadequate, and that treatment recommendations are often inexplicit and stated in vague terms (Faden, Becker, Lewis, Freeman, & Faden, 1981; Waitzkin & Stoeckle, 1976). Studies of adult patients suggest that many have little insight into why their medication is even needed, and they state that it was never explained to them (Glasgow, Wilson, & McCaul, 1985; Stanton, 1987). Insufficient time is available for patients to ask the questions necessary to support their beliefs in and positive expectations for the course of treatment (Leedham, Meyerowitz, Muirhead, & Frist, 1995; Stanton, 1987).

With pediatric chronic illness populations, the importance of knowledge in diabetes management in children and adolescents has been demonstrated extensively (Christensen, 1983). One study of pediatric adherence found that health professionals recorded the information that they provided to pediatric patients in their charts, but rarely was there evidence that health professionals addressed patients' concerns and barriers to implementing the recommendations or employed any kind of behavior modification strategies to help patients adhere (Thompson, Dahlquist, Koenning, & Bartholomew, 1995). In the treatment of asthma, Creer and Levstek (1997) noted the importance of teaching patients to take their medication as prescribed and describing the potential side effects of medications because surprise about side effects can easily lead to noncompliance. They also stressed the role of written summaries of asthma medications and methods for regular tracking and follow-up of patients' adherence. These researcher found, however, that such methods were often lacking in regular pediatric asthma treatment. Further, demonstrations of how to use inhalers and other devices correctly were found to be critically important, but rarely provided, sometimes because the medical personnel did not know how to use the devices correctly.

Certainly one of the most basic elements of communication involves finding out whether patients are, in fact, cooperating with the recommendations. One study reported that, in the pediatric setting, the accuracy of primary health providers' estimates of patient adherence was quite low, and that health professionals tended to vastly overestimate the percentage of parents that were adherent to treatment strategies for their children (Finney et al., 1993).

Trust and the Therapeutic Relationship

Trust is a critically important element of medical care. In the realm of adult adherence, patients have been found to be reluctant to take on challenging health care regimens suggested by health professionals whom they did not trust (Roter & Hall, 1992). Conversely, several studies have suggested that patient adherence is heavily dependent on patient satisfaction with the psychosocial aspects of the physician–patient relationship, including the patient's trust in the good will of the physician and the physician's positive expectations for healing (Roter & Hall, 1992). Indeed, Hazzard, Hutchinson, and Krawiecki (1990) found that adherence to care in a pediatric neurology setting was associated with parents' and children's satisfaction with the care that was delivered.

Research with adult patients suggests why trust in the physician and satisfaction with the psychosocial aspects of care may be important to adherence. Supportive health professionals may be better able than others to help patients and their families commit themselves to the efforts necessary to follow a treatment regimen (Rodin & Janis, 1979). Provider sensitivity to elements of the environment that pose limitations to patient adherence, and provider expressions of respect, rapport, empathy, understanding, and acceptance of patients' emotional experience tend to build trust and in turn enhance patient satisfaction and efforts to adhere to treatment (DiMatteo, Hays et al., 1993; DiMatteo, Hays, & Prince, 1986; DiMatteo, Linn, Chang, & Cope, 1985; Squier, 1990). Trust is built on provider empathy and attention not only to the disease, but also to the patient's and the family's distress and experiences of illness (H. Brody, 1992; Cassell, 1985).

Research on issues related to trust in the pediatric relationship paints an interesting picture. One study of physician–parent communication about psychosocial problems found that pediatricians had to depend on their own observations and judgments because parents were reluctant to bring their children's problems to the physicians' attention. Most respondent parents (81%) believed that, in theory, it was appropriate to discuss psychosocial issues with their children's physicians, but only 41% of them actually did (Horwitz, Leaf, & Leventhal, 1998). Delamater, Kurtz, White, and Santiago (1988) and Wilson and Endres (1986) reported high percentages of distorted reports by children and adolescents to health professionals about the results of their blood glucose testing, suggesting that the clinical encounter was not conducive to honest reporting and that the children may not have trusted their health professionals to be supportive of them. Further, Worchel et al. (1995) found that physicians tended to underestimate the degree to which parents desired pediatrician–parent interaction in the care of their children.

Parental comfort with disclosure of sensitive information is, not surprisingly, affected by pediatricians' own interview style. In one study, when pediatricians asked questions about psychosocial issues, made supportive statements, and listened attentively, parents were found to disclose more specific concerns relevant to their child's mental health than when those elements of communication were missing (Wissow, Roter, & Wilson, 1994). Further, Street (1991) found that parents' perceptions of physicians' informativeness, interpersonal sensitivity, and partnership-building were positively correlated with their evaluations of the quality of their children's health care. The satisfaction of anxious parents was more strongly correlated with perceptions of the physicians' interpersonal sensitivity than it was for less worried parents.

There have been a few observational studies of the process of interaction in the pediatric visit using audiotape, transcription, and content analysis. Pediatric interactions have generally been found to be highly stylized, with pediatricians taking charge of the interviews, asking more questions, and talking twice as much as parents (Arntson & Philipsborn, 1982; Sprunger, 1983). Pediatricians have also been found to use higher intonation patterns in their speech with children and lower intonations with parents, presumably to help children feel more relaxed and comfortable and to demonstrate competency to parents (Worobey, O'Hair, & O'Hair, 1987).

However, these studies did not relate interaction patterns to outcomes such as pediatric adherence to treatment. Recent changes in the delivery of health care, particularly the institution of managed care, have introduced new challenges to the building and maintenance of trust in the therapeutic relationship (Mechanic & Schlesinger, 1996). At least in the views of many adult patients, trust can be eroded when physicians operate as gatekeepers to specialists and costly services. Managed care medicine tends to come with briefer visits, the need for third party approval for diagnostic and treatment decisions, formulary controls sometimes resulting in changes of familiar medications, and limitations on access to specialists (see Walders, Nobile, & Drotar, chap. 9, this volume). Sometimes, too, continuity of care is compromised because patients are forced to switch from one primary care physician to another as physician panels change, patients change jobs, or employers respond to market pressures and change managed care plans for their employees. The implications of managed care changes for pediatric adherence are just beginning to be felt. For example, Heffer et al. (1997) recently found that lack of continuity of care and less time spent with the pediatrician were related to a greater frequency of forgotten instructions by parents.

Beliefs of the Patient and Family

In the research on adult adherence to treatment, the importance of patient beliefs is well established (Hampson, Glasgow, & Toobert, 1990). Skepticism about the regimen is one of the primary causes of reduced adherence

(Leedham et al., 1995; Stanton, 1987). Patients' beliefs in the expected efficacy and value of the treatment regimen, specifically the preponderance of treatment benefits over costs (in terms of time, attention, difficulty, and finances), help establish patient commitment to adherence behavior (DiMatteo,1995; Leedham et al., 1995; Stanton, 1987). In other words, adherence is enhanced when patients believe that the regimen is worth following. In a pediatric chronic illness population, Van Sciver, D'Angelo, Rappaport, and Woolf (1995) found that positive attitudes toward treatment were associated with better compliance behavior among boys with hemophilia. In addition, beliefs of patients and their families in the severity of a disease and their susceptibility to it have been found to enhance adherence to preventive and treatment efforts (Maiman, Becker, & Katlic, 1985). Parental beliefs that the child faces a significant mortality or morbidity risk, or has poor health status, have been shown in two studies to have a detrimental effect on adherence (Gudas, Koocher, & Wypij, 1991; Scarfone, Joffe, Wiley, Loiselle, & Cook, 1996). Further, as has been found in studies of adults with serious illnesses, such as those with vision loss due to glaucoma (Kugelmann & Bensinger, 1983; Patel & Spaeth, 1995), potentially fatal complications of end stage renal disease (Bame, Petersen, & Wray, 1993; Wolcott, Maida, Diamond, & Nissenson, 1986), and human immunodeficiency virus/AIDS (Singh et al., 1996; Slavin, 1996), nonadherence may be fostered by denial, survivor guilt, and other complex, irrational, or illogical factors (Sensky, Leger, & Gilmour, 1996).

Sociocultural Norms

To fully understand the pressures supporting or inhibiting patient adherence, researchers on adult adherence have turned to the role of sociocultural norms and constraints that guide patients' and families' responses to medical recommendations. These include specific cultural beliefs that conflict with documented medical findings, general skepticism about medical care, and embarrassment and social stigma attached to care-seeking and regimen implementation. Cultural factors strongly influence beliefs about the meaning of medication and self-care activities, as well as about the causes, symptoms, course, and treatment of the disease (Hampson et al., 1990). They also affect the individual's cognitive representations of the disease and personal metaphors of illness (e.g., that glaucoma is a normal aspect of aging or a reaction to stress or pressure [Gurwitz et al., 1993] or that chronic disease complications are a manifestation of Fate [Kimmel et al., 1995]). Despite the deficiency of pediatric research on this issue, it is reasonable to expect that pediatric adherence behavior is shaped at least partly by familial norms of health behavior, and that these norms provide clinically relevant perspectives on the meaning of illness and appropriate behavioral responses to it.

Commitment

Considerable evidence is accumulating in the study of adult adherence to treatment that commitment is a prerequisite to behavioral change. For example, the transtheoretical model notes that change does not begin with action, but rather with cognition and commitment (Prochaska et al., 1994). Relatedly, the Theory of Reasoned Action is built on the premise that intentions are necessary, but not sufficient, for behavior change (Ajzen & Fishbein, 1980). As noted in research on adult adherence to treatment, commitment is essential because it requires active analysis, in which the individual is forced to consider such issues as whether health and survival are worth the costs of adherence (Katz, 1984). Issues of free will and self-determination are brought to the forefront as patients and their families, working with their health professionals, decide whether they want to commit themselves to action. Nonadherence certainly can result from passivity, denial, laziness, or forgetfulness. However, when faced with the need to make a commitment one way or the other, patients must work actively to make a decision about what they are going to do. Reminders, supports, and other forms of practical assistance can be effective only after patients have made a commitment to action (Rivers, 1992). In adult populations, clinical recommendations have been most successful when they include questions about commitment, such as: How will you take your medication? or Will you take it? (Pozsik, 1993). In the pediatric setting, the elicitation of a parent's *promise* to the physician to give all doses of the prescribed medication to the child resulted in significantly higher adherence to an antibiotic regimen (Kulik & Carlino, 1987). Encouragement to make a behavioral commitment to others, such as family and friends, can improve adherence if that commitment is based firmly on beliefs that strongly support the behavior.

Family/Patient Habits

Of course, if commitment were all that is necessary for health behavior change, no one would ever break a New Year's resolution. Past adherence behavior (i.e., habitual behavior) is an extremely strong predictor of future adherence to treatment in adults, even independent of commitment (DiMatteo, Hays et al., 1993; DiMatteo, Sherbourne et al., 1993). Although not exactly slaves to stimulus–response patterns, most patients find that habit is a strong force in the realm of health behavior (Brownell, Marlatt, Lichtenstein, & Wilson, 1986). For this reason, effective therapeutic communication requires recognition of and work with patients' and families' habitual response patterns and the reinforcements that have maintained them.

Habits can be particularly troubling if pediatric patients and their families have had significant difficulties adhering in the past. For example, Finney and colleagues (1993) found that the application of contingency-based interventions resulted in adherence to pediatric medical regimens only as long as the contingencies were available. Once they were withdrawn, patients returned to their habits of nonadherence behaviors. Further, pediatric adherence to particular aspects of an IDDM regimen has been found to be inversely related to the degree of lifestyle habit change required by the task (Glasgow, McCaul, & Schafer, 1986; Wysocki & Greco, 1997).

Barriers Faced by Family and Patient

Effective communication is necessary if a physician is to understand what a patient and his or her family are experiencing in their attempts to cope with an illness and its treatment. Studies of adult adherence demonstrate the importance of effective physician–patient communication in assisting patients to deal with the emotional strain and physical challenges of their treatment, including exhaustion, frustration, and interference with treasured activities (Kleinman, 1988). Many pediatric chronic disease regimens are prolonged and troublesome, causing psychological stress and adversely affecting the quality of life of the patients and their families. Effective communication toward the goal of adherence includes determining the extent to which the family can cope with the complexity of the regimen (including the number of medication doses per day, medication discomfort and side effects, and financial constraints; Korsch et al., 1978; Palardy et al., 1998). In the treatment of IDDM, the number and severity of barriers were negatively related to patient adherence (Glasgow et al., 1986). Creer and Levstek (1997) have noted the particular importance in pediatric asthma care of reducing the complexity of the regimen, eliminating ineffective medications, prescribing those that cause the fewest side effects, minimizing the number of lifestyle changes, and reducing the costs of medications.

In both pediatric and adult populations, chronic daily stress in patients' and families' lives has been found to be a major barrier to adherence, and in some cases, to affect health outcomes significantly (Cox & Gonder-Frederick, 1992; Everett, Brantley, Sletten, Jones, & McKnight, 1995). For example, high stress has been strongly associated with poor glycemic control in diabetics—both because of the direct effects of stress on metabolic functioning in children and adults and, less consistently, because of a mediating effect through poor adherence (Chase & Jackson, 1981; Halford, Cuddihy, & Mortimer, 1990; Hanson et al., 1987). Bussing, Burket, and Kelleher (1996) found that psychosocial variables such as stress and anxiety also may affect the clinical course of childhood asthma.

Social Network and Social Support

A persuasive argument for the role of social support in patient adherence has been provided numerous times (Cox & Gonder-Frederick, 1992; Wolcott et al., 1986). Adherence can be greatly assisted by individuals who support the patient with both practical aid and emotional support. In the realm of pediatric care, family members who are centrally involved as cheerleaders, facilitators, and esteem builders provide the support that has been shown to have a powerful effect on adherence (Anderson, Ho, Brackett, Finkelstein, & Laffel, 1997; Irwin, Millstein, & Ellen, 1993). In IDDM, for example, supportive family relationships have been found to be strong positive predictors of adherence (Hanson et al., 1987).

One of the strongest predictors of long-term nonadherence in the treatment of IDDM is family conflict. Parents' and children's perceptions of family cohesion predicted improvement in adherence and overall higher levels of adherence, whereas family conflict has been found to be quite problematic for treatment adherence (Hauser et al., 1990).

Social support from both family and friends seems to be ideal in promoting a child's or adolescent's general and disease-specific functioning, at least in the care of IDDM. La Greca and colleagues (1995) found that family members were more likely than peers to offer tangible support, such as providing reminders and assisting with various diabetes care tasks. Peers, however, provided more companionship and emotional support than did family. In one study in a pediatric nephrology setting, the social isolation that resulted from family overprotectiveness interfered with the development of the pediatric patients' personal competency and brought about significant reductions in patient adherence (Davis, Tucker, & Fennell, 1996). Thus, as Wysocki and Greco (1997) argued, effective care of IDDM requires family acceptance of the child's/adolescent's social engagement outside the family and support of helpful peer relationships.

THE UNIQUE CHALLENGES
OF PEDIATRIC CHRONIC DISEASE CARE

There are several reasons that pediatric chronic illness may present challenges beyond those encountered in the care of chronically ill adults. First, as Glasgow and Anderson (1995) noted, child development brings changes in beliefs, attitudes, social interaction patterns, self-direction, autonomy, and dependency needs. All of these factors have implications for the clinical care of patients and their adherence to treatment recommendations. Such changes present significant challenges in clinical practice not only because children and adolescents are likely to differ from each other, but also because the same child may change drastically over time as he or she progresses from childhood to adolescence. Johnson (1995) described the role of developmental changes among children and adolescents with IDDM in terms of their knowledge and skill, attitudes toward the disease, daily management, and role of parental supervision. She also noted that hormonal changes may affect the progress of the disease. Similar fundamental issues distinguish pediatric asthma from the same illness in adults. These include different developmental and physical growth patterns, family influences, emotional precipitants, environmental risks, coping styles, and cultural influences on attributions of physical and emotional distress (Fritz & Wamboldt, 1998) .

Second, family conflict, noted earlier as a correlate of nonadherence, is often common during adolescence. When a child reaches adolescence, his or her attempts at individuation may threaten the treatment regimen and endanger his or her health (Dolgin, Katz, Doctors, & Siegel, 1986; Garrison, Biggs, & Williams, 1990; Lorenz, Christensen, & Pichert, 1985). As Wysocki and Greco (1997) noted, family functioning can be an important predictor of the family's ability to adapt to the demands of care in IDDM. Family dysfunction and the lack of family cohesiveness can interfere with the regimen (Chaney & Peterson, 1989; Hauser et al., 1990; McCaul, Glasgow, & Schafer, 1987). Further, low expectations about the ability of the patient, as well as overtly expressed worry, can weaken the patients' sense of self-efficacy and interfere with the patient's efforts at self-care (Taal, Rasker, Seydel, & Wiegman, 1993).

Third, the communication matrix in the care of pediatric chronic illness may be even more complicated than it typically is in the care of adults. For example, the message about what to do in order to be adherent to treatment must reach several people, including the child or adolescent and at least one family member (and possibly several). Opportunities for misunderstanding may be many. Further, several individuals with varying degrees of knowledge and patterns of health beliefs may need to accept the regimen and be willing and able to help the patient carry it out. Sometimes various family members will be able to work out any differences between them toward the common goal of achieving the child's treatment adherence. The danger exists, however, that disagreements resulting from complex and difficult family relationships (Hauser et al., 1990) may bring family members to undermine each other and the patient's treatment adherence (Goldenberg & Goldenberg, 1980; Minuchin, 1974; Minuchin, Rosman, & Baker, 1978). Moreover, family members who are concerned for the patient might offer suggestions to change or modify the regimen without consulting the health professionals involved (Waisbren, Hamilton, St. James, Shiloh, & Levy, 1995).

THE IMPORTANCE OF A MULTIDIMENSIONAL APPROACH
TO ADHERENCE IN THE TREATMENT OF CHRONIC ILLNESS

In research on adult populations, the need for a multilevel, multidimensional approach to adherence explanation, prediction, and change has become increasingly apparent (Agras, 1993). Over the past three decades, there have been several thousand published papers about patient adherence. Qualitative reviews and opinions abound; and empirical research, particularly on adults, is plentiful (Trostle, 1997). Most of this empirical research, however, examines one or two predictors of adherence in observational study or uses an experimental intervention to improve adherence. Not surprisingly, these studies demonstrate that doing something to help patients comply is better than doing nothing, and that compliance can usually be found to correlate with something about the patient (e.g., motivation), the regimen (e.g., complexity of dosing), or the interaction between patient and health professional (e.g., communication).

Despite this abundance of research, however, only a few studies have simultaneously examined multiple elements of the complex phenomenon of adherence (e.g., Glasgow et al., 1989). Consequently, not much is known about how the many relevant adherence predictors operate in concert or interact with one another. Understanding the multiple factors that influence pediatric adherence is particularly important because many pediatric chronic illness regimens are demanding, both behaviorally and psychologically. In the study of IDDM , for example, it has been advantageous to use a broad biopsychosocial perspective on self-management that emphasizes the interrelationships among key biological, cognitive, behavioral, and environmental factors (Cox & Gonder-Frederick, 1992; Ruggiero & Javorsky, 1999). Wysocki and Greco (1997) examined the multiple factors involved in the development of competent diabetes self-management and its effects on health status and affective adjustment to diabetes. In addition, Hanson, DeGuire, Schinkel, Henggeler, and Burghen (1992) used a multidimensional approach to compare social learning and family systems correlates of adaptation in youth with IDDM. They found that illness-specific and general family functioning (such as positive and supportive family relations, general family affection, and general family adaptability) predicted subjects' adherence to diet and their general psychosocial adaptation. Kewman, Warschausky, and Engel (1995) noted that, in the care of pediatric rheumatoid disorders and neuromuscular conditions, complex factors affect compliance including cognitive and affective development, pain, family functioning, and adaptation. Finally, Ricker, Delamater, and Hsu (1998) documented the role of age, perceived family behaviors, health locus of control, and self-competency in determining adherence to a cystic fibrosis (CF) regimen.

Multidimensional approaches to adherence are essential to successful change in adherence-related behavior. Bringing about adherence change requires designing and maintaining a treatment package that develops from an understanding of the entire picture of adherence in a given population (Dishman, 1982). "It is unlikely that any intervention attempt that ignores the multidimensionality of the problem will accomplish long run alterations of health-related behavior" (Hoover, 1989, p. 959). Unless we fully understand the phenomenon of adherence as a multidimensional construct, it is difficult to know when, where, and how best to intervene, particularly when resources are limited and choices need to be made among various possible alternatives (Martin & Dubbert, 1982). Further, unless we understand the complex elements of adherence, our efforts to change one element may result in inadvertent alteration of others (Hampson, Glasgow, & Toobert, 1990).

Therefore, research approaches and clinical suggestions to improving pediatric adherence should incorporate multiple elements of patients' lives, including their developmental level, motivations, beliefs, knowledge, barriers, norms, social support, social adjustment, and psychological history, as well as multiple aspects of communication in the clinical interaction (Sensky, Leger, & Gilmour, 1996). Both research and clinical approaches to adherence should be flexible in their incorporation of psychological, sociocultural, cognitive, and health transaction variables (Gurwitz et al., 1993).

CLINICAL APPLICATIONS

Effective practitioner–patient–family communication in the care of adult chronic illnesses involves the challenge of attending simultaneously to numerous elements in patients' lives, including the psychological, social, and behavioral. Evidence is accumulating, as described earlier, that multiple factors are also necessary to consider in any attempts to foster adherence to regimens for pediatric chronic illness. Given the many demands of the medical aspects of pediatric practice, it goes without saying that attention to psychosocial care is likely to take place only if efficient and effective methods for doing so can be suggested.

One possible efficient organizational approach derives from the following basic (almost obvious) conclusion from the copious research on adult adherence. Decades of research seem to suggest the strikingly simple conclusion that people do what they want and only what they can. Further, they typically cannot adhere to recommendations they do not understand. This summary generates three important clinical implications and three suggested (fairly easy-to-remember) corresponding components of a potential clinical checklist that is applicable to practice.

First, the clinician should be sure that patients fully understand what they are being asked to do in order to take care of themselves (see Ievers-Landis & Drotar, chap. 11, this volume). This involves encouraging patients to ask questions, fully answering those questions, and obtaining feedback from patients about what they understand about what they have been told. The clinician should provide patients with written follow-up to the verbal recommendations given in the medical visit.

Second, the clinician should determine, through sensitive questioning, whether patients have any desire and intention to follow their treatment recommendations. If they do not and the clinician wants them to, ideally he or she must determine the source of patient resistance, engage in persuasive techniques to enhance patients' beliefs in the efficacy and benefits of the regimen, and explore with patients the beliefs of influential others about the treatment regimen. This second clinical goal is intended to build patient commitment to the challenging task of adherence. Health professionals must urge patients and their families to want what is best for them, to believe in the value of treatment directives, to be motivated to follow them, and to commit to their long-term implementation. In modern popular culture, advertisers seem to define our needs and motivate our actions quite well, even in highly pervasive domains such as what we eat and how we dress. Perhaps health professionals would do well to build persuasive communication with patients and their families, making their messages clear and unambiguous, attending to patients' and families' beliefs in the efficacy and benefits of treatment, emphasizing the presence of supportive social norms, and eliciting intentions and commitment to bring about behavior change.

Third, and finally, once it is clear that patients intend to try to follow the regimen, the clinician should help them anticipate and overcome frustrating barriers and help patients and their families to be able to follow treatment recommendations. For example, the clinician should simplify the regimen, enhance its organization, and/or reduce its cost whenever possible. The clinician should eliminate unpleasant side effects or at least help make them bearable for patients. The clinician should encourage or arrange supports in the form of physical assistance and emotional nurturance (e.g., support groups, strengthening of family ties).

A related clinical issue is worthy of note. In the research literature on adult adherence and physician–patient communication, an issue arises that is deserving of careful clinical exploration in pediatric settings. It has been suggested that an inevitable concomitant of exploring the beliefs, commitments, and outcome preferences of patients and their families is conflict—between the views and opinions of the physician and those of the patient/family. Realistically, it is reasonable to expect that the several parties to clinical decisions are not always going to agree with one another, and such conflict should be expected (Brody, 1992). Although health professionals may prefer to avoid this conflict, such avoidance may actually be detrimental to the quality of care, communication, and adherence to treatment (DiMatteo & Lepper, 1998). At least in the care of adults, disagreement opens up the possibility for a process of negotiation that may ultimately lead to better outcomes. This is possible because a negotiated approach to care (cf. Speedling & Rose, 1985) allows and facilitates patients' and families' preferences for the process and outcomes of treatment to be incorporated into the decision-making process (Freidson, 1961, 1970; Lazare, Eisenthal, Frank, & Stoeckle, 1978). In the realm of pediatric care, the research evidence on this issue is simply not yet available, yet it may be worth considering and exploring. In attempts to achieve tight glycemic control in adolescent IDDM, for example, clinical exploration of what adolescents and their families are willing to do, and about what they believe they are capable of accomplishing, may open the door to a negotiated regimen that is more likely to be followed than one that is dictated. Rather than providing strict guidelines and ultimatums, it may be preferable to open up discussion and negotiation with patients and their families, seeking to surface and resolve conflicts so that noncompliance and its causes will not be hidden from the physician.

These recommendations are potentially difficult to implement, especially under the constraints of managed care. However, effective management of pediatric adherence requires attention to these issues in clinical care by physician providers and/or other members of the health care team (see Walders, Nobile, & Drotar, chap. 9, this volume).

A RESEARCH AGENDA

Several conceptual and methodological challenges arise from the multifactorial approach to pediatric adherence recommended in this chapter. First, the formulation and validation of standardized methods for quantifying both the intensity of treatments (in terms of investments of time, money, and other costs) and the developmental stages of pediatric patients are necessary for the further exploration and prediction of patient adherence. In the treatment of CF, for example, all other factors to be considered in understanding adherence are likely to be affected by the time- and labor-intensity of treatment (Miller, Jelalian, & Stark , 1999).

Second, as Glasgow and Anderson (1995) noted, it is important in research on pediatric adherence to control for demographic, developmental, and medical variables, preferably in longitudinal studies that examine the same children over time. Longitudinal research is particularly important in the study of coping and psychological adjustment, which in many pediatric diseases, such as IDDM, can evolve through various developmental stages in children and adolescents (Hauser et al., 1990).

Third, a necessary next step in fully understanding the complex elements of pediatric adherence involves fully organizing, reviewing, and summarizing the copious literature on pediatric adherence. With the research technique of meta-analysis (Rosenthal, 1991), quantitative review of the literature can be achieved. This allows for a better overall understanding of the complex relationships between adherence and characteristics of patients, their lives, their diseases, their regimens, the therapeutic relationship, and the context of medical care delivery. As an example, one study (Brown & Hedges, 1994) combined data from 17 studies published between 1982 and 1991 to test a multiple variable approach to explaining metabolic control in diabetes. Predictors of metabolic control selected for this analysis were knowledge, health beliefs, barriers, commitment, cues to action, expectancies, impact on lifestyle, support, susceptibility, and compliance/adherence.

A fourth research challenge involves the conceptualization and operationalization of adherence measurement. In practice, the majority of researchers on adherence have relied on self-report—a technique that may lead to misguided conclusions because, although patients may know their own behavior best, they may be prone to misleading self-presentation (Stanton, 1987). More technical approaches, such as pill counts, patient behavioral diaries, and electronic recording devices (e.g., MEMS units), have their own drawbacks, not the least of which may involve patients' manipulation of them when they desire to conceal their nonadherence (Granstrom, 1982).

Another important research goal involves the development and implementation of methods for building patient trust so that patients and families can be forthcoming and frank about their difficulties in following treatment suggestions (Hays & DiMatteo, 1987).

The conceptualization of adherence is an additional issue requiring further development by researchers. A common error in conceptualization (and hence assessment) of adherence involves the confusion of adherence behaviors with adherence outcomes. A patient might carry out flawlessly every behavioral expectation for his or her care, but the outcome remains disappointing. For example, despite regular glucose monitoring and active adjustment of diet, exercise, and insulin injection, an adolescent with IDDM may experience suspicious glycosolated hemoglobin results (Johnson et al., 1992). Thus, researchers should pay scrupulous attention to the accurate assessment of behavior and recognize that physiological measures should not serve as proxies for adherence (Cox & Gonder-Frederick, 1992).

Likewise, it should be recognized that biochemical markers of treatment success do not necessarily reflect better disease control and management, as well as better patient functioning and quality of life. In addition to the effect of adherence on physiological parameters, researchers should focus on the role of adherence in achieving health outcomes, health status, functional status, psychological and social functioning, and all aspects of health-related quality of life (Colaco et al., 1987; Mayer, Greco, Troncone, Auricchio, & Marsh, 1991; Murphy et al., 1997). Particularly because of the important role that day-to-day adherence management may play in the development of children and adolescents with chronic conditions, it is critically important for pediatric health professionals to consistently gather and assess data on the role of adherence in health outcomes and to determine the degree to which intensive management of the disease has enough of a positive effect on current and long-term outcomes to make adherence worth its cost (Ruggiero & Javorsky, 1999).

Finally, the ideal approach to research on multiple predictors and explanatory factors in adherence would be longitudinal studies using a causal modeling approach (Stanton, 1987). Such research requires relatively large samples (150 or more patients) to study more than a handful of variables. This might be particularly difficult in the study of diseases such as CF, for which only relatively small populations are available, especially at one site (Ricker, Delamater, & Hsu, 1998). Even when subjects may be plentiful, longitudinal data collection is time-consuming and expensive. Adequate funding for such longitudinal, multisite studies, particularly for the complexities of measurement development and subject retention, is essential.

REFERENCES

Agras, W. S. (1993). Adherence intervention research: The need for a multilevel approach. In N. A. Krasnegor, L. Epstein, S. B. Johnson, & S. J. Yaffe (Eds.), *Developmental aspects of health compliance behavior* (pp. 285–301). Hillsdale, NJ: Lawrence Erlbaum Associates.

Ajzen, I., & Fishbein, M. (1980). *Understanding attitudes and predicting social behavior.* Englewood Cliffs, NJ: Prentice-Hall.

Anderson, B., Ho, J., Brackett, J., Finkelstein, D., & Laffel, L. (1997). Parental involvement in diabetes management tasks: Relationships to blood glucose monitoring adherence and metabolic control in young adolescents with insulin-dependent diabetes mellitus. *Journal of Pediatrics, 130,* 257–265.

Arntson, P. H., & Philipsborn, H. F. (1982). Pediatrician-parent communication in a continuity-of-care setting. *Clinical Pediatrics, 21,* 302–307.

Bame, S. I., Petersen, N., & Wray, N. P. (1993). Variation in hemodialysis patient compliance according to demographic characteristics. *Social Science and Medicine, 37,* 1035–1043.

Brody, H. (1992). *The healer's power.* New Haven, CT: Yale University Press.

Brown, S. A., & Hedges, L.V. (1994). Predicting metabolic control in diabetes: A pilot study using meta-analysis to estimate a linear model. *Nursing Research, 43,* 362–368.

Brownell, K. D., Marlatt, G. A., Lichtenstein, E., & Wilson, G. T. (1986). Understanding and preventing relapse. *American Psychologist, 41,* 765–782.

Bussing, R., Burket, R. C., & Kelleher, E. T. (1996). Prevalence of anxiety disorders in a clinic-based sample of pediatric asthma patients. *Psychosomatics, 37*, 108–115.

Cassell, E. J. (1985). *Talking with patients: Vol. 1. The theory of doctor–patient communication.* Cambridge, MA: MIT Press.

Chaney, J. M., & Peterson, L. (1989). Family variables and disease management in juvenile rheumatoid arthritis. *Journal of Pediatric Psychology, 14*, 389–403.

Chase, H. P., & Jackson, G. G. (1981). Stress and sugar control in children with insulin-dependent diabetes mellitus. *Journal of Pediatrics, 98*, 1011–1013.

Christensen, K. (1983). Self management in diabetic children. *Diabetes Care, 6*, 552–555.

Colaco, J., Egan-Mitchell, B., Stevens, F. M., Fottrell, P. F., McCarthy, C. F., & McNicholl, B. (1987). Compliance with gluten free diet in coeliac disease. *Archives of Diseases in Childhood, 62*, 706–708.

Cox, D. J., & Gonder-Frederick, L. (1992). Major developments in behavioral diabetes research. *Journal of Consulting and Clinical Psychology, 60*, 628–638.

Creer, T. L., & Levstek , D. (1997). Adherence to asthma regimens. In D. S. Gochman (Ed.), *Handbook of health behavior research: II. Provider determinants* (pp. 131–148). New York: Plenum.

Davis, M. C., Tucker, C. M., & Fennell, R. S. (1996). Family behavior, adaptation, and treatment adherence of pediatric nephrology patients. *Pediatric Nephrology, 10*, 160–166.

Delamater, A. M., Kurtz, S. M., White, N. H., & Santiago, J. V. (1988). Effects of social demand on reports of self-monitored blood glucose in adolescents with Type I diabetes mellitus. *Journal of Applied Social Psychology, 18*, 491–502.

DiMatteo, M. R. (1995). Patient adherence to pharmacotherapy: The importance of effective communication. *Formulary, 30*, 596–605.

DiMatteo, M. R., & DiNicola, D. D. (1982). *Achieving patient compliance: The psychology of the medical practitioner's role.* New York: Pergamon.

DiMatteo, M. R., Hays, R. D., Gritz, E. R., Bastani, R., Crane, L., Elashoff, R., Ganz, P., Heber, D., McCarthy, W., & Marcus, A. (1993). Patient adherence to cancer control regimens: Scale development and initial validation. *Psychological Assessment, 5*, 102–112.

DiMatteo, M. R., Hays, R. D., & Prince, L. M. (1986). Relationships of physicians' nonverbal communication skill to patient satisfaction, appointment noncompliance, and physician workload. *Health Psychology, 5*, 581–594.

DiMatteo, M. R., & Lepper, H. S. (1998). Promoting adherence to courses of treatment: Mutual collaboration in the physician–patient relationship. In B. Duffy & L. Jackson (Eds.), *Health communication research* (pp. 75–86). Westport, CT: Greenwood.

DiMatteo, M. R., Linn, L. S., Chang, B. L., & Cope, D. W. (1985). Affect and neutrality in physician behavior. *Journal of Behavioral Medicine, 8*, 397–409.

DiMatteo, M. R., Sherbourne, C. D., Hays, R. D., Ordway, L., Kravitz, R. L., McGlynn, E. A., Kaplan, S., & Rogers, W. H. (1993). Physicians' characteristics influence patients' adherence to medical treatment: Results from the Medical Outcomes Study. *Health Psychology, 12*, 93–102.

Dishman, R. K. (1982). Compliance/adherence in health related exercise. *Health Psychology, 1*, 237–267.

Dolgin, M. J., Katz, E. R., Doctors, S. R., & Siegel, S. E. (1986). Caregivers' perceptions of medical compliance in adolescents with cancer. *Journal of Adolescent Health Care, 7*, 22–27.

Epstein, L. H., & Cluss, P. A. (1982). A behavioral medicine perspective on adherence to long-term medical regimens. *Journal of Consulting and Clinical Psychology, 50*, 950–971.

Everett, K. D., Brantley, P. J., Sletten, C., Jones, G. N., & McKnight, G. T. (1995). The relation of stress and depression to interdialytic weight gain in hemodialysis patients. *Behavioral Medicine, 21*, 25–30.

Faden, R., Becker, C., Lewis, C., Freeman, J., & Faden, A. (1981). Disclosure of information to patients in medical care. *Medical Care, 19*, 718–733.

Finney, J. W., Hook, R. J., Friman, P. C., & Rapoff, M. A. (1993). The overestimation of adherence to pediatric medical regimens. *Children's Health Care, 22*, 297–304.

Fox, W. (1983). Compliance of patients and physicians: Experience and lessons from tuberculosis. *British Medical Journal, 287*, 33–35.

Friedson, E. (1961). *Patients' view of medical practice*. New York: Russell Sage Foundation.

Friedson, E. (1970). *Professional dominance*. Chicago: Aldine.

Fritz, G. K., & Wamboldt, M. Z. (1998). Pediatric asthma: Psychosomatic interactions and symptom perception. In H. Kotses & A. Harver (Eds.), *Self-management of asthma* (pp. 195–230). New York: Marcel Dekker.

Garrison, W. T., Biggs, D., & Williams, K. (1990). Temperament characteristics and clinical outcomes in young children with diabetes mellitus. *Journal of Child Psychology and Psychiatry, 31*, 1079–1088.

Glasgow, R. E., & Anderson, B. J. (1995). Future directions for research on pediatric chronic disease management: Lessons from diabetes. *Journal of Pediatric Psychology, 20*, 389–402.

Glasgow, R. E., McCaul, K. D., & Schafer, L. C. (1986). Barriers to regimen adherence among persons with insulin-dependent diabetes. *Journal of Behavioral Medicine, 9*, 65–77.

Glasgow, R. E., Toobert, D. J., Riddle, M., Donnelly, J., Mitchell, D. L., & Calder, D. (1989). Diabetes-specific social learning variables and self-care behaviors among persons with Type II diabetes. *Health Psychology, 8*, 285–303.

Glasgow, R. E., Wilson, W., & McCaul, K. D. (1985). Regimen adherence: A problematic construct in diabetes adherence. *Diabetes Care, 8*, 300–301.

Goldenberg, I., & Goldenberg, H. (1980). *Family therapy: An overview*. Monterey, CA: Brooks-Cole.

Granstrom, P. (1982). Glaucoma patients not compliant with their drug therapy: Clinical and behavioural aspects. *British Journal of Ophthalmology, 66*, 464–470.

Gudas, L. J., Koocher, G. P., & Wypij, D. (1991). Perceptions of medical compliance in children and adolescents with cystic fibrosis. *Developmental and Behavioral Pediatrics, 12*, 236–242.

Gurwitz, J. H., Glynn, R. J., Monane, M., Everitt, D. E., Gilden, D., Smith, N., & Avorn, J. (1993). Treatment for glaucoma: Adherence by the elderly. *American Journal of Public Health, 83*, 711–716.

Halford, W. K., Cuddihy, S., & Mortimer, R. H. (1990). Psychological stress and blood glucose regulation in Type I diabetic patients. *Health Psychology, 9*, 516–528.

Hampson, S. E., Glasgow, R. E., & Toobert, D. J. (1990). Personal models of diabetes and their relations to self-care activities. *Health Psychology, 9*, 632–646.

Hanson, C., DeGuire, M. J., Schinkel, A. M., Henggeler, S. W., & Burghen, G. A. (1992). Comparing social learning and family systems correlates of adaptation in youths with IDDM. *Journal of Pediatric Psychology, 17*, 555–572.

Hanson, C. L., Henggeler, S. W., & Burghen, G. (1987). Social competence and parental support as mediators of the link between stress and metabolic control in adolescents with insulin-dependent diabetes mellitus. *Journal of Consulting and Clinical Psychology, 55*, 529–533.

Hauser, S. T., Jacobson, A. M., Lavori, P., Wolfsdorf, J. I., Herskowitz, R. D., Milley, J. E., Bliss, R., Wertlieb, D., & Stein, J. (1990). Adherence among children and adolescents with insulin-dependent diabetes mellitus over a four-year longitudinal follow-up: II. Immediate and long-term linkages with the family milieu. *Journal of Pediatric Psychology, 15*, 527–542.

Hays, R. D., & DiMatteo, M.R. (1987). Key issues and suggestions, sources of information, focus of measures, and nature of response options. *Journal of Compliance in Health Care, 2*, 37–53.

Hazzard, A., Hutchinson, S. J., & Krawiecki, N. (1990). Factors related to adherence to medication regimens in pediatric seizure patients. *Journal of Pediatric Psychology, 15,* 543–555.

Heffer, R. W., Worchel-Prevatt, F., Rae, W. A., Lopez, M. A., Young-Saleme, T., Orr, K., Aikman, G., Krause, M., & Weir, M. (1997). The effects of oral versus written instructions on parents' recall and satisfaction after pediatric appointments. *Journal of Developmental and Behavioral Pediatrics, 18,* 377–382.

Hoover, H. (1989). Compliance in hemodialysis patients: A review of the literature. *Journal of the American Dietetic Association, 89,* 957–959.

Horwitz, S. M., Leaf, P. J., & Leventhal, J. M. (1998). Identification of psychosocial problems in pediatric primary care: Do family attitudes make a difference? *Archives of Pediatrics and Adolescent Medicine, 152,* 367–371.

Irwin, C. E., Millstein, S. G., & Ellen, J. M. (1993). Appointment-keeping behavior in adolescents: Factors associated with follow-up appointment-keeping. *Pediatrics, 92,* 20–23.

Johnson, S. B. (1995). Managing insulin-dependent diabetes mellitus in adolescence: A developmental perspective. In J. L. Wallander & L. J. Siegel (Eds.), *Adolescent health problems: Behavioral perspectives. Advances in pediatric psychology* (pp. 265–288). New York: Guilford.

Johnson, S. B., Kelly, M., Henretta, J. C., Cunningham, W. R., Tomer, A., & Silverstein, J. H. (1992). A longitudinal analysis of adherence and health status in childhood diabetes. *Journal of Pediatric Psychology, 17,* 537–553.

Katz, J. (1984). *The silent world of doctor and patient.* New York: The Free Press.

Kewman, D. G., Warschausky, S. A., & Engel, L. (1995). Juvenile rheumatoid arthritis and neuromuscular conditions: Scoliosis, spinal cord injury, and muscular distrophy. In M. C. Roberts (Ed.), *Handbook of pediatric psychology* (2nd ed., pp. 384–402). New York: Guilford.

Kimmel, P. L., Peterson, R. A., Weihs, K. L., Simmens, S. J., Boyle, D. H., Verme, D., Umana, W. O., Veis, S., & Cruz, I. (1995). Behavioral compliance with dialysis prescription in hemodialysis patients. *Journal of the American Society of Nephrology, 5,* 1826–1834.

Kleinman, A. (1988). *The illness narratives: Suffering, healing, and the human condition.* New York: Basic Books.

Korsch, B. M., Fine, R. N., & Negrete, V. F. (1978). Noncompliance in children with renal transplants. *Pediatrics, 61,* 872–876.

Kugelmann, R., & Bensinger, R. E. (1983). Metaphors of glaucoma. *Culture, Medicine, and Psychiatry, 7,* 313–328.

Kulik, J. A., & Carlino, P. (1987). The effect of verbal commitment and treatment choice on medication compliance in a pediatric setting. *Journal of Behavioral Medicine, 10,* 367–376.

La Greca, A. M., Auslander, W. F., Greco, P., Spetter, D., Fisher, E. B., & Santiago, J. V. (1991). Adolescents with IDDM: Family and peer support of diabetes care. *12th Annual Proceedings of the Society of Behavioral Medicine, 110* (Abstract).

Lazare, A., Eisenthal, S., Frank, A., & Stoeckle, J. (1978). Studies on a negotiated approach to patienthood. In E. B. Gallagher (Ed.), *The doctor–patient relationship in a changing health scene* (NIH No. 78-189, pp. 119–139). Washington, DC: U.S. Department of Health, Education, and Welfare.

Leedham, B., Meyerowitz, B. E., Muirhead, H., & Frist, W. H. (1995). Positive expectations predict health after heart transplantation. *Health Psychology, 14,* 74–79.

Ley, P. (1979). Memory for medical information. *British Journal of Social & Clinical Psychology, 18,* 245–255.

Lorenz, R. A., Christensen, N. K., & Pichert, J. W. (1985). Diet-related knowledge, skill, and adherence among children with insulin-dependent diabetes mellitus. *Pediatrics, 75,* 872–876.

Maiman, L. A., Becker, M. H., & Katlic, A. W. (1985). How mothers treat their children's physical symptoms. *Journal of Community Health, 10,* 136–155.

Martin, J. E., & Dubbert, P. M. (1982). Exercise applications and promotion in behavioral medicine: Current status and future directions. *Journal of Consulting and Clinical Psychology, 50,* 1004–1017.

McCaul, K. D., Glasgow, R. E., & Schafer, L. C. (1987). Diabetes regimen behaviors: Predicting adherence. *Medical Care, 25,* 868–881.

Mechanic, D., & Schlesinger M. (1996). The impact of managed care on patients' trust in medical care and their physicians. *Journal of the American Medical Association, 275,* 1693–1697.

Meichenbaum, D., & Turk, D. C. (1987). *Facilitating treatment adherence: A practitioner's guidebook.* New York: Plenum.

Miller, D. L., Jelalian, E., & Stark, L. J. (1999). Cystic fibrosis. In A. J. Goreczny & M. Hersen (Eds.), *Handbook of pediatric and adolescent health psychology* (pp. 127–139). Boston, MA: Allyn & Bacon.

Minuchin, S. (1974). *Families and family therapy.* Cambridge, MA: Harvard University Press.

Minuchin, S., Rosman, B. L., & Baker, L. (1978). *Psychosomatic families: Anorexia nervosa in context.* Cambridge, MA: Harvard University Press.

Murphy, L. M. B., Thompson, R. J., Jr., & Morris, M. A. (1997). Adherence behavior among adolescents with Type I insulin-dependent diabetes mellitus: The role of cognitive appraisal processes. *Journal of Pediatric Psychology, 22,* 811–825.

Mayer, M., Greco, L., Troncone, R., Auricchio, S., & Marsh, M. N. (1991). Compliance of adolescents with coeliac disease with a gluten free diet. *Gut, 32,* 881–885.

Palardy, N., Greening, L., Ott, J., Holderby, A., & Atchison, J. (1998). Adolescents' health attitudes and adherence to treatment for insulin-dependent diabetes mellitus. *Developmental and Behavioral Pediatrics, 19,* 31–37.

Parsons, T. (1951). *The social system.* New York: The Free Press.

Patel, S. C., & Spaeth, G. L. (1995). Compliance in patients prescribed eyedrops for glaucoma. *Ophthalmic Surgery, 26,* 233–236.

Pozsik, C. J. (1993). Compliance with tuberculosis therapy. *Medical Clinics of North America, 77,* 1289–1301.

Prochaska, J. O., Velicer, W. F., Rossi, J. S., & Goldstein, M. G. (1994). Stages of change and decisional balance for twelve problem behaviors. *Health Psychology, 13,* 39–46.

Ricker, J. H., Delamater, A. M., & Hsu, J. (1998). Correlates of regimen adherence in cystic fibrosis. *Journal of Clinical Psychology in Medical Settings, 5,* 159–172.

Rivers, P. H. (1992). Compliance aids—do they work? *Drugs and Aging, 2,* 103–111.

Rodin, J., & Janis, I. L. (1979). The social power of health-care practitioners as agents of change. *Journal of Social Issues, 35,* 60–81.

Rosenthal, R. (1991). *Meta-analytic procedures for social research.* Newbury Park, CA: Sage.

Roter, D. L., & Hall, J. A. (1992). *Doctors talking with patients/patients talking with doctors.* Westport: Auburn House.

Ruggiero, L., & Javorsky, D. (1999). Diabetes self-management in children. In A. J. Goreczny & M. Hersen (Eds.), *Handbook of pediatric and adolescent health psychology* (pp. 49–70). Boston, MA: Allyn & Bacon.

Scarfone, R. J., Joffe, M. D., Wiley, J. F., Loiselle, J. M., & Cook, R. T. (1996). Noncompliance with scheduled revisits to a pediatric emergency department. *Archives of Pediatric and Adolescent Medicine, 150,* 948–953.

Sensky, T., Leger, C., & Gilmour, S. (1996). Psychosocial and cognitive factors associated with adherence to dietary and fluid restriction regimens by people on chronic hemodialysis. *Psychotherapy and Psychosomatics, 65,* 36–42.

Singh, N., Squier, C., Sivek, M., Wagener, M., Nguyen, M. H., & Yu, V. L. (1996). Determinants of compliance with antiretroviral therapy in patients with immunodeficiency virus: Prospective assessment with implications for enhancing compliance. *AIDS Care, 8,* 261–269.

Slavkin, H. C. (1996). An update on HIV/AIDS. *Journal of the American Dental Association,*
    127, 1401–1404.
Speedling, E. J., & Rose, D. N. (1985). Building an effective doctor–patient relationship: From
    patient satisfaction to patient participation. *Social Science & Medicine, 21,* 115–120.
Sprunger, L. W. (1983). An analysis of physician–parent communication in pediatric prena-
    tal interviews. *Clinical Pediatrics, 22,* 553–558.
Squier, R. W. (1990). A model of empathic understanding and adherence to treatment regi-
    mens in practitioner–patient relationships. *Social Science & Medicine, 30,* 325–339.
Stanton, A. L. (1987). Determinants of adherence to medical regimens by hypertensive
    patients. *Journal of Behavioral Medicine, 10,* 377–394.
Street, R. L. (1991). Physicians' communication and parents' evaluations of pediatric con-
    sultations. *Medical Care, 29,* 1146–1152.
Taal., E., Rasker, J. J., Seydel, E. R., & Wiegman, O. (1993). Health status, adherence with
    health recommendations, self-efficacy and social support in patients with rheumatoid
    arthritis. *Patient Education and Counseling, 20,* 63–76.
Thompson, S., Dahlquist, L., Koenning, G. M., & Bartholomew, L. K. (1995). Adherence-facil-
    itating behaviors of a multidisciplinary pediatric rheumatology staff. *Journal of Pediatric*
    Psychology, 20, 291–297.
Trostle, J. A. (1997). Patient compliance as an ideology. In D. S. Gochman (Ed.), *Handbook*
    of health behavior research: II. Provider determinants (pp. 109–122). New York:
    Plenum.
Van Sciver, M. M., D'Angelo, E. J., Rappaport, L., & Woolf, A. D. (1995). Pediatric compliance
    and the roles of distinct treatment characteristics, treatment attitudes, and family stress:
    A preliminary report. *Journal of Developmental and Behavioral Pediatrics, 16,* 350–358.
Waisbren, S. E., Hamilton, B. D., St. James, P. J., Shiloh, S., & Levy, H. L. (1995). Psychosocial
    factors in maternal phenylketonuria: Women's adherence to medical recommendations.
    American Journal of Public Health, 85, 1636–1641.
Waitzkin, H., & Stoeckle, J. (1976). Information control and the micropolitics of health care:
    Summary of an ongoing research project. *Social Science and Medicine, 10,* 263–276.
Wilson, D. P., & Endres, R. K. (1986). Compliance with blood glucose monitoring in children
    with Type I diabetes mellitus. *Journal of Pediatrics, 108,* 1022–1024.
Wissow, L. S., Roter, D. L., & Wilson, M. E. (1994). Pediatrician interview style and mothers'
    disclosure of psychosocial issues. *Pediatrics, 93,* 289–295.
Wolcott, D. L., Maida, C. A., Diamond, R., & Nissenson, A. (1986). Treatment compliance in
    end-stage renal disease patients on dialysis. *American Journal of Nephrology, 6,*
    329–338.
Worchel, F. F., Prevatt, B. C., Miner, J., Allen, M., Wagner, L., & Nation, P. (1995). Pediatri-
    cian's communication style: Relationship to parent's perceptions and behaviors. *Journal*
    of Pediatric Psychology, 20, 633–644.
Worobey, J., O'Hair, H. D., & O'Hair, M. C. (1987). Pediatrician–parent–patient communica-
    tions: A descriptive analysis. *Language and Communication, 7,* 293–301.
Wysocki, T., & Greco, P. (1997). Self-management of childhood diabetes in family context. In
    D. S. Gochman (Ed.), *Handbook of health behavior research: II. Provider determinants*
    (pp. 169–187). New York: Plenum.

CHAPTER ELEVEN

Parental and Child Knowledge of the Treatment Regimen for Childhood Chronic Illnesses: Related Factors and Adherence to Treatment

Carolyn E. Ievers-Landis
Dennis Drotar
Rainbow Babies and Children's Hospital, Cleveland, OH

Knowledge of the treatment regimen has been identified as a prerequisite for the child and family to manage the treatment-related tasks of a chronic illness (Ievers et al., in press; Johnson, 1984; La Greca & Schuman, 1995; Rusakow et al., 1998). Nevertheless, knowledge of the specific tasks of recommended treatments is not in itself sufficient for successful management of illness-related medical tasks because other factors may impede the ability of children with a chronic illness and their parents to adhere to the treatment regimen (Johnson, 1984). Despite this, parents of children with chronic illnesses cannot be expected to responsibly oversee the day-to-day administration of medical treatments for their children unless they are fully versed in the specifics of what has been prescribed. Knowledge of the treatment regimen is therefore a necessary if not sufficient ingredient for successful adherence for children with a chronic illness. Consequently, parents and children must be thoroughly educated about medically recommended treatments.

In marked contrast to the potential importance of knowledge of the treatment regimen to adherence, this component has been understudied and not well defined by researchers (Ievers et al., in press). Moreover, inadequate definitions of knowledge have limited scientific understanding of (a) the magnitude of the problem of gaps or inaccuracies in parental or child knowledge of the treatment regimen, and (b) the relationship of this type of knowledge to adherence to prescribed treatments for children with chronic illnesses and their parents. To address these needs, this chapter defines knowledge and understanding of the treatment regimen for childhood chronic illnesses, reviews and critiques the relevant empirical literature on this topic, and describes the implications for research and clinical care concerning treatment adherence.

DEFINING KNOWLEDGE

Knowledge of the Illness

In research on adherence to medical treatments for childhood chronic illnesses, *knowledge* has usually been conceptualized as children's or parents' grasp of factual information about the illness and their understanding of the purpose of treatments. For instance, studies of knowledge for children with asthma have employed measures of children's knowledge of the basic principles of asthma and asthma control, including understanding of the purpose of medications (Rubin, Bauman, & Lauby, 1989; Smith et al., 1986); asthma-related symptoms, triggers, and treatments (Fitzclarence & Henry, 1990); appropriate responses to hypothetical scenarios of asthma attacks (Kolbe, Vamos, James, Elkind, & Garrett, 1996); and the majority of these (Tehan, Sloane, Walsh-Robart, & Chamberlain, 1989). For children and young adults diagnosed as having cystic fibrosis (CF) and their parents, measurement of knowledge has encompassed a wide range of areas, including understanding of disease pathophysiology, treatment (i.e., reason for certain therapies), genetics and reproduction, as well as the possible effects of short- versus long-term treatment cessation and the seriousness of various symptoms (e.g., coughing blood; Nolan, Desmond, Herlich, & Hardy, 1986). The diabetes literature includes measurement of various aspects of children's general knowledge of their condition (e.g., causes and complications) and daily management skills (e.g., Collier & Etzwiler, 1971; Hamburg & Inoff, 1982; Hess & Davis, 1983; Johnson et al., 1982). Diabetes-related research has led to the conclusion that knowledge in one area (e.g., skill at insulin injection) is not necessarily related to knowledge in others (e.g., skill at urine testing; Johnson, 1984). Knowledge measures employed with children who have cancer have included such components as the incidence, prevalence, warning signs, chances for recovery, methods of treatment, and ways to avoid getting cancer (e.g., Michielutte, Diseker, & Hayes, 1979; Tamaroff, Festa, Adesman, & Walco, 1992).

Limitations in Operational Definitions of Knowledge in Childhood Chronic Illness

The definition of *knowledge* that has been used in adherence research for childhood chronic illness has several important limitations. First, the marked variations in operational definitions of *knowledge of the illness* limit examination of findings across studies of the relationship of knowledge to adherence from different illness groups and hence restrict generalizability of available findings. Similarly, because different measures of knowledge have also been used in research within specific chronic illnesses, it is difficult to ascertain the specific deficits in knowledge most commonly occurring among children with each chronic condition and their parents.

Current definitions of knowledge also have limited implications for interventions. First, due to the numerous different measures of *knowledge of the illness* used within the same chronic illness groups, it is difficult to ascertain whether educational interventions have successfully enhanced children's knowledge. As an example of this problem, a meta-analysis of teaching interventions for children with asthma could not consider knowledge as an outcome variable due to the incomparability of the scales of measurement of knowledge from one study to another (Bernard-Bonnin, Stachenko, Bonin, Charette, & Rousseau, 1995). Second, some educational interventions targeting certain pediatric illness groups (e.g., asthma and diabetes) improved child and family knowledge of disease, but these interventions have not always led to demonstrable improvements in the management of these illnesses or in disease control (Brandt & Magyary, 1993; Etzwiler & Robb, 1972; Howland et al., 1988). Although certain educational interventions designed to increase disease-related knowledge in children or adolescents with asthma and diabetes have been shown to improve adherence (e.g., Da Costa et al., 1997; Epstein et al., 1981; Smith et al., 1986; Tehan et al., 1989), these interventions have also included behavioral strategies (e.g., token systems, supervision of compliance, tailoring the drug regimen to the subjects' daily routines) and did not evaluate the specific effects of the educational components.

Operational Definitions of Knowledge of the Treatment Regimen

To address these limitations, we believe a shift in focus and a more precise operational definition of *knowledge* for adherence research in childhood chronic illness is necessary to advance scientific understanding. For this reason, in this chapter, *knowledge* is defined as the following: (a) the understanding of the specifics of the treatment regimen (e.g., what are the prescribed treatments and how often these treatment should be performed), (b) the ability to accurately recall the prescribed treatments over the course of the illness, and (c) knowledge about how to implement the treatment regimen (i.e., treatment-related skills). We believe that this latter point is particularly important.

Depending on the specific chronic illness, knowledge could include what is recommended and what is not, including guidelines for exercise frequency and caloric consumption, the name and dose of any medications, the frequency of these treatments, the duration of treatments, the order of administration of treatments, and any special techniques that are required to administer treatments. Using CF as an example, an assessment of *knowledge of the treatment regimen* based on our recommended operational definition would include asking the child with CF and his or her parents to indicate which treatments have been prescribed (e.g., chest physical therapy, pancreatic enzymes, antibiotics, aerosol medications, vitamins, etc.), the name and dose of any prescribed medications or nonprescribed vitamins and medications (e.g., ibuprofen), the frequency prescribed for each treatment (e.g., how often to take antibiotics, how often to perform chest physical therapy), the duration of treatments (e.g., minutes to perform chest physical therapy), the order of administration of treatments (e.g., whether to take pancreatic enzymes before, during, or after eating), as well as the special techniques needed to perform treatments (e.g., the recommended procedures for using a flutter device for airway clearance or for inhaling aerosolized medications). See Table 11.1 for an outline of the most important elements required to sufficiently assess knowledge of the treatment regimen.

Knowledge needed to implement the treatment regimen for a chronic illness is qualitatively quite different from knowledge of the illness. Knowledge of the treatment regimen includes basic information about the medical recommendations for the day-to-day management of the illness and therefore is an obvious prerequisite for adherence. Although knowledge of

TABLE 11.1
Assessment of Knowledge of the Treatment Regimen

1. Survey of all prescribed or recommended treatments (e.g., medications, exercise frequency, dietary recommendations)
2. Names and doses of any prescribed or nonprescribed medications
3. Frequency of treatments
4. Duration of treatments (i.e., minutes to perform treatment, days to take medication)
5. Order of administration of treatments
6. Special techniques required to perform treatments
7. Action plans

factual information about the illness or the purpose of treatments (e.g., the reason to take pancreatic enzymes) may indeed relate to adherence, a child and his or her parents do not necessarily have to be educated about the disease or purpose of treatments to adhere to the prescribed treatment regimen. First and foremost, they need to understand and remember over time what the child's medical caregivers have recommended to have the highest likelihood for successful adherence to these recommendations. Although it makes intuitive sense that children and parents cannot adhere to a treatment that they do not clearly understand or remember, few studies exist to demonstrate this association (Ievers et al., in press).

Assessment of Knowledge of the Treatment Regimen

How does one assess children's and parents' knowledge of the treatment regimen for a chronic illness? The goal of a comprehensive assessment of knowledge of the treatment regimen is to determine how well parents and children are able to recall and report the specifics of all facets of the prescribed treatment regimen. Consequently, assessment should involve asking children with a chronic illness and their parents what has been prescribed by their medical providers rather than what they are currently doing, which is a proxy for their adherence behaviors. For example, the question might be worded as: How often does your medical provider suggest that your child perform chest physical therapy? rather than How often does your child perform chest physical therapy? This assessment could include queries of parents and their children with a chronic illness of such information as a prescribed medication's name and dose, when the medication was originally prescribed, for how long the medication should be taken, and what the medical caregiver said should be done when a dose has been missed.

Another useful knowledge of the treatment question is whether a treatment was prescribed as PRN and what this means to the parents and to the child (e.g., take only when the child has certain symptoms). To determine the accuracy of parents' and children's knowledge, this information should be compared to physician prescriptions either taken from a medical chart or via interviews with involved clinical caregivers (e.g., nurses, dieticians, respiratory therapists).

Furthermore, child patients' or parents' skills at performing special techniques for prescribed treatments should be assessed to more comprehensively evaluate their knowledge of prescribed treatments. Observational assessments have been conducted for peak flow meter and inhaler technique for children with asthma (e.g., Christiansen et al., 1997) and for urine testing and self-injection skills for children with diabetes (e.g., Johnson et al., 1982). For each of these, the children were either given points or pass–fail scores on a series of steps to obtain a quantitative index of their skills at performing the treatment-related task. Further work is needed to establish scoring criteria for treatment-related tasks performed by children with other chronic illnesses (e.g., flutter technique for children with CF).

EMPIRICAL FINDINGS CONCERNING CHILD AND PARENT KNOWLEDGE OF THE TREATMENT REGIMEN

Little research exists to describe the adequacy of knowledge of the treatment regimen as defined herein for children with various chronic illnesses and their parents. Although multiple studies have assessed knowledge of the illness and have included questions related to the child patients' or parents' knowledge of prescribed treatments, the majority have failed to examine knowledge of how to apply these treatments. Therefore, these studies do not describe child patients' or parents' knowledge about the treatment regimen apart from their general understanding of the illness. Thus, significant gaps across many illness groups exist in the research literature on child and family knowledge regarding the application of the treatment regimen for childhood chronic illnesses (Ievers et al., in press).

Parental Knowledge of Pediatricians' Recommendations

When assessing knowledge of the treatment regimen in childhood chronic illnesses, inclusion of data from parents or other caregivers in research studies in this area is vital to obtain a more comprehensive view of the level of knowledge for the management of children's conditions. Parents must necessarily take a primary role in administering or supervising their children's treatments and keeping track of any changes in the regimens. Moreover, even as children become adolescents, most parents remain involved in their medical care in one form or another (Drotar & Ievers, 1994). Therefore, parental knowledge is of continuing importance for optimal adherence for children at all developmental levels.

Research findings have consistently demonstrated that parents of child patients in primary care pediatric settings often do not accurately recall what the medical provider has told them. As an example, parents who were interviewed 5 to 7 days after a visit to their child's pediatrician recalled 75% of prescribed medications but only 29% of nonprescription recommendations (e.g., restrict the child's diet, use a vaporizer; Heffer et al., 1997). Mothers of infants recalled approximately 88% of what doctors told them (Hulka et al., 1975).

Relatively few studies have been conducted to assess knowledge of treatment with parents of children with chronic conditions. In a study of parents of children with CF, 14% reported that chest physical therapy was only necessary when their child was not feeling well, and the majority were not aware that pancreatic enzymes should be taken with snacks as well as meals (Henley & Hill, 1990). In a sample of 93 parents of children with CF (ages 5–18), Gudas, Koocher, and Wypiz (1991) discovered that parents did not accurately report the specific elements of their children's treatment regimens. For example, nearly half of parents (47%) did not agree with medical providers as to whether a formal diet had been prescribed, and approximately 9% did not agree with providers about whether chest physical therapy was a recommended treatment. Likewise, a recent study by Rusakow et al. (1998) of 47 patients with CF (ages 1–26) and their parents found that 19% of the sample were not taking their pancreatic enzymes as recommended or suspected by their physicians (i.e., exclusively after eating meals). Of particular note, only 25% had discussed the recommended dose or order of administration of enzymes (i.e., before, during, or after eating) with their medical caregivers within the previous 6 months although they had two clinic visits within that time period.

Ievers et al. (in press) interviewed 45 mothers of children with CF (ages 6–12) to determine the accuracy of their knowledge of their children's prescribed treatment regimen. As part of this study, mothers were asked to indicate what they believed to be the prescribed frequency of their child's treatments on a 6-point Likert scale (0 = *not at all*; 1 = *2 to 3 times per month*; 3 = *3 to 4 times per week*; 4 = *once per day*; 5 = *twice per day*; and 6 = *three times or more per day*); their responses were compared to the prescribed treatments recorded in the children's medical charts. The findings were that one fifth of the sample could not report the prescribed frequency of airway clearance treatments and nearly one third could not accurately report the prescribed frequency of aerosol medications.

Similar findings have been reported for parents of children with other chronic illnesses. For instance, parents of children with diabetes recalled only two of seven recommendations for diabetes care made by providers during a clinic visit (Page, Verstraete, Robb, & Etzwiler, 1981). Also, insufficient or incorrect information about the treatment regimen was identified as a contributor to nonadherence among families of children with asthma (Alexander, 1983).

Children's Knowledge of Medical Recommendations

Although the assessment of parental knowledge is of great importance, children's level of knowledge of their own treatment regimen for a chronic illness should also be assessed. As children develop, they assume more responsibility for administering their own treatments (Drotar & Ievers, 1994). Consequently, any errors or limitations in their knowledge of the specifics of treatments could result in poor adherence to medical recommendations described as *inadvertent nonadherence* by Johnson (1984).

Research on children's knowledge of medical treatments has identified significant problems with recall of physician prescriptions as well as inaccurate knowledge about their recommended treatments. For example, children ranging in age from 6 to 17 years recalled about half (47%) of medication-related information and only one third (32%) of the total recommendations made by their physician in a primary care setting immediately after the visit (Lewis, Pantell, & Sharp, 1991). In a study of children receiving growth hormone (GH) therapy, 40% of the sample did not know the prescribed volume to inject, and the majority did not know the volume of water that should be added to the GH powder prior to injection (Lopez Siquero, Martinez Aedo, Lopez Moreno, & Martinez Valverde, 1995).

Twenty-two percent of a sample of children diagnosed as having CF thought they only needed to perform chest physical therapy when they were not feeling well, and the majority of the sample did not know that pancreatic enzymes should be taken with snacks (Henley & Hill, 1990). In a sample of 100 patients with CF (ages 5–20), 40% did not agree with medical providers as to whether a formal diet was prescribed, and approximately 12% did not agree with providers about whether chest physical therapy was recommended (Gudas, Koocher, & Wypiz, 1991). In an investigation of children with CF (ages 6–12, $n = 45$) by Ievers et al. (in press), the children reported the frequency of prescribed medical treatments on a 6-point Likert scale (0 = *not at all*; 1 = *2 to 3 times per month*; 3 = *3 to 4 times per week*; 4 = *once per day*; 5 = *twice per day*; and 6 = *three times or more per day*); their responses were compared to the prescribed treatments recorded in their medical charts. Findings were that 45% of the sample could not report the prescribed frequency of airway clearance treatments, and 53% could not report the prescribed frequency of aerosol medications. Not surprisingly, child patients were found to have less accurate knowledge of medical information than did their mothers.

For children with other chronic illnesses, more than 80% of a sample of children with insulin-dependent diabetes made one or more serious errors on a skills demonstration test of urine testing (e.g., incorrect timing); 40% made serious errors on the self-injection test (e.g., bubbles in the insulin to be injected; Johnson et al., 1982). Older children demonstrated greater skills than younger children.

RELATIONSHIP BETWEEN KNOWLEDGE ABOUT TREATMENT
AND TREATMENT ADHERENCE

In studies conducted with parents of child patients in primary care pediatric settings, recall of the specific treatment regimen has been associated with better medical adherence (Becker et al., 1972; Mattar et al., 1975).

Some evidence also exists for a relationship between incorrect and insufficient information about illness management and poor adherence in pediatric chronic illness populations such as asthma (e.g., Alexander, 1983), diabetes (Page, Verstraete, Robb, & Etzwiler, 1981), and cancer (Tebbi, Richards, Cummings, Zevon, & Mallon, 1988). For example, in a sample of adolescents with cancer and their parents, higher parent–child agreement about prescribed treatments (e.g., number of medications, time of day for taking medications, and dose required at each administration) was related to greater self-reported compliance with treatments (Tebbi et al., 1988). Additional evidence for the association between knowledge of the treatment regimen and adherence for children with CF has been gathered by Ievers et al. (in press). A sample of 45 children with CF (ages 6–12) and their mothers were interviewed during a specialty clinic visit to determine the association of their knowledge of the specifics of the prescribed treatment regimen to the child's reported level of treatment adherence. The measure completed by mothers and children was the Treatment Adherence Questionnaire–Cystic Fibrosis (TAQ–CF; Quittner et al., 1996). The TAQ–CF measures parent and child report of adherence to three central domains of the CF treatment regimen (airway clearance, aerosol treatments, and pancreatic enzymes) in addition to parent and child report of physicians' treatment recommendations for the three domains (i.e., knowledge of prescribed treatments). A second measure, the Treatment Adherence Questionnaire–Cystic Fibrosis: Physician Version (TAQ–CF: Physician Version; Ievers et al., in press), was created by the author as a parallel form of the TAQ–CF. The Physician Version of the TAQ–CF measures the recommended treatment regimen, including prescribed frequency and duration of airway clearance techniques, frequency of aerosol treatments, and pancreatic enzyme use from medical providers or the patient's medical chart. See Table 11.2 for examples of parallel items from each of the versions of the TAQ–CF (i.e., parent, child, and physician).

To determine the relationship of knowledge of the treatment regimen to reported adherence to prescribed treatments, six hierarchical regression equations were performed using child and maternal reports of treatment-related behaviors across the three domains of treatments from the TAQ–CF as the dependent variables. For each regression analysis, the physician's prescription for that aspect of treatment from the TAQ–CF: Physician Version was forced into the equation as the first independent variable to statistically control for individual differences in the child's prescribed treatment. An examination of the significance of the change in R^2 was conducted to determine whether knowledge was predictive of reported treatment-related behaviors after controlling for the prescribed treatments (Ievers et al., in press).

TABLE 11.2
Selected Parallel Items From the Parent,[a] Child,[a] and Physician[b] Versions
of the Treatment Adherence Questionnaire–Cystic Fibrosis: Knowledge
of the Prescribed Frequency of Airway Clearance Treatments[c]

Version	Items
Parent	
How often does the CF medical staff (e.g., physician, respiratory therapist, nurse) suggest that your teen do airway clearance? (Circle one.)	0 = not at all 1 = occasionally (2–3 times/month) 2 = once or twice a week 3 = every other day (3–4 times/week) 4 = once/day 5 = twice/day 6 = 3 or more times a day PRN = as often as needed
Child	
How often does the CF medical staff (e.g., physician, respiratory therapist, nurse) suggest that you do airway clearance? (Circle one.)	0 = not at all 1 = occasionally (2–3 times/month) 2 = once or twice a week 3 = every other day (3–4 times/week) 4 = once/day 5 = twice/day 6 = 3 or more times a day PRN = as often as needed
Physician	
How often do you suggest that this child do airway clearance? (Circle one.)	0 = not at all 1 = occasionally (2–3 times/month) 2 = once or twice a week 3 = every other day (3–4 times/week) 4 = once/day 5 = twice/day 6 = 3 or more times a day PRN = as often as needed

[a] The Parent and Child Versions of the TAQ–CF were developed by Quittner et al. (1996).

[b] The Physician Version of the TAQ–CF was based on the Parent/Child Versions and was created for an investigation by Ievers et al. (in press).

[c] These items illustrate how knowledge of the treatment regimen may be assessed by comparing parent or child reports of their prescribed treatments to the actual prescriptions.

For mothers, knowledge of the prescribed treatment accounted for a significant amount of the variance in reported treatment-related behaviors for frequency of airway clearance treatments and aerosol medications. Children's knowledge of prescribed treatments accounted for a significant amount of the variance in self-reported treatment-related behaviors in frequency of airway clearance treatments, aerosol medications, and enzyme use. Thus, mothers' and children's knowledge of the treatment regimen for CF predicted reported adherence behaviors even when controlling for individual differences in the prescribed treatments (Ievers et al., in press).

One implication of these findings is that both children's and parents' inaccurate knowledge of the treatment regimen may disrupt their adherence to treatments for a chronic illness. Even if families of children with chronic illnesses have the best intentions to administer recommended treatments, adherence is not possible if they do not have an accurate understanding of the clinically relevant details of their treatment regimen (e.g., what is recommended for treatments, including such factors as frequency, duration, order of administration, etc.).

FACTORS THAT INFLUENCE KNOWLEDGE OF THE TREATMENT REGIMEN

The contributing factors to the understanding of the specifics of the recommended treatment regimen by children with a chronic illness and their parents are not well documented. Among the factors that have been proposed to account for level of knowledge of the treatment regimen are the quality of provider–patient communication, the complexity of treatment regimens for chronic conditions, and the child patient's cognitive developmental level.

Quality of Provider–Patient Communication

One factor that may serve to impact patients' and their families' knowledge of medical treatment regimens is the quality of clinical care providers' communication of prescribed treatments. Due to increasing demands from managed care and pressures from competing hospitals and clinics in the same geographical location, physicians must necessarily see more patients in less amounts of time (Gordon, Baker, & Levinson, 1995). Consider the potential impact of the fact that the usual time allotted for a return visit in many managed care settings is 10 minutes (Gordon, Baker, & Levinson, 1995). Shorter visits translate into less medical information about treatment being communicated to child patients and their parents, and a relative absence of this information obviously leads to poorer recall. In fact, in studies of adult patients, the amount of medical information imparted by physicians is associated with patient recall of this information (e.g., Roter, Hall, & Katz, 1987). Additionally, the amount of time physicians spent with adult patients discussing adherence-related issues has been found to be positively related to patient recall of medical advice (Kravitz et al., 1993). There is no reason to believe that these findings would be any different for parents of child patients and children with chronic illnesses who must follow a complex daily treatment regimen.

Complexity of Treatments

A second set of factors that may serve to undermine child and parent knowledge of the details of treatments involves the number and complexity of treatments prescribed for childhood chronic illnesses (La Greca & Schuman, 1995). However, although the complexity of treatments (i.e., prescriptions of more than one medication on different administration schedules) has indeed been found to be related to lower adherence rates (Francis et al., 1969; Markello, 1985; Mattar et al., 1975), less is known about how increased treatment complexity relates to patient recall of this information. As an example of a study addressing this question in an adult population, patients' knowledge of prescribed medications was inversely related to the number of medications prescribed by their physicians (Fletcher et al., 1979). In this sample, only 58% knew the dosage schedule of all of their medications. Additional research is needed to better determine the relationship of complexity of treatments to level of recall or knowledge of physicians' prescriptions among children with a chronic illness and their parents.

Child Patients' Cognitive Developmental Level

The developmental level of the child with a chronic illness is a third factor that has been proposed to relate to child patients' level of knowledge about the medical treatment regimen and skill at administering recommended treatments (Johnson, 1984). For example, intervention studies with children who have diabetes have found that older children know more about their diabetes care and benefit more from educational programs to increase their skill at administering their own treatments than do their younger counterparts (e.g., Gilbert et al., 1982; Harkavy et al., 1983; Heston & Lazar, 1980). Additionally, a study assessing knowledge of the treatment regimen for mothers and their children with cancer (9–19 years old) found that child age was positively correlated with level of child–parent agreement concerning medical instruction (i.e., older children were more likely to agree with their mothers about prescribed treatments such as medication dose, frequency, and number; Tebbi et al., 1988). However, the child's age has not consistently been found to relate to accuracy of knowledge about prescribed treatments in studies of other childhood chronic illness groups, such as CF (Ievers et al., in press), so further study of this relationship would be valuable.

EMPIRICAL STUDIES OF INTERVENTIONS TO IMPROVE PARENTS' AND CHILDREN'S KNOWLEDGE OF TREATMENTS

One viable means to raise adherence rates may be to increase parent and child knowledge of each and every treatment recommended by their medical caregivers. By encouraging parents and their children with a chronic condition to become more aware of expectations for medical care, it may be possible to decrease nonadherence rates due to inaccurate knowledge of the treatment regimen. In terms of the potential efficacy of any of these interventions to increase medical adherence, a caveat should be raised. As Ley (1982) noted, the effectiveness of increasing understanding of and memory for medical information depends on the reason for the patient's nonadherence. Through his review of experimental studies of primarily adult patients, Ley recognized that interventions to improve patient recall of medical information and/or patient–physician communication have a large effect on involuntary noncompliers who have insufficient information about their prescribed treatments. However, the same types of interventions have no effect on voluntary noncompliers who already have adequate information concerning the specifics of their medical treatments. Likewise, Hulka et al. (1975) used the terms *scheduling misconception* to describe compliance problems due to a lack of communication between physician and patient on medication dose and/or frequency and the term *scheduling noncompliance* to identify poor compliance when the patient is correctly informed but chooses not to take medications as prescribed.

Historically, interventions aimed at increasing recall of medical advice have been targeted primarily at adult patient populations, and many have focused on changing the medical provider's communication style (for reviews, see Ley, 1979, 1982). Six suggestions have emerged from experimental studies to improve patients' recall of medical information. These include: (a) present the most important information first; (b) emphasize key instructions and information; (c) use short words and sentences and minimize medical terminology; (d) organize information for patients by stating explicit categories; (e) make specific, definite, and concrete statements; and (f) use repetition within the appointment and over several appointments (Ley, 1979; Schraa & Dirks, 1982). Ley tested these techniques by studying recall of medical information in the patients of four primary care practitioners. Results suggest that, by using the previous suggestions, physicians increased the amount of information recalled by their pediatric, adult, and elderly patients (Ley, 1979). In a sample of 79 adult patients, more drug information given during the end of the medical appointment was related to poorer recall (Rost, Roter, Bertakis, & Quill, 1990). However, this relationship reversed as physician–patient familiarity increased.

More recently, some promising interventions to improve patients' or parents' knowledge of medical recommendations have been developed and empirically validated for child patients and their parents in primary care pediatric settings (Heffer et al., 1997; Lewis, Pantell, & Sharp, 1991). These interventions have consisted of the following: (a) brief education of patients and parents to improve their understanding of treatment recommendations for primarily minor childhood illnesses and recall of this information, and (b) providers giving written instructions to patients during office visits.

A randomized clinical trial with 141 children ranging in age from 5 to 15 years old was conducted to determine a brief educational intervention's effectiveness on medical communication in general pediatric practices (Lewis, Pantell, & Sharp, 1991). The intervention consisted of three videotapes for parents, physicians, and child patients that emphasized building skills and motivation for increased child competence and participation during pediatric medical visits. Children were given workbooks and encouraged to write down questions they had for their physicians and to record information presented during the visit. Physicians were provided with research articles related to health consequences of effective communication and cognitively appropriate interviewing techniques for children of different ages. Results show that physicians included children more frequently in discussions of medical recommendations in the intervention than in the control group, and children recalled more recommendations about medication in the intervention group. Because the authors did not provide any information about the children's medical conditions, it is not known whether any children with chronic illnesses were represented in the sample.

In another intervention study, written instructions given to 96 parents at appointments with their child's pediatrician were associated with greater parental satisfaction and recall of instructions for primarily minor conditions of childhood (e.g., colds and ear infections) than oral presentation of instructions alone (Heffer et al., 1997). This was particularly true for parents having less previous experience with the pediatrician. Physician instructions included such information as dosage, frequency, and duration of prescription and nonprescription medications, as well as recommendations for follow-up visits and medical consultations. It should be noted that only one child included in this intervention had a chronic illness.

Some educational interventions with various childhood chronic illness groups that included interventions to increase child patients' and/or their parents' knowledge of the illness to improve adherence or self-management behaviors have also included a component that addressed knowledge of the treatment regimen (e.g., Bartholomew et al., 1991; Brazil, McLean, Abbey, & Musselman, 1997; Tehan et al., 1989). Unfortunately, the efficacy of such components have rarely been tested alone. Moreover, whether these interventions were successful in increasing the child patient's or parents' understanding of the specifics of prescribed treatment-related tasks is not known. However, adherence is such a challenging target to change that multidimensional approaches are often needed. Consequently, the efficacy of increasing knowledge of the treatment regimen for improving adherence has not been established for children with chronic illnesses and their parents.

CLINICAL INTERVENTIONS TO INCREASE KNOWLEDGE OF THE TREATMENT REGIMEN

Clinical interventions designed to increase knowledge of the treatment regimen may have different targets depending on the particular chronic illness that children and their families must manage. In some pediatric illness groups, prevention to either minimize exacerbations or retard the course of the illness may be the key component of treatment (i.e., sickle cell disease, CF). Cure of the illness might be the focus of treatment for other illness groups, such as achieving remission for children with cancer. Children in these illness groups may require a day-to-day medical regimen that is complex but fairly routine barring any serious complications (e.g., pneumonia for a child with CF, a pain crisis for a child with sickle cell disease, relapse for a child with cancer). For these children and their parents, interventions to increase knowledge of the specifics of the treatment regimen, such as dosage and timing of medications and other recommendations for a healthy lifestyle (e.g., avoiding extreme temperatures for children with sickle cell disease), may be supplied to enable them to be optimally adherent to their prescribed treatment regimen and enjoy the best possible health.

However, children whose illnesses potentially have a more variable day-to-day course (e.g., diabetes or asthma) may experience frequent fluctuations in their condition that require specific actions for optimal treatment. For these children and their parents, interventions to increase knowledge of the treatment regimen would necessarily include the teaching of self-management strategies to prevent or limit illness-related problems. This type of knowledge would appear to be much more complex than the mere recall of the prescribed treatment regimen from the previous clinic visit. As is already being attempted in some education programs for children with asthma, *action plans* devised by medical caregivers and taught to child patients and their parents that address the most common illness-related events may help ensure adequate knowledge of treatments in these populations (e.g., Gillies et al., 1996).

Provide Written Instructions

One relatively simple suggestion for increasing children's and parents' recall of prescribed treatments and other recommendations is for providers to give families written instructions for treatments at each clinic visit. Explicit written instructions have already been found to be effective for enhancing drug therapy compliance in pediatric populations (Mattar, Markello, & Yoffee, 1975) and increasing parental recall of medical recommendations in general pediatric settings (Heffer et al., 1997).

Written instructions can also take the form of self-management plans to assist parents of children diagnosed with a chronic illness to determine intervention needs, such as for changing medications or obtaining further medical assistance. An example of this is the development and empirical evaluation of an action plan for children with mild to moderate asthma (Gillies et al., 1996). Families of 102 children with asthma were given written guidelines, and parents were asked to bring this action plan to all of their children's subsequent medical appointments. The action plan was found to be both effective and acceptable for home management of children with asthma. Significant improvements noted over the 4-month intervention included decreases in nights awakened from asthma from 30.4% to 16.9% and in *days out of action* from 3.8 to 1.7. The authors hypothesized that the success of the action plan may have been partially due to increases in children's and families' knowledge of the treatment regimen for asthma and improved communication with general practitioners. A similar written self-management plan could be developed for children with other chronic conditions and readily lends itself to individualized treatment plans required for many children with chronic conditions.

Review the Treatment Plan at Each Clinic Visit

Another important suggestion for clinical intervention is for medical caregivers to review the child's treatment plan with the child patient and parent(s) at each clinic visit to maximize their knowledge of the treatment regimen. In addition to the problem of children and their parents forgetting treatment-related information over time, all of the caregivers (parents, stepparents, grandparents) are not necessarily present at each visit or hospitalization. Thus, reviewing this material helps the child patient and parents learn successful medical management skills and increases the likelihood that all involved caregivers are personally educated about the specifics of the treatment regimen.

To further illustrate the need for frequent review of the child's treatment regimen, consider the following interchange among a 12-year-old female with CF, her parents, and the senior author of this chapter during an intervention session designed to increase adherence to treatments. This videotaped session occurred approximately 2 years after the child had been prescribed the flutter device for airway clearance. When asked "How long do you have to do the flutter?", the child replied, "About 5 minutes . . . 10 . . . around there." Her mother interjected, "You never do no 10." The child said, "Well, he (the physician) tells me to do five sets; that's only five blows per set. That don't take long." The father then asked, "What did the videotape (on the use of the flutter device) say to do?" The child said, "Yeah, what did the videotape say?" The father then said, "We got the videotape at home. You ever watched it?" The child answered, "No." The father said, "I'll have to show it to you. Maybe all three of us should sit down and view this videotape so we can make sure you're doing it correctly, and then you'll know how long you're supposed to be doing it." In a later session on the same subject discussing the child's original training to use the flutter, the mother admitted, "It's been awhile, and I can truthfully say I don't remember how long he (the respiratory therapist) told her to do it."

Improve the Frequency and Quality of Physician Communication With Child and Adolescent Patients Concerning the Treatment Regimen

To encourage greater independence in the management of a condition, many physicians who care for children and adolescents with chronic illnesses begin to see child patients alone for their medical visits as they grow older. Based on our clinical experience, the timing of this transition varies considerably by physician and by child and family. Unfortunately, there is little available research to provide guidance to medical providers as to when children may be competent enough to assume responsibility for independently discussing the status of their current treatment regimen or any recommended changes in treatments with their medical caregivers. Specifically, it is not yet known at what age children can adequately recall the clinically relevant details of conversations with their medical caregivers about treatment recommendations, although available data indicate that children have even more difficulty recalling medical recommendations than their parents (e.g., Ievers et al., in press). However, information concerning age-related patterns of responsibility for illness management, at least for some clinical conditions such as diabetes and CF, suggests that adolescents continue to require supervision and help from their parents in managing their chronic illness (Drotar & Ievers, 1994). Consequently, although medical caregivers may prefer to spend some time alone with older children discussing their condition and adjustment, any recommended changes in treatment-related tasks need to be reviewed with the child's parents.

FUTURE DIRECTIONS

Research Recommendations

Measurement. Many limitations exist with regard to the current measurement of knowledge of the treatment regimen for childhood chronic illnesses. Some of the currently existing measures of knowledge in these populations mix items that assess components of knowledge of the illness, such as the purpose of treatments and understanding of genetics and reproduction with a few items assessing knowledge of the treatment regimen (i.e., what the physician recommended to the patient for certain treatments; e.g., Fitzclarence & Henry, 1990; Tamaroff, Festa, Adesman, & Walco, 1992; Tebbi et al., 1988). Such instruments may not detect clinically relevant deficits in knowledge about actions required for implementation of the treatment regimen. In addition, the majority of studies of knowledge in childhood chronic illnesses have usually lumped all knowledge-related items together for a total *knowledge* score and thus have failed to examine the various components of knowledge separately.

Another limitation is that previous research has failed to differentiate what children and parents know to be the recommended treatments from their actual treatment-related behaviors. Parents and/or their children with chronic illnesses are often asked to describe what their children are doing with respect to their treatments. This information is then equated with their knowledge of what the physician prescribed. However, this method may be misleading because children and parents may not be performing their treatments according to their physician's prescription. Some may choose to perform treatments more or less often than as prescribed, and therefore their descriptions of children's treatment-related behaviors would differ from their reports of prescribed treatments. In the case of the Rusakow et al. (1998) study, children with CF and their parents were asked to report when the children took their pancreatic enzymes (e.g., before, during, or after meals). It was not determined whether those who were taking their enzymes after meals knew that this was not recommended by their medical caregivers. This is important information to obtain because the reason for noncompliance could be ascertained (i.e., a lack of knowledge of physician recommendations vs. some other factor such as the child's forgetfulness—he or she may not remember to take enzymes until after finishing a meal or snack). Thus, measurement of knowledge of the treatment regimen should inquire about the child patient and parents' understanding of what specific treatments were recommended to them by medical personnel, rather than what the child patient is currently doing with respect to his or her treatment.

With some notable exceptions (Gudas, Koocher, & Wypiz, 1991; Ievers et al., in press), few measures containing items assessing knowledge of the treatment regimen compared child and parent reports of treatment-related recommendations with actual medical prescriptions taken from medical charts or interviews with physicians, nurses, dieticians, and so on. Instead, a usual standard of care is employed to determine level of knowledge of the treatment regimen. This method is problematic because children with the same chronic illness can have different treatment regimens. Using CF as an example, some physicians may recommend that children with few symptoms perform chest physical therapy on an as-needed basis (i.e., PRN) rather than routinely, which is a much more typical or standard regimen. In these PRN cases, children with CF and their parents who report that they were told to do chest physical therapy only when the child is ill are actually exhibiting adequate knowledge of medical recommendations. Making assumptions about individual children's and parents' level of knowledge of treatment based on the standard or usual treatments for illnesses neglects important individual differences in medical care due to treatment severity, physician beliefs about appropriate treatment, and so on.

Consequently, we recommend that measurement of knowledge of the treatment regimen should include the administration of a questionnaire to assess the child patient's or parents' understanding of the child's prescribed treatments, the name and dose of prescribed and nonprescribed medications, the duration and frequency of treatments, and the order of administration of treatments if applicable. The measurement of knowledge of the treatment regimen should also include an assessment of the actual medical recommendations obtained from the medical chart or interviews with their medical caregivers. These medical recommendations should then be compared to the child patient's or parents' responses on the knowledge measure to determine the accuracy of their understanding of the treatment regimen. Most important, the questions and scales employed on both assessment devices must be equated so as to ensure that a direct comparison is possible. As an example of parallel items from such a measure, refer to Table 11.2.

Finally, to compare findings within chronic illness groups (i.e., between studies and among the various treatment domains) and across illness groups, the percentage of child patients and parents who demonstrate accurate knowledge of prescribed treatments (i.e., scaled scores on the knowledge of treatment questionnaire that correspond closely to scaled scores on the physician treatment questionnaire) could be reported as in Ievers et al. (in press). These percentages would enable researchers to determine not only which treatment domains are associated with the poorest knowledge within a particular illness group, but also may indicate which chronic illness groups might benefit the most from interventions to increase their knowledge of prescribed treatments.

One challenge of this method that needs to be addressed in future research is this: The subsequent evaluation of the clinical significance of varying levels of child patients' and parents' accuracy about prescribed treatments—whether small discrepancies between patient and/or parent knowledge of treatments and physician recommendations constitute a threat to the child's health. Often the clinical significance of inaccurate knowledge of the treatment regimen is not clear (Ievers et al., in press).

Interventions. Although interventions to increase recall of treatment recommendations have been conducted in primary care pediatric care settings, these have yet to be empirically validated in children with chronic conditions attending specialty clinics (Heffer et al., 1997; Lewis, Pantell, & Sharp, 1991). For example, in a recent intervention that involved physicians providing parents and their children with written instructions, only one child in this sample had a chronic illness (Heffer et al., 1997). A similar study is warranted for parents of children diagnosed as having chronic illnesses to determine the benefits of providing written instructions, as did Gillies and colleagues (1996) with their action plans for children with asthma.

Educational interventions should be developed to enhance child and parental knowledge of treatment regimens for chronic illnesses and to determine whether and to what extent improved knowledge of treatment is associated with treatment adherence. One possibility is to test the efficacy of specific treatment components designed to increase knowledge of the treatment regimen in existing educational intervention programs developed for children with chronic illnesses. For example, the Bartholomew et al. (1991) Family Education Program for children with CF includes a session to teach children and their parents about communicating with medical providers about treatments. This session could be expanded and employed as an intervention to increase children's and parents' communication skills during clinic visits with their medical caregivers to enhance their understanding of treatments.

Another recommendation is to conduct a randomized controlled trial of the intervention suggested by Rusakow et al. (1998): to give patients and/or their parents a written test of their knowledge of their medical treatment regimen. Parents and children could be given a test of the child's treatment regimen to be completed prior to the medical visit. For the experimental group, this test could be reviewed by medical caregivers to correct any misconceptions or omissions of treatments. A follow-up assessment could then be conducted immediately following the visit and at longer intervals to determine the effectiveness of this intervention in increasing parents' and children's knowledge of the treatment regimen.

Finally, an intervention study with child patients who have a chronic illness and their parents could be developed to test the efficacy of alternative methods of physicians' and/or the treatment team's presentation of information about medical treatments using the communication strategies suggested by Ley (1979). In the experimental group, pediatricians or other medical caregivers could be trained in communication strategies that have been found to enhance patient recall of medical information (e.g., present the most important information first, emphasize key instructions and information, use short words and sentences, and minimize medical terminology). Accuracy of knowledge of the treatment regimen and recall of medical information from the previous clinic visit could be compared for child patients and parents in the experimental and control groups to determine the efficacy of these strategies. To ensure that medical caregivers in the experimental group were indeed employing the strategies appropriately, physician/patient communication during clinic visits could be audiotaped and analyzed to attest to the integrity of the intervention. A great deal needs to be learned about child and family knowledge of chronic illness treatment regimens and the relationship to treatment adherence. Additional research on this topic would have clinical relevance in that it would help physicians clarify key elements of treatment for their patients and reduce misunderstandings among children, parents, and physicians concerning recommended treatments.

ACKNOWLEDGMENT

Supported in part by NIH HL 47064 Trial of Family Intervention in Cystic Fibrosis.

REFERENCES

Alexander, A. B. (1983). The nature of asthma. In P. J. McGrath & P. Firestone (Eds.), *Pediatric and adolescent behavioral medicine: Issues in treatment* (pp. 28–66). New York: Springer.

Bartholomew, L. K., Parcel, G. S., Seilheimer, D. K., Czyzewski, D., Spinelli, S. H., & Congdon, B. (1991). Development of a health education program to promote the self-management of cystic fibrosis. *Health Education Quarterly, 18*(4), 429–443.

Becker, M. H., Drachman, R. H., & Kirscht, J. P. (1972). Predicting mothers' compliance with pediatric medical regimens. *Journal of Pediatrics, 81,* 843–854.

Bernard-Bonnin, A. C., Stachenko, S., Bonin, D., Charette, C., & Rousseau, E. (1995). Self-management teaching programs and morbidity of pediatric asthma: A meta-analysis. *Journal of Allergy and Clinical Immunology, 95,* 34–41.

Brandt, P. A., & Magyary, D. L. (1993). The impact of a diabetes education program on children and mothers. *Journal of Pediatric Nursing, 8*(1), 31–40.

Brazil, K., McLean, L., Abbey, D., & Musselman, C. (1997). The influence of health education on family management of childhood asthma. *Patient Education and Counseling, 30,* 107–118.

Christiansen, S. C., Martin, S. B., Schleicher, N. C., Koziol, J. A., Mathews, K. P., & Zuraw, B. L. (1997). Evaluation of a school-based asthma education program for inner-city children. *Journal of Allergy and Clinical Immunology, 100,* 613–617.

Collier, B. N., & Etzwiler, D. D. (1971). Comparative study of diabetes knowledge among juvenile diabetics and their parents. *Diabetes, 20*(1), 51–57.

Da Costa, I. G., Rapoff, M. A., Lemanek, K., & Goldstein, G. L. (1997). Improving adherence to medication regimens for children with asthma and its effect on clinical outcome. *Journal of Applied Behavior Analysis, 30*(4), 687–691.

Drotar, D., & Ievers, C. (1994). Age differences in parent and child responsibilities for management of cystic fibrosis and insulin-dependent diabetes mellitus. *Journal of Developmental and Behavioral Pediatrics, 15*(4), 265–272.

Epstein, L. H., Beck, S., Figueroa, J., Farkas, G., Kasdin, A. E., Daneman, D., & Becker, D. (1981). The effects of targeting improvements in urine glucose on metabolic control in children with insulin-dependent diabetes. *Journal of Applied Behavior Analyasis, 14*, 365–375.

Etzwiler, D. D., & Robb, J. R. (1972). Evaluation of programmed education among juvenile diabetics and their families. *Diabetes Care, 21*, 967–971.

Fitzclarence, C. A. B., & Henry, R. L. (1990). Validation of an asthma knowledge questionnaire. *Journal of Pediatric Child Health, 26*, 200–204.

Fletcher, S. W., Fletcher, R. H., Thomas, D. C., & Hamann, C. (1979). Patients' understanding of prescribed drugs. *Journal of Community Health, 4*(3), 183–189.

Francis, V., Korsch, B. M., & Morris, M. J. (1969). Gaps in doctor-patient communication: Patients' response to medical advice. *New England Journal of Medicine, 280*, 535–540.

Gilbert, B. O., Johnson, S. B., Spillar, R., McCallum, M., Silverstein, J. H., & Rosenbloom, A. (1982). The effects of a peer-modeling film on children learning to self-inject insulin. *Behavior Therapy, 13*, 186–193.

Gillies, J., Barry, D., Crane, J., Jones, D., MacLennan, L., Pearce, N., Reid, J., Toop, L., & Wilson, B. (1996). A community trial of a written self-management plan for children with asthma. *New Zealand Medical Journal, 109*, 30–33.

Gordon, G. H., Baker, L., & Levinson, W. (1995). Physician-patient communication in managed care. *Western Journal of Medicine, 163*(6), 527–531.

Gudas, L. J., Koocher, G. P., & Wypiz, D. (1991). Perceptions of medical compliance in children and adolescents with cystic fibrosis. *Journal of Developmental and Behavioral Pediatrics, 12*(4), 236–242.

Hamburg, B., & Inoff, G. E. (1982). Relationships between behavioral factors and diabetic control in children and adolescents: A camp study. *Psychosomatic Medicine, 44*(4), 321–339.

Harkavy, J., Johnson, S. B., Silverstein, J., Spillar, R., McCallum, M., & Rosenbloom, A. (1983). Who learns what at diabetes summer camp. *Journal of Pediatric Psychology, 8*, 143–153.

Heffer, R. W., Worchel-Prevatt, F., Rae, W. A., Lopez, M. A., Young-Saleme, T., Orr, K., Aikman, G., Krause, M., & Weir, M. (1997). The effects of oral versus written instructions on parents' recall and satisfaction after pediatric appointments. *Journal of Developmental and Behavioral Pediatrics, 18*(6), 377–382.

Henley, L. D., & Hill, I. D. (1990). Global and specific disease-related information needs of cystic fibrosis patients and their families. *Pediatrics, 85*(6), 1015–1021.

Hess, G. E., & Davis, W. K. (1983). The validation of a diabetes patient knowledge test. *Diabetes Care, 6*, 591–596.

Heston, J. V., & Lazar, S. J. (1980). Evaluating a learned device for juvenile diabetic children. *Diabetes Care, 3*, 668–671.

Howland, J., Bauchner, H., & Adair, R. (1988). The impact of pediatric asthma education on morbidity: Assessing the evidence. *Chest, 94*, 964–969.

Hulka, B., Kupper, L., Cassel, J., Elfird, R., & Burdette, J. (1975). Medication use and misuse: Physician-patient discrepancies. *Journal of Chronic Diseases, 28*, 7–21.

Ievers, C. E., Brown, R. T., Drotar, D., Caplan, D., Pishevar, B. S., & Lambert, R. G. (in press). Knowledge of physician prescriptions and adherence to treatment among children with cystic fibrosis and their mothers. *Journal of Developmental and Behavioral Pediatrics.*

Johnson, S. B. (1984). Knowledge, attitudes, and behavior: Correlates of health in childhood diabetes. *Clinical Psychology Review, 4*, 503–524.

Johnson, S. B., Pollak, T., Silverstein, J. H., Rosenbloom, A. L., Spillar, R., McCallum, M., & Harkavy, J. (1982). Cognitive and behavioral knowledge about insulin dependent diabetes among children and parents. *Pediatrics, 69,* 708–713.

Kolbe, J., Vamos, M., James, F., Elkind, G., & Garrett, J. (1996). Assessment of practical knowledge of self-management of acute asthma. *Chest, 109*(1), 86–90.

Kravitz, R. L., Hays, R. D., Sherbourne, C. D., DeMatteo, R., Rogers, W. H., Ordway, L., & Greenfield, S. (1993). Recall of recommendations and adherence to advice among patients with chronic medical conditions. *Archives of Internal Medicine, 153,* 1869–1878.

La Greca, A. M., & Schuman, W. B. (1995). Adherence to prescribed medical regimens. In M. C. Roberts (Ed.), *Handbook of pediatric psychology* (2nd ed., pp. 55–83). New York: Guilford.

Lewis, C. C., Pantell, R. H., & Sharp, L. (1991). Increasing patient knowledge, satisfaction, and involvement: Randomized trial of a communication intervention. *Pediatrics, 88*(2), 351–358.

Ley, P. (1979). Memory for medical information. *British Journal of Social and Clinical Psychology, 18*(2), 245–255.

Ley, P. (1982). Satisfaction, compliance, and communication. *British Journal of Social and Clinical Psychology, 21,* 241–254.

Lopez Siquero, J. P., Martinez Aedo, M. J., Lopez Moreno, M. D., & Martinez Valverde, A. (1995). Treatment with growth hormone. What do children know and how do they accept it? *Hormone Research, 44*(3), 18–25.

Markello, J. R. (1985). Factors influencing pediatric compliance. *Pediatric Infectious Disease, 4*(5), 579–583.

Mattar, M. F., Markello, J., & Yaffe, S. J. (1975). Pharmaceutic factors affecting pediatric compliance. *Pediatrics, 55,* 101–108.

Michielutte, R., Diseker, R., & Hayes, D. (1979). Knowledge of cancer: A cross-cultural comparison among students in the US and the UK. *International Journal of Health Education, 22,* 242–248.

Nolan, T., Desmond, K., Herlich, R., & Hardy, S. (1986). Knowledge of cystic fibrosis in patients and their parents. *Pediatrics, 77*(2), 229–235.

Page, P., Verstraete, D., Robb, J. R., & Etzwiler, D. D. (1981). Patient recall of self-care recommendations in diabetes. *Diabetes Care, 4*(1), 96–98.

Quittner, A. L., Tobert, V. E., Regoli, M. J., Orenstein, D. M., Hollingsworth, J. L., & Eigen, H. (1996). Development of the role play inventory of situations and coping strategies for parents of children with cystic fibrosis. *Journal of Pediatric Psychology, 21,* 209–235.

Rost, K., Roter, D., Bertakis, K., & Quill, T. (1990). Physician–patient familiarity and patient recall of medication changes. *Family Medicine, 22*(6), 453–457.

Roter, D. L., Hall, J. A., & Katz, N. R. (1987). Relations between physicians' behaviors and analogue patients' satisfaction, recall, and impressions. *Medical Care, 25*(5), 437–451.

Rubin, D. H., Bauman, L. J., & Lauby, J. L. (1989). The relationship between knowledge and reported behavior in childhood asthma. *Journal of Developmental and Behavioral Pediatrics, 10*(6), 307–312.

Rusakow, L. S., Miller, T., McCarthy, C. A., Gershan, W. M., & Splaingard, M. L. (1998). Unsuspected nonadherence with recommended pancreatic enzyme administration in patients with cystic fibrosis. *Children's Health Care, 27*(4), 259–264.

Schraa, J. C., & Dirks, J. F. (1982). Improving patient recall and comprehension of the treatment regimen. *Journal of Asthma, 19*(3), 159–162.

Smith, N. A., Seale, J. P., Ley, P., Shaw, J., & Bracs, P. U. (1986). Effects of intervention on medication compliance in children with asthma. *The Medical Journal of Australia, 144,* 119–122.

Tamaroff, M. H., Festa, R. S., Adesman, A. R., & Walco, G. (1992). Therapeutic adherence to oral medication regimens by adolescents with cancer: II. Clinical and psychologic correlates. *Journal of Pediatrics, 120,* 812–817.

Tebbi, C. K., Richards, M. E., Cummings, K. M., Zevon, M. A., & Mallon, J. C. (1988). The role of parent-adolescent concordance in compliance with cancer chemotherapy. *Adolescence, 23*(91), 599–611.

Tehan, N., Sloane, B. C., Walsh-Robart, N., & Chamberlain, M. D. (1989). Impact of asthma self-management education on the health behavior of young adults. *Journal of Adolescent Health Care, 10,* 513–519.

PART VI

IMPACT OF TREATMENT ADHERENCE ON CHILD HEALTH OUTCOMES AND RESEARCH FINDINGS

Contributors to this section consider the implications of the impact of treatment noncompliance on children's health and well-being as well as research findings. Although the prevalence of treatment nonadherence in populations of children with chronic health conditions has been documented, the impact of treatment adherence on children's health and quality of life is much less understood. In chapter 12, Varni and his colleagues present a conceptual model to guide understanding of the impact of patient adherence on children's health-related quality of life. In this model, background factors such as age, gender, family composition, and illness-related factors such as diagnosis and severity are hypothesized to contribute to the development of health-related quality of life and skills in problem solving and coping.

Varni et al. (chap. 12) derive the hypothesis that adherence to chronic treatment is affected by health-related knowledge, attitudes and skills, and problem solving. One of the specific contributions of this model is to highlight the importance of practices of the health care team, including communication, quality improvement strategies, and treatment care paths and management plans. Children's quality of life is expected to be influenced by their physical symptoms as well as the practices of the health care team. Varni and colleagues articulate the importance of health-related quality of life as an indicator of child health. They argue that it may be a more important outcome measure of treatment effectiveness than either clinical or biomedical outcomes. In this model, one of the goals of health care is to improve patients' health-related quality of life by enhancing symptom management, treatment adherence, and ability to cope with the impact of their physical condition on their daily functioning.

To address the problem of limited measures of the measurement of health-related quality of life in pediatric populations, Varni and colleagues have developed the Pediatric Quality of Life–Version 3. This is a pediatric quality of life inventory that can be used across multiple chronic conditions and has generic core scales and disease-specific modules. Potential applications of this measure in different illness groups, including diabetes and asthma, are described.

Varni and colleagues underscore the need for additional empirical studies to establish the link between treatment adherence for chronic illness and health outcomes in children. They also recommend that specific interventions (e.g., problem solving concerning illness management) be designed to enhance health-related quality of life outcomes and improve health care utilization. Health-related quality of life measures provide a way to assess the potential impact of such interventions on symptom management and on patients' perceptions of the impact of their illness.

In chapter 13, Johnson contributes an interesting analysis of the impact of noncompliance on data that are obtained from clinical trials evaluating the effects of medication and/or other medical interventions. She notes that noncompliance with treatment traditionally has been viewed as a source of error that must be controlled or minimized by careful subject selection procedures and/or intention-to-treat analyses. Johnson argues convincingly that the traditional scientific perspective of viewing noncompliance as error has severely restricted the nature of the information that is collected, created problems with interpretation of data, and limited the significance of results. Johnson questions the assumption that there are sufficient numbers of highly compliant individuals available for study to allow investigators to accurately identify these compliant individuals prior to study initiation. Moreover, there is no solid evidence that compliant patients can be accurately identified.

Johnson presents data from various clinical trials that question the practice of using a prerandomization run-in period to identify and exclude potentially noncompliant persons from trial participation. She notes that exclusion of patients who did not comply with run-in procedures would not only limit the ability to compare study effects across ethnic groups, but limit generalization of study findings. Johnson also critically examines the impact of intent-to-treat analyses, which are predicated on the assumption that eliminating noncompliant participants may introduce unwanted bias.

As an alternative to these practices, she argues that inclusion of compliance behavior in statistical analyses would permit potential estimates of therapeutic thresholds and address the important need to determine how much medication or other treatments are necessary to yield clinically meaningful results. Although patients are instructed to take all of their medication, it is quite possible that less medication would be equally effective. In the absence of assessments of compliance behavior, one cannot determine whether patients who took less medication did as well as those who took all of it.

Johnson describes several promising applications of compliance behavior research (e.g., longitudinal studies of disease onset and prevention), which typically require large numbers of persons who are monitored over long periods of time and afford opportunities to identify the factors that contribute to participation versus nonparticipation in clinical trials. Other opportunities include genetic testing studies, where the expertise of behavioral scientists can be used to enhance participant compliance in genetic testing, and effectiveness research, which offers opportunities to examine patient compliance behavior within known treatments in clinical practice and to assess treatment acceptability.

Johnson notes that it is important to develop effective intervention strategies to assist those who initially may not be good candidates for clinical trials to participate more effectively in research. Moreover, a detailed assessment on compliance behavior can also provide critical information that is relevant to a demonstration of treatment threshold effects (e.g., what level of compliance is necessary to achieve a satisfactory effect of medical treatment).

CHAPTER TWELVE

Treatment Adherence as a Predictor of Health-Related Quality of Life

James W. Varni
*Children's Hospital and Health Center, San Diego, CA,
and University of California, San Diego, School of Medicine*

Jenifer R. Jacobs
Michael Seid
Children's Hospital and Health Center, San Diego, CA

Strategies to measure and enhance adherence to treatment regimens have received increasing prominence as biomedical science and technology have developed interventions deemed worthy to be followed. It has long been assumed that patient nonadherence to prescribed treatment regimens seriously undermines the effectiveness of interventions in both preventive and curative situations and results in unnecessary morbidity, mortality, and cost. For pediatric chronic health conditions, symptom management rather than cure is the potentially achievable goal of treatment (Varni, 1983; Wallander & Varni, 1998). However, symptom management typically requires extensive family involvement and patient self-management over extended periods, often for life (Varni & Wallander, 1984). Given the complexities and duration of most pediatric chronic health conditions, the prevalence of nonadherence is significant, and the impact of nonadherence can have direct effects on the management of patient symptoms.

Although strict adherence to some treatment regimens may have a salutary effect on specific disease-related symptoms, it may also have an untoward impact on overall patient-perceived health-related quality of life (HRQOL). A more comprehensive, integrative perspective of the relationship between therapeutic adherence and health status, including a broader view beyond disease-specific symptoms, may ultimately lead to more tailored interventions to enhance HRQOL, with therapeutic adherence being one component of the conceptual framework. Figure 12.1 repre-

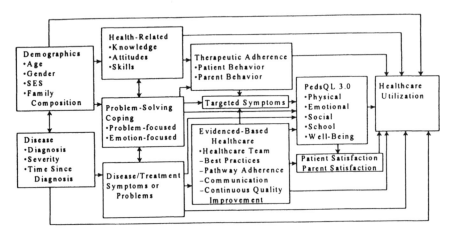

FIG. 12.1. Integrated conceptual model of therapeutic adherence and health related quality of life (adapted from Varni, 1998).

sents our integrative conceptual model at this stage of development. We describe specific aspects of this heuristic conceptual framework as they relate to therapeutic adherence and HRQOL, and we succinctly review the extant literature in adults and children to illustrate the hypothesized measurement and structural components of the path model. Diabetes and asthma are utilized as exemplary disease models where applicable.

We begin with the standardized measurement of HRQOL outcomes using the PedsQL™ (Pediatric Quality of Life Inventory) as an example: We predict HRQOL by disease-specific symptoms, discuss findings on the relationship between therapeutic adherence and HRQOL from the available literature, and present the concept of tailoring interventions, including those for enhancing therapeutic adherence, based on PedsQL™ computer-assisted assessment as an exemplary illustration.

THE HEALTH-RELATED QUALITY OF LIFE CONSTRUCT

The accurate, comprehensive measurement of health outcomes in pediatric chronic health conditions requires a multidimensional approach (Varni, Pruitt, & Seid, 1998). *Quality of life, functional status,* or *health status* are terms frequently used interchangeably in the assessment of the impact of a physical disorder, although health-related quality of life is the more comprehensive concept (Guyatt, Feeny, & Patrick, 1993). Similar to laboratory tests for biological disease, screening for HRQOL morbidity in a patient population requires a standardized test with established reliability and validity (Varni & Setoguchi, 1992). As a broad measure of health, HRQOL is a multidimensional construct that includes primary domains of physical and mental health functioning, social and role functioning, disease- and treatment-related symptoms, and general perceptions of well-being (Varni, Seid, & Kurtin, 1999). Traditional biomedical outcomes often lack the ability to assess the full impact of chronic conditions. Consequently, HRQOL may be a more important health outcome measure of treatment effectiveness than clinical or biomedical outcomes for many nonfatal diseases and chronic disorders. With these chronic health conditions, the main goal of health care may best be to improve the patient's HRQOL by enhancing symptom management, treatment adherence, and ability to cope with the impact of his or her physical condition on daily functioning.

Measurement of HRQOL in pediatric populations is especially challenging because of several factors, including the importance of developmental considerations and questions regarding the best respondent for HRQOL assessment. The circumstances under which proxies' ratings of patients' quality of life are accurate and acceptable have been a topic of growing empirical scrutiny. Imperfect concordance has been consistently noted in adult HRQOL research between adult patients' self-reports of their HRQOL and the ratings of both health care providers and significant others (e.g., spouses; Sprangers & Aaronson, 1992). In pediatrics, a lack of ideal congruence has been documented among child/adolescent, parent, teacher, and health care professionals' reports in the assessment of physically healthy children's adjustment (Achenbach, McConaughy, & Howell, 1987). Agreement among observers has been found to be lower for internalizing problems (e.g., depression, anxiety, pain, nausea) than for externalizing problems (e.g., hyperactivity, aggression, physical functioning). This discordance or lack of agreement among reporters of child/adolescent adjustment has been termed *cross-informant variance* (Varni, Katz, Colegrove, & Dolgin, 1995). It has been demonstrated in the HRQOL assessment of children with asthma (Guyatt, Juniper, Griffith, Feeny, & Ferry, 1997), cancer (Varni, Katz, Seid, Quiggins, Friedman-Bender, & Castro, 1998), and other pediatric chronic health conditions. Given that HRQOL derives from a person's perceptions of the impact of disease and treatment (Schipper, Clinch, & Olweny, 1996), the presence of cross-informant variance indicates a critical need to develop pediatric patient self-report HRQOL instruments to ensure that the child's perceptions are accurately measured.

The development of a reliable and valid parent proxy-report of HRQOL to supplement pediatric patient self-report is important in at least two ways. First, children are rarely in the position to refer themselves for treatment even when they are experiencing symptoms and problems. It is the parents' perceptions of the child's HRQOL that influence the likelihood that care will be sought. Thus, the parents' perception of HRQOL, although not necessarily reflecting the patient's experience with complete accuracy, is important in seeking treatment for the child. Second, the use of a proxy rater to estimate patient HRQOL may be necessary when the patient is either unable or unwilling to complete the HRQOL measure. Given these considerations, the evaluation of HRQOL with parallel pediatric patient self-report and parent proxy-report forms is essential (Varni, Seid, & Rode, 1999).

THE PEDSQL™ MEASUREMENT MODEL

The PedsQL™ 3.0 (Pediatric Quality of Life Inventory, Version 3.0) builds on and expands a programmatic measurement research instrument development effort in pediatric chronic health conditions by Varni and his associates during the past 15 years. Specifically, standardized measurement of pain, coping, and functional status in pediatric arthritis (Varni, Thompson, & Hanson, 1987; Varni et al., 1996; Varni, Wilcox, Hanson, & Brik, 1988) and functional status and health care satisfaction in pediatric limb deficiency (Pruitt, Seid, Varni, & Setoguichi, 1999; Pruitt, Varni, Seid, & Setoguchi, 1997, 1998; Pruitt, Varni, & Setoguchi, 1996) provided the empirical experience for the development of pediatric patient self-report and parent proxy-report HRQOL measurement instruments across a wide age range. A disease-specific HRQOL instrument, the Pediatric Cancer Quality of Life Inventory (PCQL), was first developed and field tested with 291 pediatric cancer patients and their parents (Varni, Katz, Seid, Quiggins, Friedman-Bender, & Castro, 1998), followed by the development of the 32-item PCQL–32 short form and health care satisfaction module (Varni, Katz, Seid, Quiggins, & Friedman-Bender, 1998; Varni, Quiggins, & Ayala, in press; Varni, Rode, Seid, Katz, Friedman-Bender, & Quiggins, 1999).

The PedsQL™ 1.0, originally derived from the PCQL pediatric cancer database, is a generic pediatric quality of life inventory designed to be utilized noncategorically (i.e., across multiple pediatric chronic health conditions) with generic core scales and disease-specific modules (Varni, Seid, & Rode, 1999). Given that instrument development is an iterative process, the PedsQL™ 2.0 was a further advancement in our measurement model, including additional constructs and items, a more sensitive scaling range, and a broader age range for patient self-report and parent proxy-report. The PedsQL™ 2.0 five generic core scales were field tested in pediatric asthma and arthritis, along with the development of the PedsQL™ Asthma and Arthritis Disease-Specific Modules (Varni, Seid, Jacobs, & Rode, 1999).

The development and field testing of the PedsQL™ 3.0 further enhances the measurement properties of the PedsQL™ within our planned methodology, whereby we constantly upgrade and enhance the measurement instrument to be consistent with state-of-the-art measurement and computer technology. The pediatric self-report (ages 5–18) and parent proxy-report (ages 2–18) multidimensional 30-item PedsQL™ 3.0 encompasses essential core domains for pediatric HRQOL: (a) Physical Functioning (eight items), (b) Emotional Functioning (five items), Social Functioning (five items), (d) School Functioning (five items), (e) Well-Being (six items), and (f) a global perception of overall health status (one item). The PedsQL™ 3.0 is currently being field tested with several thousand children and adolescents in pediatrician offices, hospital specialty clinics, community settings, and schools (for healthy population norms). The PedsQL™ 3.0 has been translated into Spanish and can be computer administered utilizing Audio-CASI (computer-assisted self-administered interview).

COMPUTER-ASSISTED SELF-ADMINISTERED ASSESSMENT

Health status survey research methods have traditionally relied on paper-and-pencil procedures administered by interviewers or self-administered by respondents (Fowler, 1993). Technological advances in the past decade have facilitated the development of interviewer-administered computer-assisted telephone interviewing (CATI) and computer-assisted personal (face-to-face) interviewing (CAPI). With CATI and CAPI, the questions appear on a computer screen and are read to the respondent by the interviewer either in person or over the telephone. The interviewer then enters the response directly into the computer after each question. The newer generation of laptop and palmtop lightweight computers has now enabled computer-assisted assessment technology to encompass the self-administered interview. The computer-assisted self-administered interview (CASI) involves the respondent interacting directly with the computer. With CASI, the interviewer merely enters the respondent's identification number at the outset and gives the respondent some brief instructions about how to complete the interview directly on the computer through self-administration (Couper & Rowe, 1996). Computer-assisted self-administered health status survey technologies have the potential to adjust the language of questions to the language of the respondent, as well as read questions out loud for those who have difficulty reading (Fowler, 1993).

The audio computer-assisted self-administration interview (Audio–CASI) offers the advantages of CASI without limiting data collection to the literature segment of the population (O'Reilly, Hubbard, Lessler, Biemer, & Turner, 1994). Additionally, Audio–CASI has been demonstrated to increase the reporting of sensitive health-related information in comparison with more traditional self-administered paper-and-pencil questionnaires (Turner et al., 1998). The application of this technology to the measurement of patient self-report and parent proxy-report of adherence to treatment regimens may provide a more accurate measure of this health behavior, as well as the measurement of HRQOL.

THE PEDSQL™ DISEASE-SPECIFIC MODULES

The concept of integrating into one assessment instrument both generic core HRQOL scales and disease-specific modules was influenced by the measurement research conducted by the European Organization for Research and Treatment of Cancer (EROTC) study group (Sprangers, Cull, Bjordal, Groenvold, & Aaronson, 1993). Generic HRQOL measures permit comparisons across different diseases, between acutely and chronically ill patient populations, and between ill and healthy individuals. Because generic measures can be administered to a broad array of patients and populations, they can be particularly instrumental in making health policy decisions, such as the allocation of resources related to health, education, or social services (Varni, Seid, & Kurtin, 1999). The supplemental modules are intended to assess disease and treatment effects and other relevant HRQOL issues not sufficiently covered in the generic core measure.

The PedsQL™ 3.0 generic core scales are designed to enable comparisons across patient populations, including healthy populations. The goal of the chronic health condition-specific modules is to assess functioning specifically related to disease or treatment effects within a circumscribed clinical sample. Disease-specific measures are presumed to be more sensitive to changes in disease states and consequently may be more useful in comparing treatments within a disease. However, disease-specific measures are limited in their usefulness for comparison across different patient populations and with healthy population norms for benchmarking purposes. Thus, the PedsQL™ measurement model combines the strengths of both assessment strategies: the clinical utility and sensitivity of a disease-specific measure, and the applicability of generic core scales across healthy and patient populations required for standardized comparisons among different groups. Measurement of disease- and treatment-specific symptoms and problems by the PedsQL™ 3.0 chronic health condition-specific modules is illustrated using diabetes and asthma as exemplary models.

Diabetes

The PedsQL™ 3.0 Diabetes Module is in its first of several iterations. The module was developed from a review of the literature and focus interviews with youngsters (ages 5 to 18) with diabetes and their families. The measure focuses on issues relevant to the disease and treatment of diabetes. The module is composed of questions related to symptoms such thirst, hunger, fatigue, or frequent urination. Also the effects associated with hypoglycemia, such as shaking, sweating, headaches, and irritability, are included. Treatment variables include acute pain associated with finger sticks for blood glucose monitoring and insulin shots, planning meals, limiting intake of food, and monitoring exercise. Worry about the long-term complications of diabetes is also assessed. Finally, items measuring adherence to the prescribed regimen are imbedded in the module.

Asthma

The PedsQL™ 3.0 Asthma Module consists of items measuring disease-specific symptoms (e.g., feel wheezy, out of breath) and treatment-related problems (e.g., side effects, difficulties with self-management). The Asthma Module was developed through focus groups and individual interviews of pediatric asthma patients and their parents. In a recent study, the pediatric patient self-report and parent proxy-report Asthma Module predicted the PedsQL™ generic core scales in the hypothesized direction (Varni, Seid, Jacobs, & Rode, 1999).

HEALTH-RELATED KNOWLEDGE, ATTITUDES, AND SKILLS

Disease-specific knowledge, attitudes, skills, and health behavior have been investigated in multiple disease prevention and symptom management studies. They are prototypically integrated within one of the major stage theories of health behavior, such as the Health Belief Model, Transtheoretical Model, and Theory of Reasoned Action (cf. Curry & Emmons, 1994; Weinstein, Rothman, & Sutton, 1998, for reviews). Patient and parent knowledge of the disease and acquisition of the skills required for implementing the disease-specific symptom management regimen are best viewed as necessary but insufficient conditions for improving therapeutic adherence (Gilbert & Varni, 1988; Greenan-Fowler, Powell, & Varni, 1987; Sergis-Deavenport & Varni, 1983).

Attitudes develop out of a system of beliefs, which are the generalized expectancies and perceptions of health and illness (Holden & Edwards, 1989). Attitudes are hypothesized to lead to intentions to perform specific health behaviors (Box & Anderson, 1997). The empirically observed interrelationships among knowledge, attitudes, skills, and health behavior are hypothesized to inform the development of interventions to enhance therapeutic adherence (e.g., Aiken, West, Woodward, & Reno, 1994; Bond,

Aiken, & Somerville, 1992; Putnam, Finney, Barkley, & Bonner, 1994; Wiebe & Christensen, 1997).

Diabetes

Knowledge is an important variable in pediatric diabetes for a variety of reasons. Families and children with diabetes must fully understand their disorder to begin to cope with it. They must understand the relationships among calories, sugar, insulin, exercise, and stress, and they must recognize the signs and symptoms of hypoglycemia. They need to understand the rationale for frequent blood glucose monitoring and injections. They need to see the *big picture*. The literature has generally found knowledge to be a necessary but insufficient condition of good metabolic control. Although some studies find that more knowledgeable children and adolescents are more adherent (Lorenz et al., 1985), others find no clear relationship between diabetes knowledge and HRQOL. In a study by Johnson et al. (1992), linear structural equation modeling was utilized with a large longitudinal sample to test the effects of mother and child knowledge about diabetes and past adherence to the diabetes regimen. Although maternal and child knowledge were found to be inconsistent predictors of adherence, better maternal knowledge was associated with more frequent blood glucose tests, and better child knowledge was associated with a low-fat, high-carbohydrate diet. Thus, the findings to date are inconsistent.

Attitudes have also been examined in relation to adherence for pediatric diabetes. In a study testing the constructs of the Health Belief Model, Palardy et al. (1998) found that *health attitudes* (defined as self-efficacy for treatment management, response efficacy of treatment, and response costs of adherence) were strongly related to adolescents' self-report of adherence. The authors concluded that appraisals of the benefits of adherence are important predictors of what adolescents actually do in terms of self-care behaviors.

Asthma

In a study of young children with asthma, Eiser, Town, and Tripp (1988) found that most children (ages 7–16 years) had a poor understanding of asthma in general. Over 50% of the children could not answer questions about what happened inside their bodies to provoke an asthma attack, and about a third of the children not only failed to understand specific precipitants of their own attacks, but also displayed a lack of intentional behavior to avoid attacks (Eiser et al., 1988). A study by Rubin et al. (1989) found that the relationship between knowledge and behavior (adherence to asthma management) was not a linear one; accurate knowledge was related to engaging in more of the recommended behaviors, but only up to the point of moderate knowledge. It appears that, once youngsters have acquired a moderate level of knowledge, more education alone will not increase adherence.

THERAPEUTIC ADHERENCE AS A PREDICTOR OF DISEASE-SPECIFIC SYMPTOMS

The hypothesized interrelationships between health behavior and health status, although assumed to be highly interconnected, have not been unequivocally supported by the research evidence for many chronic health conditions (cf. Johnson, 1994, for a review).

Diabetes

For pediatric diabetes, daily adherence behaviors have been determined, with specific guidelines for treatment (American Diabetes Association, 1998). Because the use of injected insulin only crudely approximates the function of the healthy human pancreas, recommendations for maintaining adequate levels of blood glucose are rather definitive. Specifically, adherence behaviors include insulin injections once or twice a day in a timed relationship with meals. Small meals should be eaten frequently throughout the day (25% of calories at breakfast, 25% at lunch, 30% at dinner, and 20% by snacks), and meals and snacks should be void of concentrated sweets and low in fats. Regular exercise is also part of the recommended regimen for diabetes, but must be done in conjunction with food intake and blood glucose tests to maintain a balance in glycemic levels.

Many studies have documented a small relationship between diabetes adherence and metabolic control (Davis et al., 1995; Hanson et al., 1996; Johnson, Freund, Silverstein, Hansen, & Malone, 1990; Johnson et al., 1992). However, the relationship between adherence and specific symptoms has remained largely unexamined. Further, it is unclear whether a relationship exists between metabolic control and other measures of morbidity, such as sick days, school absences, and emergency room visits (Johnson, 1994). One study of adults found that higher HbA_{1c} levels were significantly associated with higher number of symptoms (thirst, polyuria, weight loss, and neuropathic symptoms; Van der Does et al., 1996). However, this finding may not apply to children who have not yet begun to experience long-term complications of diabetes. In a study examining the Health Belief Model in 56 adolescents with IDDM, no relationship between adherence (measured by 24-hour recall interviews) and metabolic control was found (Bond et al., 1992).

Asthma

The suggested treatment of asthma consists of four main components: (a) objective measures of lung function, (b) pharmacological therapy, (c) environmental control, and (d) specific immunotherapy (see Bender et al., chap. 7, this volume). Objective measurement of lung function includes spirometry and regular peak flow monitoring for all children over age 5. Environmental control involves avoidance of dust mites, cigarette smoke, and cleaning, cooking, and cosmetic fumes. Pharmacological management involves assessment of severity and drug treatment for chronic and/or acute symptoms. Immunotherapy, or specific inoculation, has been found to be helpful if children are allergic to pollen or dust mites (Boner, 1989).

It is a logical assumption that better adherence with the asthma medical regimen should lead to better control of the disease. However, a careful review of the literature suggests that the relationship between adherence and health status in asthma is tenuous at best. This may be due to the variable nature of the disease in general, as well as flaws in the research designs. The relationship between adherence and health status is typically examined using two different methods. In the first method, a correlational design is used: Both adherence data and health status data are recorded, and the relationship between the two is examined. In the second method, a group design is used and participants are divided into groups. One group receives an intervention to increase adherence and the other group receives no such intervention. If, at postintervention, there are advantages in health status between the intervention and the no intervention (control) groups, it is suggested that increasing adherence had a positive effect on health status.

The majority of correlational studies, with both children and adults suffering from asthma, have failed to find support for the hypothesis that adherence is related to decreased morbidity (Gibson et al., 1995; Kelloway, Wyatt, & Adlis, 1994; Laird, Chamberlain, & Spicer, 1994; Pinzone, Carlson, Kotses, & Creer, 1991). However, several studies of children with asthma have found a significant relationship between good adherence and better health status (Chryssanthopoulos, Laufer, & Torphy, 1983; Cluss, Epstein, Galvis, Fireman, & Friday, 1984; Mazon et al., 1994).

The majority of group design intervention studies have found indirect support for the hypothesis that adherence is related to decreased morbidity (see Walders et al., chap. 9, this volume, for a description of intervention studies with asthma). The intervention studies that have targeted self-

management and adherence education have found significant health outcome benefits for their intervention groups as compared with control
groups (Bailey et al., 1990; Bolton, Tilley, Kuder, Reeves, & Schultz, 1991;
Lewis, Rachelefsky, Lewis, de la Sota, & Kaplan, 1984; Muhlhauser, Kraut,
Weske, Worth, & Berger, 1991). However, studies by Mitchell et al. (1986),
Rakos et al. (1985), Whitman et al. (1985), and Clark et al. (1986) found
that education in asthma self-management did not significantly affect
health care use or asthma morbidity in pediatric populations. These intervention studies typically did not assess adherence rates in either the control or intervention groups, so the link between adherence and health outcome in these studies is implied, but not directly tested. Although a
randomized intervention study by Hughes and associates (Hughes,
McLeod, Garner, & Goldbloom, 1991) with 95 children with asthma found
significantly better health outcomes for the group that received nursing
visitations and special health education, this effect was not present at a 1-
year follow-up assessment. This finding underscores the need for follow-
up studies to determine whether the health benefits reported in the
majority of the previous studies are only temporary effects.

THERAPEUTIC ADHERENCE AS A PREDICTOR OF HRQOL

Within the conceptual model, symptoms targeted for treatment adherence are hypothesized to directly affect HRQOL (i.e., targeted symptoms
are hypothesized to be causal indicators of HRQOL). Thus, in structural
equation terminology (Loehlin, 1998), disease- and treatment-related
symptoms or problems are hypothesized to be causal indicators of the
HRQOL construct, whereas physical, emotional, social, school functioning, and well-being are hypothesized to be effect indicators or outcomes
(Fayers & Hand, 1997). For example, in a recent study with the PedsQL™,
higher levels of asthma and arthritis disease-specific symptoms were
causal indicators of lower levels of the five PedsQL™ generic core scales
(Physical, Emotional, Social, School, Well-Being), which are effect indicators of generic HRQOL (Varni, Seid, Jacobs, & Rode, 1999). This provides
initial empirical support for the conceptual model in terms of disease-specific symptoms predicting generic HRQOL.

Stronger causal evidence would result from an intervention study, in
which an intervention designed to enhance adherence to an asthma or
arthritis disease management regimen resulted in lower asthma or arthritis
disease-related symptoms or problems (such as pain in arthritis or breathing difficulties in asthma), further resulting in higher PedsQL™ generic core
scale scores. In a 4-year longitudinal, observational study of 2,125 adult
patients with chronic health conditions (hypertension, diabetes, recent

myocardial infarction, congestive heart failure), conducted as an analysis of the Medical Outcomes Study (MOS) database, the relationship between adherence to medical recommendations and the measure of HRQOL (SF-36) was more complex than has often been assumed (Hays et al., 1994). Clearly integrative models that take into account variables beyond the assumed direct relationship between adherence and generic HRQOL are needed to further explicate these now recognized complex interrelationships. Research evidence of this relationship is a high priority for enhancing the health and well-being of pediatric patients with chronic conditions.

TAILORING INTERVENTIONS TO ENHANCE HRQOL AND THERAPEUTIC ADHERENCE

Given the research to date suggesting that adherence and HRQOL are related, albeit in a complex and as yet not fully understood way, it is important to understand the effect that increasing adherence will have on HRQOL. In particular, it is important to review the specific interventions that have the greatest documented impact on increasing both adherence and HRQOL to best understand what works in which situations. This can then lead to a tailoring of interventions for specific diseases, patients, and circumstances.

Results from the adult health education research literature provide emerging evidence for the advantages of tailored instruction (Campbell et al., 1994; Dijkstra, DeVries, Roijackers, & van Breukelen, 1998; Prochaska, DiClemente, Velicer, & Rossi, 1993; Skinner, Strecher, & Hospers, 1994). These investigations may be instructive in the design of the next generation of pediatric therapeutic adherence intervention research studies. For example, Prochaska et al. (1993) applied the stages of change model to develop a tailored intervention for enhancing adherence to a smoking cessation program based on the following five stages: (a) *Precontemplation* is the period preceding thinking about making a health behavior change; (b) *Contemplation* is the period of time during which an individual seriously thinks about making a health behavior change; (c) *Preparation* is defined as the period during which individuals who have tried to adhere to health behavior change in the past year and are seriously thinking about adhering in the next month; (d) *Action* is the period ranging from 0 to 6 months and occurs after an individual has made the overt change to adhere to a prescribed regimen; and (e) *Maintenance* is defined as the period beginning 6 months after the action stage has started and continuing as long as adherence is indicated, which may be for life in some pediatric chronic health conditions. Results of the Prochaska et al. (1993) study suggest that individualized manuals matched to stage-related variables plus interactive expert-system computer reports outperformed the best self-help programs previously available; in addition, they were delivered in a more cost-effective manner than trained counselors who provided personalized feedback.

Given the wide variation in both the problems encountered and HRQOL outcomes among pediatric patients with chronic health conditions (Wallander & Varni, 1998), computer-assisted tailored health interventions hold the promise of individualizing treatment strategies to maximize efficacy across multiple behavioral, psychosocial, and health domains. For instance, in adults with arthritis and diabetes, it has been found that depressive symptoms and social relationships predict HRQOL and health care utilization outcomes (Kohen, Burgess, Catalan, & Lant, 1998; Patterson et al., 1993; Vali & Walkup, 1998). These findings have implications for tailoring interventions to enhance HRQOL outcomes and health care utilization by identifying factors other than disease-specific symptoms that might respond to cognitive-behavioral intervention, and thereby potentially optimizing disease-related outcomes.

Many authors have stressed the importance of using theory to drive research and interventions. The model described herein suggests ways in which the complex constructs of adherence and HRQOL might be related. Other interrelated variables that have been identified by previous research have also been included in the model. After testing the model with specific pediatric chronic health conditions, we can potentially have a clearer understanding of the predictors of adherence and HRQOL and their interrelationships, which may allow us to better tailor our interventions to enhance treatment efficacy and effectiveness. Problem-solving therapy is an illustration of an empirically derived generic intervention that can be tailored for specific pediatric chronic health conditions. For instance, if the PedsQL™ Social Functioning Scale indicates problems in social relationships with peers for pediatric cancer patients, a tailored social-cognitive problem-solving intervention could be implemented.

PROBLEM-SOLVING COPING STRATEGIES

D'Zurilla and Goldfried (1971) first conceptualized problem-solving theory and research as a five-stage process: (a) Problem Orientation, (b) Problem Definition and Formulation, (c) Generation of Alternative Solutions, (d) Decision Making, and (e) Solution Implementation and Verification. Subsequently, D'Zurilla described in detail the specific techniques in the problem-solving therapy approach to stress management and prevention (D'Zurilla, 1986, 1990). Explicative theoretically driven analyses and treatment research studies have demonstrated the hypothesized relationships among problem-solving skills and emotional distress, knowledge acquisition, and health-related quality of life (D'Zurilla, Nezu, & Maydeu-Olivaries, in press). The application of this approach in teaching problem-solving skills to enhance HRQOL constructs in pediatric cancer patients and maternal caregivers of pediatric cancer patients has been encouraging (Varni, Katz, Colegrove, & Dolgin, 1993; Varni et al., 1999) and may provide a useful treatment model for tailored interventions to enhance HRQOL and adherence to treatment regimens. For example, problem-solving techniques might be used to identify and resolve barriers to optimal adherence, including emotional distress, social incompetence, and other comorbid conditions. Further research is required to determine the efficacy of this approach in improving therapeutic adherence and HRQOL outcomes.

SUMMARY AND CONCLUSIONS

In a recent meta-analysis of the extant empirical literature on the effectiveness of interventions to improve patient adherence, it was concluded that more comprehensive interventions combining cognitive, behavioral, and affective components were more effective than interventions with one only component (Roter et al., 1998). Roter et al. (1998) further suggested that the adherence research intervention studies conducted thus far have been too narrow in focus and would benefit from a broader view of treatment outcomes, including HRQOL. Assessing HRQOL and then tailoring interventions based on these findings would enhance adherence to treatment regimens by taking into account not only the potential symptom management benefits of treatment adherence, but also patient-centered management of the possible side effects of strict adherence.

It is proposed that the next generation of treatment adherence research studies begin with health-related quality of life assessment and then integrate the adherence enhancement intervention within a broader, more comprehensive tailored intervention designed to maximize HRQOL outcomes, rather than simply targeting disease-related symptoms. The integration of multidimensional assessment with multifactorial interventions may result in an enhanced health behavior change and subsequently greater HRQOL outcomes. A programmatic clinical research agenda is needed to determine the efficacy, effectiveness, and ultimate cost–benefit of this interactive, tailored intervention treatment model.

REFERENCES

Achenbach, T. M., McConaughy, S. H., & Howell, C. T. (1987). Child/adolescent behavioral and emotional problems: Implications of cross-informant correlations for situational specificity. *Psychological Bulletin, 101*, 213–232.

Aiken, L. S., West, S. G., Woodward, C. K., & Reno, R. R. (1994). Health beliefs and compliance with mammography-screening recommendations in asymptomatic women. *Health Psychology, 13,* 122–129.

American Diabetes Association. (1998). Standards of medical care for patients with diabetes mellitus. *Diabetes Care, 21,* S23–S31.

Bailey, W. C., Richards, J. M., Jr., Brooks, C. M., Soong, S., Windsor, R. A., & Manzella, B. A. (1990). A randomized trial to improve self-management practices of adults with asthma. *Archives of Internal Medicine, 150,* 1664–1668.

Bolton, M. B., Tilley, B. C., Kuder, J., Reeves, T., & Schultz, L. R. (1991). The cost and effectiveness of an educational program for adults who have asthma. *Journal of General Internal Medicine, 6,* 401–407.

Bond, G. G., Aiken, L. S., & Somerville, S. (1992). The Health Belief Model and adolescents with insulin-dependent diabetes mellitus. *Health Psychology, 11,* 190–198.

Boner, A. L. (1989). Therapy of asthma in children. *European Respiratory Journal, 2*(Suppl.), 545s–550s.

Box, V., & Anderson, Y. (1997). Cancer beliefs, attitudes and preventive behaviours of nurses working in the community. *European Journal of Cancer Care, 6,* 192–208.

Campbell, M. K., DeVellis, B. M., Strecher, V. J., Ammerman, A. S., DeVellis, R. F., & Sandler, R. S. (1994). Improving dietary behavior: The effectiveness of tailored messages in primary care settings. *American Journal of Public Health, 84,* 783–787.

Chryssanthopoulos, C., Laufer, P., & Torphy, D. E. (1983). Assessment of acute asthma in the emergency room: Evaluation of compliance and combined drug therapy. *Journal of Asthma, 20,* 35–38.

Clark, N. M., Feldman, C. H., Evans, D., Levison, M. J., Wasilewski, Y., & Mellins, R. B. (1986). The impact of health education on frequency and cost of health care use by low income children with asthma. *Journal of Allergy and Clinical Immunology, 78,* 108–115.

Cluss, P. A., Epstein, L. H., Galvis, S. A., Fireman, P., & Friday, G. (1984). Effect of compliance for chronic asthmatic children. *Journal of Consulting and Clinical Psychology, 52,* 909–910.

Couper, M. P., & Rowe, B. (1996). Evaluation of a computer-assisted self-interview component in a computer-assisted personal interview survey. *Public Opinion Quarterly, 60,* 89–105.

Curry, S. J., & Emmons, K. M. (1994). Theoretical models for predicting and improving compliance with breast cancer screening. *Annuals of Behavioral Medicine, 16,* 302–316.

Davis, W. B., Coon, H., Whitehead, P., Ryan, K., Burkley, M., & McMahon, W. (1995). Predicting diabetic control from competence, adherence, adjustment, and psychopathology. *Journal of the American Academy of Child and Adolescent Psychiatry, 34,* 1629–1636.

Dijkstra, A., DeVries, H., Roijackers, J., & vanBreukelen, G. (1998). Tailored interventions to communicate state-matched information to smokers in different motivational stages. *Journal of Consulting and Clinical Psychology, 66,* 549–557.

D'Zurilla, T. J. (1986). *Problem-solving therapy: A social competence approach to clinical intervention.* New York: Springer.

D'Zurilla, T. J. (1990). Problem-solving training for effective stress management and prevention. *Journal of Cognitive Psychotherapy, 4,* 327–355.

D'Zurilla, T. J., & Goldfried, M. (1971). Problem-solving and behavior modification. *Journal of Abnormal Psychology, 78,* 107–126.

D'Zurilla, T. J., Nezu, A. M., & Maydeu-Olivaries, A. (in press). *Social problem-solving inventory.* North Tonawands, NY: Multi-Health Systems.

Eiser, C., Town, C., & Tripp, J. H. (1988). Illness experience and related knowledge amongst children with asthma. *Child Care, Health, and Development, 14,* 11–24.

Fayers, P. M., & Hand, D. J. (1997). Factor analysis, causal indicators, and quality of life. *Quality of Life Research, 6,* 139–150.

Fowler, F. J., Jr. (1993). *Survey research methods* (2nd ed.). Newbury Park, CA: Sage.

Gibson, P. G., Wlodarczyk, J., Hensley, M. J., Murree-Allen, K., Olson, L. G., & Saltos, N. (1995). Using quality-control analysis of peak expiratory flow recordings to guide therapy for asthma. *Annals of Internal Medicine, 123,* 488–492.

Gilbert, A., & Varni, J. W. (1988). Behavioral treatment for improving adherence to factor replacement therapy by children with hemophilia. *Journal of Compliance in Health Care, 3,* 67–76.

Greenan-Fowler, E., Powell, C., & Varni, J. W. (1987). Behavioral treatment of adherence to therapeutic exercise by children with hemophilia. *Archives of Physical Medicine and Rehabilitation, 68,* 846–849.

Guyatt, G. H., Feeny, D. H., & Patrick, D. L. (1993). Measuring health-related quality of life: Basic science review. *Annals of Internal Medicine, 70,* 225–230.

Guyatt, G. H., Juniper, E. F., Griffith, L. E., Feeny, D. H., & Ferry, P. J. (1997). Children and adult perceptions of childhood asthma. *Pediatrics, 99,* 165–168.

Hanson, C. L., De Guire, M. J., Schinkel, A. M., Kolterman, O. G., Goodman, J. P., & Buckingham, B. A. (1996). Self-care behaviors in insulin-dependent diabetes: Evaluative tools and their associations with glycemic control. *Journal of Pediatric Psychology, 21,* 467–482.

Hays, R. D., Fravitz, R. L., Mazel, R. M., Sherbourne, C. D., DiMatteo, M. R., Rogers, W. H., & Greenfield, S. (1994). The impact of patient adherence on health outcomes for patients with chronic disease in the Medical Outcomes Study. *Journal of Behavioral Medicine, 17,* 347–360.

Holden, G. W., & Edwards, L. A. (1989). Parental attitudes toward child rearing: Instruments, issues, and implications. *Psychological Bulletin, 106,* 29–58.

Hughes, D. M., McLeod, M., Garner, B., & Goldbloom, R. B. (1991). Controlled trial of a home and ambulatory program for asthmatic children. *Pediatrics, 87,* 478–486.

Johnson, S. B. (1994). Health behavior and health status: Concepts, methods, and applications. *Journal of Pediatric Psychology, 19,* 128–141.

Johnson, S. B., Freund, A., Silverstein, J. H., Hansen, C. A., & Malone, J. (1990). Adherence-health status relationships in childhood diabetes. *Health Psychology, 9,* 606–631.

Johnson, S. B., Kelly, M., Henretta, J. C., Cunningham, W. R., Tomer, A., & Silverstein, J. H. (1992). A longitudinal analysis of adherence and health status in childhood diabetes. *Journal of Pediatric Psychology, 17,* 537–553.

Kelloway, J. S., Wyatt, R. A., & Adlis, S. A. (1994). Comparison of patients' compliance with prescribed oral and inhaled asthma medications. *Archives of Internal Medicine, 154,* 1349–1352.

Kohen, D., Burgess, A. P., Catalan, J., & Lant, A. (1998). The role of anxiety and depression in quality of life and symptom reporting in people with diabetes mellitus. *Quality of Life Research, 7,* 197–204.

Laird, R., Chamberlain, K., & Spicer, J. (1994). Self-management practices in adult asthmatics. *New Zealand Medical Journal, 107,* 73–75.

Lewis, C. E., Rachelefsky, G. S., Lewis, M. A., de la Sota, A., & Kaplan, M. (1984). A randomized trial of ACT (Asthma Care Training) for kids. *Pediatrics, 74,* 478–486.

Loehlin, J. C. (1998). *Latent variable models: An introduction to factor, path, and structural analysis* (3rd ed.). Hillsdale, NJ: Lawrence Erlbaum Associates.

Lorenz, R., Christensen, N. K., & Pichert, J. (1985). Diet-related knowledge, skill, and adherence among children with insulin dependent diabetes mellitus. *Pediatrics, 75,* 872–876.

Mazon, A., Nieto, A., Nieto, F. J., Menendez, R., Boquete, M., & Brines, J. (1994). Prognostic factors in childhood asthma: A logistic regression analysis. *Annals of Allergy, 72,* 455–461.

Mitchell, E. A., Ferguson, V., & Norwood, M. (1986). Asthma education by community child health nurses. *Archives of Disease in Childhood, 61,* 1184–1189.

Muhlhauser, L. R. B., Kraut, D., Weske, G., Worth, H., & Berger, M. (1991). Evaluation of a structured treatment and teaching programme on asthma. *Journal of Internal Medicine, 230*, 157–164.

O'Reilly, J. M., Hubbard, M. L., Lessler, J. T., Biemer, P. P., & Turner, C. F. (1994). Audio and video computer assisted self-interviewing: Preliminary tests of new technologies for data collection. *Journal of Official Statistics, 10*, 197–214.

Palardy, N., Greening, L., Ott, J., Holderby, A., & Atchison, J. (1998). Adolescents' health attitudes and adherence to treatment for insulin-dependent diabetes mellitus. *Journal of Developmental and Behavioral Pediatrics, 19*, 31–37.

Patterson, G. R., Connis, R. T., Broadhead, W. E., Patrick, D. L., Taylor, T. R., & Tse, C. K. (1993). Disease-specific versus generic measurement of health-related quality of life in insulin-dependent diabetic patients. *Medical Care, 31*, 629–639.

Pinzone, H. A., Carlson, B. W., Kotses, H., & Creer, T. L. (1991). Prediction of asthma episodes in children using peak expiratory flow rates, medication compliance, and exercise data. *Annals of Allergy, 67*, 481–486.

Prochaska, J. O., DiClemente, C. C., Velicer, W. F., & Rossi, J. S. (1993). Standardized, individualized, interactive, and personalized self-help programs for smoking cessation. *Health Psychology, 12*, 399–405.

Pruitt, S. D., Seid, M., Varni, J. W., & Setoguchi, Y. (1999). Toddlers with limb deficiency: Conceptual basis and initial application of a functional status outcome measure. *Archives of Physical Medicine and Rehabilitation, 80*, 819–824.

Pruitt, S. D., Varni, J. W., Seid, M., & Setoguchi, Y. (1997). Prosthesis satisfaction outcome measurement in pediatric limb deficiency. *Archives of Physical Medicine and Rehabilitation, 78*, 750–754.

Pruitt, S. D., Varni, J. W., Seid, M., & Setoguchi, Y. (1998). Functional status in limb deficiency: Development of an outcome measure for preschool children. *Archives of Physical Medicine and Rehabilitation, 79*, 405–411.

Pruitt, S. D., Varni, J. W., & Setoguchi, Y. (1996). Functional status in children with limb deficiency: Development and initial validation of an outcome measure. *Archives of Physical Medicine and Rehabilitation, 77*, 1233–1238.

Putnam, D. E., Finney, J. W., Barkley, P. L., & Bonner, M. J. (1994). Enhancing commitment improves adherence to a medical regimen. *Journal of Consulting and Clinical Psychology, 62*, 191–194.

Rakos, R. F., Grodek, M. V., & Mack, K. K. (1985). The impact of a self-administered behavioral intervention program on pediatric asthma. *Journal of Psychosomatic Research, 29*, 101–108.

Roter, D. L., Hall, J. H., Merisca, R., Nordstrom, B., Cretin, D., & Svarstad, B. (1998). Effectiveness of interventions to improve patient compliance: A meta-analysis. *Medical Care, 36*, 1138–1161.

Rubin, D. H., Bauman, L. J., & Lauby, J. L. (1989). The relationship between knowledge and behavior in childhood asthma. *Journal of Developmental and Behavioral Pediatrics, 10*, 307–312.

Schipper, H., Clinch, J. J., & Olweny, C. L. M. (1996). Quality of life studies: Definitions and conceptual issues. In B. Spilker (Ed.), *Quality of life and pharmacoeconomics in clinical trials* (2nd ed., pp. 11–23). Philadelphia: Lippincott-Raven.

Sergis-Deavenport, E., & Varni, J. W. (1983). Behavioral assessment and management of adherence to factor replacement therapy in hemophilia. *Journal of Pediatric Psychology, 8*, 367–377.

Skinner, C. C., Strecher, V. J., & Hospers, H. (1994). Physicians' recommendations for mammography: Do tailored messages make a difference? *American Journal of Public Health, 84*, 43–49.

Sprangers, M. A. G., & Aaronson, N. K. (1992). The role of health care providers and significant others in evaluating the quality of life of patients with chronic disease: A review. *Journal of Clinical Epidemiology, 45,* 743–760.

Sprangers, M. A. G., Cull, A., Bjordal, K., Groenvold, M., & Aaronson, N. K. (1993). The European Organization for Research and Treatment of Cancer approach to quality of life assessment: Guidelines for developing questionnaire modules. *Quality of Life Research, 2,* 287–295.

Turner, C. F., Ku, L., Rogers, S. M., Lindberg, L. D., Pleck, J. H., & Sonenstein, F. L. (1998). Adolescent sexual behavior, drug use, and violence: Increased reporting with computer survey technology. *Science, 280,* 867–873.

Vali, F. M., & Walkup, J. (1998). Combined medical and psychological symptoms: Impact on disability and health care utilization of patients with arthritis. *Medical Care, 7,* 1073–1084.

Van der Does, F. E. E., Grootenhuis, P. A., De Neeling, J. N. D., Bouter, L. M., Snoek, F. J., Heine, R. J., & Kostense, P. J. (1996). Symptoms and well-being in relation to glycemic control in Type II diabetes. *Diabetes Care, 19,* 204–210.

Varni, J. W. (1983). *Clinical behavioral pediatrics: An interdisciplinary biobehavioral approach.* New York: Pergamon.

Varni, J. W. (March, 1998). *Pediatric health-related quality of life: Patient-based health outcomes.* Visiting scholar invited presentation at the Center for Pediatric Outcomes Research, Childrens Hospital, Los Angeles.

Varni, J. W., Katz, E. R., Colegrove, R., & Dolgin, M. (1993). The impact of social skills training on the adjustment of children with newly diagnosed cancer. *Journal of Pediatric Psychology, 18,* 751–767.

Varni, J. W., Katz, E. R., Colegrove, R., & Dolgin, M. (1995). Adjustment of children with newly diagnosed cancer: Cross-informant variance. *Journal of Psychosocial Oncology, 13,* 23–38.

Varni, J. W., Katz, E. R., Seid, M., Quiggins, D. J. L., & Friedman-Bender, A. (1998). The Pediatric Cancer Quality of Life Inventory-32 (PCQL-32): I. Reliability and validity. *Cancer, 82,* 1184–1196.

Varni, J. W., Katz, E. R., Seid, M., Quiggins, D. J. L., Friedman-Bender, A., & Castro, C. M. (1998). The Pediatric Cancer Quality of Life Inventory (PCQL): I. Instrument development, descriptive statistics, and cross-informant variance. *Journal of Behavioral Medicine, 21,* 179–204.

Varni, J. W., Pruitt, S. D., & Seid, M. (1998). Health-related quality of life in pediatric limb deficiency. In S. A. Herring & J. G. Birch (Eds.), *The child with a limb deficiency* (pp. 457–473). Rosemont, IL: American Academy of Orthopaedic Surgeons.

Varni, J. W., Quiggins, D. J. L., & Ayala, G. X. (in press). Development of the Pediatric Hematology-Oncology Parent Satisfaction survey. *Children's Health Care.*

Varni, J. W., Rode, C. A., Seid, M., Katz, E. R., Friedman-Bender, A., & Quiggins, D. J. L. (1999). The Pediatric Cancer Quality of Life Inventory–32 (PCQL–32): II. Feasibility and range of measurement. *Journal of Behavioral Medicine, 22,* 397–406.

Varni, J. W., Sahler, O. J., Katz, E. R., Mulhern, R. K., Copeland, D. R., Noll, R. B., Phipps, S., Dolgin, M. J., & Roghmann, K. (1999). Maternal problem-solving therapy in pediatric cancer. *Journal of Psychosocial Oncology, 16,* 41–71.

Varni, J. W., Seid, M., Jacobs, J. R., & Rode, C. A. (1999). *The PedsQL^{TM}: II. Development of the Asthma and Arthritis Disease-Specific Modules for the Pediatric Quality of Life Inventory.* Submitted for publication.

Varni, J. W., Seid, M., & Kurtin, P. S. (1999). Pediatric health-related quality of life measurement technology: A guide for health care decision makers. *Journal of Clinical Outcomes Management, 6,* 33–40.

Varni, J. W., Seid, M., & Rode, C. A. (1999). The PedsQL^{TM}: Measurement model for the Pediatric Quality of Life Inventory. *Medical Care, 37,* 126–139.

Varni, J. W., & Setoguchi, Y. (1992). Screening for behavioral and emotional problems in children and adolescents with congenital or acquired limb deficiencies. *American Journal of Diseases of Children, 146*, 103–107.

Varni, J. W., Thompson, K. L., & Hanson, V. (1987). The Varni/Thompson Pediatric Pain Questionnaire: I. Chronic musculoskeletal pain in juvenile rheumatoid arthritis. *Pain, 28*, 27–38.

Varni, J. W., Waldron, S. A., Gragg, R. A., Rapoff, M. A., Bernstein, B. H., Lindsley, C. B., & Newcomb, M. D. (1996). Development of the Waldron/Varni Pediatric Pain Coping Inventory. *Pain, 67*, 141–150.

Varni, J. W., & Wallander, J. L. (1984). Adherence to health-related regimens in pediatric chronic disorders. *Clinical Psychology Review, 4*, 585–596.

Varni, J. W., Wilcox, K. T., Hanson, V., & Brik, R. (1988). Chronic musculoskeletal pain and functional status in juvenile rheumatoid arthritis: An empirical model. *Pain, 32*, 1–7.

Wallander, J. L., & Varni, J. W. (1998). Effects of pediatric chronic physical disorders on child and family adjustment. *Journal of Child Psychology and Psychiatry, 39*, 29–46.

Weinstein, N. D., Rothman, A. J., & Sutton, S. R. (1998). Stage theories of health behavior: Conceptual and methodological issues. *Health Psychology, 17*, 290–299.

Whitman, N., West, D., Brough, F. K., & Welch, M. (1985). A study of self-care rehabilitation program in pediatric asthma. *Health Education Quarterly, 12*, 333–342.

Wiebe, J. S., & Christensen, A. J. (1997). Health beliefs, personality, and adherence in hemodialysis patients: An interactional perspective. *Annuals of Behavioral Medicine, 19*, 30–35.

CHAPTER THIRTEEN

Compliance Behavior in Clinical Trials: Error or Opportunity?

Suzanne Bennett Johnson
University of Florida, Gainesville, FL

Clinical trials are an important component of the National Institutes of Health's (NIH) research mission and are an essential step in the development of new agents by the pharmaceutical industry. Usually biological interventions (e.g., an experimental medication for the treatment of hyperactivity) are the focus of such trials, but occasionally behavioral interventions (e.g., use of behavior therapy for the treatment of hyperactivity) are tested often in conjunction with a biological intervention (e.g., medication plus behavior therapy). Compliance is critical because it influences the investigator's ability to detect true treatment effects. From this perspective, noncompliance is viewed as an annoying source of error—something that must be controlled or minimized. Historically, two methods have been used to control or minimize this source of error: (a) careful subject selection procedures, and (b) reliance on intent-to-treat analyses.

In this chapter, each of these methods of controlling or minimizing error is carefully examined. I argue that the error perspective has severely restricted the nature of the scientific information we collect, created problems with data interpretation, and limited the significance of our results. In other words, the error perspective has resulted in numerous missed opportunities to collect meaningful scientific information as part of a clinical trial. I argue that an alternative framework, in which compliance behavior is viewed as a central component of clinical trial research rather than solely as an annoying source of error, provides investigators

307

with an important opportunity to enhance both the scientific quality and clinical relevance of the data obtained.

CONTROLLING ERROR BY CAREFUL SUBJECT SELECTION

There are, of course, good reasons why noncompliance has been viewed as a source of error rather than opportunity in clinical trials. If the experimental group does not take the experimental medication as prescribed, the true effects of the medication cannot be observed. Consequently, by studying only participants who are highly compliant over the time frame of the clinical trial, and rejecting those who are noncompliant from further study, one can reasonably conclude that any difference between the experimental and comparison groups is the result of the experimental treatment. This approach assumes that: (a) there are sufficient numbers of highly compliant individuals available for study, and (b) the investigator can accurately identify and successfully recruit these highly compliant individuals prior to study initiation. Both of these assumptions are problematic.

Are There Sufficient Numbers of Compliant Patients Available?

If most patients were compliant with their medical regimens, the availability of sufficient numbers of highly compliant individuals for clinical trials would be of little concern. However, the empirical literature suggests quite the opposite is the case: Noncompliance is so common that it is considered a major health care problem. For example, Dunbar-Jacob, Dunning, and Dwyer (1993) reviewed the compliance literature published from 1970 to 1989 that focused specifically on pediatric and adolescent populations. Ninety-one published research studies were identified. Although compliance rates varied somewhat across studies, populations, and behaviors, overall compliance rates remained comparable to the 54% weighted mean reported by Haynes, Taylor, and Sacket (1979) in their earlier review. There was no evidence that compliance rates have improved in the last 20 years.

Can Compliant Patients Be Accurately Identified?

Even when there are sufficient numbers of highly compliant patients available, it is unclear that such patients can be accurately identified. The most common approach is to have the investigator exclude those individuals with certain characteristics thought to be associated with poor compliance (e.g., current drug or alcohol abusers or those with a history of such abuse, persons with psychiatric histories, those with minimal education). Unfortunately, exclusionary criteria are often based on investigator beliefs rather than scientific evidence (Hughes, 1993). Such an approach assumes that people have noncompliant or compliant personalities—a popular belief, but one with little empirical foundation. Research has shown that patients exhibit highly variable behavior across different components of a medical regimen (Gross, Samson, Sanders, & Smith, 1988; Johnson, Silverstein, Rosenbloom, Carter, & Cunningham, 1986; Johnson, Tomer, Cunningham, & Henretta, 1990; Orme & Binik, 1989; Rudd et al., 1989). For example, some patients may take their medications but not follow their diet, whereas others may exhibit the reverse constellation of behaviors. Knowing a patient's level of compliance with one component of a treatment regimen does not predict level of compliance with a different component of the same medical regimen. Patients do not have compliant or noncompliant personalities, nor is there any scientific evidence that investigator beliefs about who would and would not be compliant in a clinical trial are valid predictors of patient behavior during a trial.

Although nonempirically based investigator-initiated methods of compliant patient selection are common, more behavioral approaches have been used as well. The use of a prerandomization run-in period is an example of such a behaviorally based method to identify and exclude potentially noncompliant persons from trial participation. In this approach, the patient may be given a placebo, active medication or some other study-related task during a time period of several weeks to months. Only those who are adherent during this run-in are permitted to subsequently enter the clinical trial. Although this approach may have some intuitive appeal, there are few empirical studies addressing its validity or impact on study conclusions. In an interesting report, Davis, Applegate, Gordon, Curtis, and McCormick (1995) described their study of a placebo run-in for 3 weeks as part of an investigation assessing the effect of medication on cholesterol reduction in older adults. Subsequent to the run-in, all persons, regardless of their compliance during the run-in, were included in the clinical trial. Using pill counts, persons who took at least 80% of the placebo during the run-in were labeled *compliers*; approximately 85% of those studied met this criterion. Run-in compliers differed from run-in noncompliers in both race (33% of the run-in noncompliers were African American compared with only 19% of the run-in compliers) and education (noncompliers were less educated). Differences between the run-in compliers and noncompliers during the clinical trial are depicted in Table 13.1.

Although persons who were not compliant during the run-in were also less compliant during the clinical trial, the differences were not large and did not predict well for individual cases. In fact, over 70% who failed to meet the compliance criteria ($\geq$ 80% medication taken) during the run-in

TABLE 13.1
A Comparison of Run-In Compliers Versus Noncompliers
on Subsequent 3-Month Clinical Trial Outcomes

Trial Outcomes	Run-In Noncompliers (n = 66)	Run-In Compliers (n = 365)	Total Sample (n = 431)
Adherence			
Mean	80.4%	90.9%	89.3%
≥ 80%	71.2%	88.8%	86.1%
LDL Change			
Placebo	−3.3	1.5	.7
20 mg	−42.1	−47.3	−46.5
40 mg	−44.7	−57.7	−55.6

Note. From Davis et al. (1995).

met this same criterion during the clinical trial. Further, the effect of the medication was similar for both groups, although, as expected, it was somewhat larger in the more compliant group. However, a comparison of the total sample to the compliant group indicates that inclusion of the run-in noncompliers had minimal impact on study findings.

Further, exclusion of the run-in noncompliers would have meant eliminating large numbers of African-American patients because they composed a larger proportion of the run-in noncompliers.[1] This would have limited the investigators' abilities to compare study effects across ethnic groups. The authors appropriately caution against the use of prerandomization run-ins in clinical trials where there is an absence of empirical data as to their impact on study recruitment, outcome, and interpretation of study findings. Consequently, even behavioral methods to identify and exclude noncompliant persons using pretrial behavior tasks are likely to be inaccurate and may result in missed opportunities to learn important information relevant to the patient population excluded by such procedures.

Problems With Data Interpretation
and Generalization of Study Findings

The highly restrictive sample selection practices currently in use in most clinical trials lack empirical justification and can be criticized for this reason alone. However, an equally serious problem is the inherent limitation such an approach places on any attempt to generalize study findings

---

[1]Multivariate analyses indicated that education, not race, was the strongest predictor of run-in compliance.

beyond the narrow group selected for study. For example, suppose an investigator excludes persons with only a high school education (or less) from a study protocol because the investigator believes that such persons will be noncompliant during the clinical trial. Because U.S. African Americans and Hispanics often have poorer educational attainment than Whites, this exclusion is likely to result in low numbers of minority participants in the study; the investigator will be unable to ascertain whether the treatment worked equally well across all ethnic groups and will be forced to limit conclusions to White Americans only. In this example, like the Davis et al. (1995) study, an investigator's attempt to minimize error through a restrictive selection procedure would result in a lost opportunity to learn more about the effects of the experimental treatment on persons other than White Americans.

Investigator-initiated restriction of samples to purportedly compliant patients also places severe limitations on our ability to learn about a particular experimental procedure's acceptability to a patient population. For example, the Diabetes Control and Complications Trial (DCCT) was conducted with a highly select sample of predominantly adult patients with Type 1 diabetes. Care of their diabetes was intensified through increased frequency of daily insulin injections, blood glucose monitoring, and insulin adjustment (DCCT Research Group, 1993). Although Type 1 diabetes is almost always diagnosed in childhood or adolescence, few youngsters were asked to join the trial because investigators believed adolescents would not comply with the trial's requirements.

Nevertheless, the National Diabetes Information Clearinghouse currently recommends intensive therapy for all youngsters 13 years or older (U.S. Department of Health and Human Services, 1994). Because of its nonrepresentative sample selection procedures, the DCCT could provide no information as to who or how many Type 1 patients would agree to such a procedure. Subsequently, Thompson, Cummings, Chalmer, Gould, and Newton (1996) distributed the results of the DCCT to a large sample of insulin-treated patients ranging in age from 15 to 60 years. They ascertained each patient's interest in initiating intensive therapy to improve his or her glycemic control. Counter to physician beliefs, younger patients expressed a greater interest. Nevertheless, only 37% of interested patients were willing to take three or more insulin injections per day, and only 18% were willing to come to clinic every month as required by intensive therapy. Tercyak, Johnson, Kirkpatrick, and Silverstein (1998) conducted a similar study with a nonselect sample of adolescents with Type 1 diabetes. Nearly half of those approached declined to participate, citing an unwillingness to take more injections, come to clinic more often, or blood glucose test more often. The DCCT's highly restrictive sample selection methods, a product of an attempt to reduce error associated with noncompliance, resulted in a missed opportunity to collect important information on the acceptability of intensive therapy procedures to the Type 1 patient population at large. Consequently, we have yet to learn for whom this approach is a truly viable treatment option.

INTENT-TO-TREAT ANALYSES

As mentioned previously, the potential problems induced by noncompliance in clinical trials have primarily been addressed by highly restrictive subject selection procedures and intent-to-treat analyses. Although true treatment effects should only occur in patients who are adherent to the treatment protocol, intent-to-treat analyses are predicated on the assumption that eliminating noncompliant participants may introduce unwanted bias. Persons may be noncompliant in the experimental and control groups for different reasons. If so, eliminating noncompliant participants may result in experimental versus control group differences that are the result of these peculiar subject characteristics rather than the experimental manipulation. For this reason, intent-to-treat analyses require that no subject be eliminated due to noncompliance (Friedman, Furberg, & DeMets, 1996). Unfortunately, this approach has often resulted in a failure to consider compliance behavior in the analysis at all. From a behavioral scientist's point of view, both the experimental manipulation and the participants' compliance behavior should be included in the analysis. Currently available multivariate statistical methods make this quite possible. Both the main effect of the experimental treatment (intent to treat) as well as any main effect of compliance and the interaction between the two can be ascertained. True treatment effects can be better estimated when compliance behavior is known (Mark & Robins, 1993).

Intent-to-Treat Analyses Ignore Treatment
Threshold Effects

Further, inclusion of compliance behavior in the analysis would permit an estimate of therapeutic thresholds. Currently we rarely know how much medication, weight change, exercise, or dietary modification is necessary to yield clinically meaningful results. Patients are instructed to take all of their medication, but it is quite possible that less medication (e.g., 75% of the dose prescribed) would be equally effective. Rarely are threshold effects studied in clinical trials. Because compliance behavior is not assessed, we are unable to examine whether patients who took less medication did as well as those who took all of the medication. Failure to assess compliance behavior per se results in a missed opportunity to collect important, initial estimates of therapeutic threshold effects that could guide subsequent research and, ultimately, clinical practice.

Intent-to-Treat Analyses Ignore Reasons for Noncompliance

The availability of compliance behavior data may be particularly important for the interpretation of failure to find treatment effects in intent-to-treat analyses. Some would argue that the reasons underlying a treatment failure (no true treatment effect vs. high noncompliance with the treatment) have no practical import. If the treatment fails because study participants would not comply with its demands, the treatment has no value because it cannot be tolerated by most persons. However, this view fails to consider the reasons for the participants' noncompliance and whether these reasons are modifiable (e.g., subsequent research could focus on reducing the specific side effects of an otherwise promising treatment). Further, this view ignores the substantial effects that clinical trial results' disclosure can have on patients' subsequent attitudes and behavior—an important but understudied area of research (e.g., Buchwald et al., 1993).

Intent-to-Treat Analyses Ignore Compliance Main Effects

Although compliance behavior is usually seen as a source of error in clinical trials, there is some interesting evidence that compliance behavior per se is associated with important health outcomes. Although intent-to-treat analyses are testing for treatment main effects (independent of compliance), a number of studies have documented compliance main effects (independent of drug or placebo assignment). Two examples are provided in Table 13.2.

In both of these studies, the overall intent-to-treatment analyses yielded no differences between the test medication and placebo. However, noncompliant participants experienced significantly greater mortality than compliant subjects, regardless of whether they were randomly assigned to the test drug or placebo. This phenomenon was first noted by Epstein in 1984 and has been reconfirmed since (Friedman et al., 1996). After conducting an extensive review of over 500 studies, Epstein (1984) was able to locate only six studies that tested for compliance main effects (e.g., compliant vs. noncompliant patients) and treatment main effects (e.g., drug vs. placebo), as well as the interaction between the two. In five of the six studies, a main effect of compliance was confirmed; in many cases, the compliance effect was stronger than the treatment effect. Epstein argues that this is an important phenomenon in its own right and not just a methodological problem to be addressed solely by intent-to-treatment

TABLE 13.2
Compliance Main Effects: Two Examples

Study	Percentage Mortality		
	Overall	Compliant	Noncompliant
Coronary Drug Project (1980)			
Clofibrate	18.2	15.0	24.6
Placebo	19.4	15.1	28.2
Aspirin Myocardial Infarction Study (1984)			
Aspirin	10.9	6.1	21.9
Placebo	9.7	5.1	22.0

Note. Adapted from Friedman et al. (1996).

comparisons. Unfortunately, it has been difficult to study this phenomenon because compliance behavior is so rarely analyzed in clinical trials.

COMPLIANCE BEHAVIOR IN CLINICAL TRIALS HAS NOT BEEN VIEWED AS A TOPIC WORTHY OF STUDY IN ITS OWN RIGHT

Although compliance behavior is acknowledged to be a critical component of clinical trials because it has been conceptualized solely as a source of error, it has rarely been studied in its own right. Further, when compliance has been assessed, biological rather than behavioral measures have typically been used. For example, Besch (1995) reviewed published reports of prospective, randomized, multicenter HIV clinical trials evaluating antiretroviral agents since 1987; 12 were identified. In four, no definition or description of compliance was given. In one study, *compliance* was defined as study visit attendance, with no effort to measure medication compliance. Six studies measured compliance using a biological assay—either a measure of serum drug level or a measure of health status. Biological measures provide a crude index of patient compliance behavior that is often inaccurate. Only one study attempted to ascertain compliance by patient interview; none took advantage of the more sophisticated behavioral measurement strategies currently available (e.g., Johnson, 1993; Rudd, 1993).

Although clinical trials have been primarily concerned with ensuring compliance behavior in the experimental group through highly restrictive subject selection procedures, the behavior of the control group has generally been ignored. This is unfortunate because control group behavior can easily wreak havoc on clinical trial results. For example, if persons in the control group attempt to mimic the experimental group, the true effects of the experimental treatment will go undetected. This is a real problem in any trial where an experimental treatment is compared to no treatment, standard care, or a placebo and the experimental treatment is readily available outside of the clinical trial.

The Diabetes Prevention Trial for Type 1 Diabetes (DPT-1) is an example. This multicenter trial identifies children and adults at high risk for Type 1 diabetes prior to disease onset. These at-risk persons are then randomly assigned to daily insulin injections or no treatment (both groups also receive frequent observation). Prior research has shown that a substantial number of these at-risk persons report engaging in a variety of lifestyle behavior changes subsequent to at-risk notification in an effort to delay or prevent disease onset. Further, more anxious at-risk persons are more likely to report behavior change (Johnson & Tercyak, 1995). Because almost all of the high-risk participants in the DPT-1 come from families that include a member with Type 1 diabetes, insulin is readily available to the no-treatment controls. Further, through the informed consent process, the controls are well aware that insulin is being administered to persons in the experimental group. At-risk persons are likely to join the DPT-1 trial because they hope to prevent diabetes onset, and their willingness to engage in behavior change subsequent to at-risk notification has been documented. Because all participants are told that they are at high risk for diabetes and that insulin injection is the experimental treatment to be tested in the trial, the likelihood of crossover (the control group initiating the experimental treatment on their own) seems high. Unfortunately, compliance behaviors of both the experimental and control groups in the DPT-1 are not being carefully monitored.

In other studies, the use of placebos may attenuate this effect, but participants have been known to have their medication tested to ascertain whether they have been given a placebo (Besch, 1995). Unless the compliance behavior of both the experimental and control groups is assessed, interpretation of study findings will remain compromised.

EMERGING OPPORTUNITIES FOR COMPLIANCE BEHAVIOR RESEARCH

Although clinical trials have historically failed to consider compliance behavior as a topic worth of study in its own right, there are a number of areas where compliance behavior research may enjoy greater acceptability. I have labeled these areas as *emerging opportunities* because the value of compliance behavior research may not be established but neither is it devalued on a priori grounds. In many cases, behavioral scientists still have to educate others as to the value of their behavioral expertise and the importance of assessing compliance behavior per se as part of the larger research enterprise.

Longitudinal Studies of Disease Onset and Prevention

There is currently great interest in understanding the natural history of disease development. Studies of this type require large numbers of persons who are monitored over long periods of time. Issues of subject recruitment and maintenance are paramount; both are essentially behavioral phenomena. Physician investigators, who are usually the principal investigators in research of this type, are quickly learning that recruitment and maintenance of participants in the study protocol is difficult. If behavioral scientists come forward and can offer their expertise, they may be welcomed with open arms. Prevention trials offer similar opportunities. These trials require identification of high-risk persons before disease onset, an experimental treatment of some type aimed at preventing or delaying disease onset, and random assignment to the experimental intervention or to no treatment. The psychological issues involved are many: heightened anxiety in response to at-risk notification, difficulty following an aversive experimental procedure, unwillingness to accept no treatment, engagement in alternative treatments by the no-treatment group, and difficulty maintaining patient cooperation over long periods of time. Although these psychological issues may not be initially apparent to the naive medical investigator, it will not take long before they become so great as to threaten the viability of the trial. In such cases, the expertise of a behavioral scientist may be more than welcome.

Many natural history and prevention trials differ from traditional clinical trials because large sample sizes are required and investigators cannot afford to exclude large numbers of persons because they may not be compliant. At-risk persons are often expensive to locate, sometimes requiring thousands of persons to be screened to find one at-risk person. A protypical at-risk person is valuable and every effort will be made to recruit and retain such an individual in the trial. Investigators cannot afford to rely on traditional clinical trial methods of screening out anyone with some particular characteristic that the investigator finds questionable. Consequently, they may value behavioral scientists' assistance in data analysis and interpretation where patient compliance behavior can be factored into the results. Further, behavioral scientists' expertise may prove equally valuable in the participant recruitment and maintenance aspects of the research enterprise.

Genetic Testing Studies

The NIH, in collaboration with the Department of Energy, expects to map the human genome by the year 2005. The NIH already recognizes the importance of behavioral and psychosocial factors to this enterprise and has established the Ethical, Legal, and Social Issues Program of the National Center for Human Genome Research at NIH (http://www. nhgri.nih.gov/About_NHGRI/Der/elsi_res). It funds research relevant to: (a) communicating information about genetic testing to affected persons, health providers, as well as the lay public; (b) behavioral, social, and emotional impact of genetic testing results on the affected person as well as family members; (c) uptake or refusal of genetic testing procedures; and so on. Obviously all of these issues are well within the behavioral scientist's domain and represent opportunities to study participant compliance relevant to genetic testing.

Effectiveness Research

Because most clinical trials are conducted with a highly restricted sample, there is a clear need for research that examines the uptake and impact of a treatment, deemed effective in a clinical trial, with a more general patient population. Effectiveness research is supported by the NIH, the Agency for Health Care Policy and Research (AHCPR; http://www. ahcpr.gov), among others. It offers opportunities to examine patient compliance behavior within the context of a known treatment, helping to answer important questions about acceptability (who will accept and comply with the treatment) and effectiveness within the context of a everyday patient care.

When compliance behavior becomes a focus of effectiveness research, a number of important questions can be asked and answered. For example, perhaps a complex medical regimen, such as the use of intensive therapy for the treatment of Type 1 diabetes, has proved effective in the context of a traditional clinical trial, such as the DCCT. Because trials of this type typically involve a highly select sample of patients, it remains unclear how many patients can actually benefit from the trial's findings. In effectiveness research, the investigator could ascertain the pretreatment characteristics of those patients most likely to succeed. This may be particularly critical when there are limited health care resources. Intensive therapy for Type 1 diabetes not only places increased demand on the patient, but places large time demands on the medical staff as well. The prospect of accurately identifying good candidates for intensive therapy prior to the initiation of such extremely labor-intensive intervention means better use of health care dollars. In most instances, the identification of good candidates requires considerable behavioral expertise because the patient's behavioral, social, and psychological characteristics are likely to be the best predictors of who can successfully comply with an intensive therapy regimen.

In some situations, the identification of good candidates prior to treatment initiation has far more than economic implications. This is particularly true when treatment noncompliance threatens the health of the patient or, in extreme cases, the society at large. For example, current treatments for the HIV/AIDS virus require expensive, complex multidrug regimens that involve numerous side effects. Not only is compliance with such regimens difficult and costly, but failure to comply can result in new drug-resistant strains that threaten not only the patient, but the health of the society at large (Wainberg & Friedland, 1998). At issue is how to accurately identify those who can comply with such a difficult treatment regimen. This is a particular challenge because HIV/AIDS populations are often characterized by poverty, low educational attainment, and minority status (all characteristics that would typically result in exclusion from a traditional clinical trial). Once again, the identification of good candidates requires careful behavioral and psychological assessment.

A focus on compliance behavior in effectiveness research need not be restricted to identification of good candidates prior to treatment initiation. Equally important is the development of effective intervention strategies to assist those who initially may not be good candidates. For example, an adolescent with Type 1 diabetes who receives little family support for his diabetes care may be a poor candidate for intensive therapy. An intervention that increases diabetes-related family support may enable the youngster to succeed, opening up opportunities for youngsters who would normally be excluded from treatment.

Finally, a focus on compliance behavior as part of effectiveness research can provide important information relevant to treatment threshold effects. Many treatments for chronic disease are exceedingly complex, involving multiple medications and behaviors, often with particular timing requirements (e.g., the medication must be taken on an empty stomach four times a day with at least 4 hours between administrations). Frequently, we do not know which particular components of the treatment regimen are most critical for success. For example, although the DCCT demonstrated that intensive therapy was more effective than standard care for the management of Type 1 diabetes, it did not tell us which components of intensive therapy (more frequent insulin injections, increased daily blood glucose testing, daily insulin adjustment, frequent provider contact) were most critical for its success (DCCT Research Group, 1993). Within the context of an effectiveness trial, a focus on compliance behavior will enable the investigator to gain some important insights as to which components of the intervention seem most powerful. With this information, the investigator may be able to develop a simpler, more streamlined treatment regimen to be tested in a subsequent clinical trial.

Health Care Systems' Studies

Health care systems, including private managed care programs as well as public health care systems, are often interested in provider compliance with treatment guidelines, patient behavior change subsequent to educational programs, and ways in which provider behavior can influence patient behavior. Medical procedures and treatments recommended to patients by providers, as well as uptake of those treatments (as well as other treatments) by patients, all have financial implications. In the private health care marketplace, patient satisfaction can further influence selection of health care programs. Behavioral scientists can bring to the table expertise in the measurement of provider as well as patient behavior that may prove useful to health care systems' planning and outcomes evaluation.

Inclusion of Pediatric Populations
in NIH-Supported Research

In March 1998, the NIH released new guidelines on the inclusion of children as participants in research involving human subjects. Historically, children have been excluded from much NIH research as well as research conducted by the pharmaceutical industry out of concern for their welfare. This has had the unfortunate consequence of severely limiting our knowledge of pediatric disease and its treatment. The American Academy of Pediatrics has reported that few drugs used with children have any pediatric research basis, having been developed almost exclusively with adults. As of October 1, 1998, the NIH now requires that all applications involving human subjects include children unless there are scientific and ethical reasons to exclude them, which must be fully justified by the investigator (see http://www4.od.nih.gov/ocm/contracts/rfps/childpol for NIH guideline text). The required inclusion of pediatric patients in NIH-supported research is likely to have ramifications well beyond the NIH research portfolio. For example, the Food and Drug Administration (FDA) has published (http://www.fda.gov) a proposed regulation calling for a change in the pharmaceutical industry's tests of prescription drugs to specifically examine their impact on children. Consequently, the impact of the NIH guideline is likely to be widespread, affecting private as well as government-supported research activities.

These changes pose considerable opportunities for scientists, with behavioral expertise. Issues of parental informed consent and child assent are expected to become more salient as investigators are forced to include children in their research activities. Little is actually known about the best methods to ensure true understanding and assent in young children. Further, the inclusion of children complicates the experimental protocol because, in most cases, both parents and the child are involved in the delivery of the experimental medication/procedure to the child. There may be greater interest in measuring compliance per se as the investigators try to sort out which children actually received the experimental medication/procedure as prescribed.

Because historically children have not been the focus of clinical trials, a new set of investigators—those with pediatric expertise—are likely to enter the clinical trial enterprise for the first time. These investigators may not bring to the research enterprise the same biases common to clinical trial investigators of the past. Indeed, psychologists have had a long, successful history working with pediatricians in the treatment of medical as well as behavioral disorders of childhood. Consequently, pediatric investigators may be more willing to accept clinical-trial compliance behavior as a topic worthy of study in its own right. However, this is unlikely to happen unless behavioral scientists take the opportunity to educate their pediatric colleagues as to the advantages of good compliance behavior assessment within the context of any clinical trial.

ACKNOWLEDGMENT

Supported in part by National Institutes of Health Grant RO1-HD13820.

REFERENCES

Besch, C. (1995). Compliance in clinical trials. *AIDS, 9,* 1–10.

Buchwald, H., Fitch, L., Matts, J., Johnson, J., Hansen, B., Stuenkel, M., & Brooks, H. (1993). Perception of quality of life before and after disclosure of trial effects: A report from the Program on the Surgical Control of the Hyperlipidemias. *Controlled Clinical Trials, 14,* 500–510.

Davis, D., Applegate, W., Gordon, D., Curtis, C., & McCormick, M. (1995). An empirical evaluation of the placebo run-in. *Controlled Clinical Trials, 16,* 41–50.

DCCT Research Group. (1993). The effect of intensive treatment of diabetes on the development and progression of long-term complications in insulin-dependent diabetes mellitus. *New England Journal of Medicine, 329,* 977–986.

Dunbar-Jacob, J., Dunning, E., & Dwyer, K. (1993). Compliance research in pediatric and adolescent populations: Two decades of research. In N. Krasnegor, L. Epstein, S. B. Johnson, & S. Yaffee (Eds.), *Developmental aspects of health compliance behavior* (pp. 29–51). Hillsdale, NJ: Lawrence Erlbaum Associates.

Epstein, L. (1984). The direct effects of compliance on health outcome. *Health Psychology, 3,* 385–393.

Friedman, L., Furberg, C., & DeMets, D. (1996). *Fundamentals of clinical trials.* St. Louis, MO: Mosby-Year Book.

Gross, A., Samson, G., Sanders, S., & Smith, C. (1988). Patient noncompliance: Are children consistent? *American Journal of Orthodontics and Dentofacial Orthopedics, 93*, 518–519.

Haynes, R., Taylor, D., & Sackett, D. (Eds.). (1979). *Compliance in health care*. Baltimore, MD: Johns Hopkins University Press.

Hughes, J. (1993). Exclusion of "noncompliant" individuals from clinical trials. *Controlled Clinical Trials, 13*, 176–177.

Johnson, S. B. (1993). Chronic diseases of childhood: Assessing compliance with complex medical regimens. In N. Krasnegor, L. Epstein, S. B. Johnson, & S. Yaffee (Eds.), *Developmental aspects of health compliance behavior* (pp. 157–184). Hillsdale, NJ: Lawrence Erlbaum Associates.

Johnson, S. B., Silverstein, J., Rosenbloom, A., Carter, R., & Cunningham, W. (1986). Assessing daily management of childhood diabetes. *Health Psychology, 5*, 545–564.

Johnson, S. B., & Tercyak, K. (1995). Psychological impact of islet cell antibody screening for IDDM in children, adults, and their family members. *Diabetes Care, 18*, 1370–1372.

Johnson, S. B., Tomer, A., Cunningham, W., & Henretta, J. (1990). Adherence in childhood diabetes: Results of a confirmatory factor analysis. *Health Psychology, 9*, 493–501.

Mark, S., & Robins, J. (1993). A method for the analysis of randomized trials with compliance information: An application to the Multiple Risk Factor Intervention Trial. *Controlled Clinical Trials, 14*, 79–97.

Orme, C., & Binik, Y. (1989). Consistency of adherence across regimen demands. *Health Psychology, 8*, 27–43.

Rudd, P. (1993). The measurement of compliance: Medication taking. In N. Krasnegor, L. Epstein, S. B. Johnson, & S. Yaffee (Eds.), *Developmental aspects of health compliance behavior* (pp. 185–213). Hillsdale, NJ: Lawrence Erlbaum Associates.

Rudd, P., Byyny, R., Zachary, V., LoVerde, M., Titus, C., Mitchell, W., & Marshall, G. (1989). The natural history of medication compliance in a drug trial: Limitations on pill counts. *Clinical Pharmacology and Therapeutics, 46*, 169–176.

Tercyak, K., Johnson, S. B., Kirkpatrick, K., & Silverstein, J. (1998). Offering a randomized trial of intensive therapy for IDDM to adolescents. *Diabetes Care, 21*, 213–215.

Thompson, C., Cummings, J., Chalmer, J., Gould, C., & Newton, R. (1996). How have patients reacted to the implications of the DCCT? *Diabetes Care, 19*, 876–879.

U.S. Department of Health and Human Services. (1994). *Diabetes Control and Complications Trial (DCCT)*. Washington, DC: U.S. Government Printing Office.

Wainberg, M., & Friedland, G. (1998). Public health implications of antiretroviral therapy and HIV drug resistance. *Journal of the American Medical Association, 279*, 1977–1983.

INTERVENTIONS TO PROMOTE TREATMENT ADHERENCE IN CHILDHOOD CHRONIC ILLNESS

The development of empirically supported intervention to promote adherence to treatment in pediatric chronic illness is an important research need. Section VII showcases the efforts of investigators who are conducting such research.

In chapter 14, Rapoff describes adherence to medical treatment regimens for pediatric rheumatoid diseases (PRD), reviews previous studies designed to improve adherence to treatment regimens for these conditions, and proposes a prevention model to facilitate adherence to treatment for PRD. Rapoff and colleagues' research has documented the different patterns of problems experienced by children with PRD in following various elements of treatment regimens, such as medications, therapeutic exercises, and wearing joint splints to prevent contractures.

Rapoff describes the findings from his and his colleagues' single-subject designs and recently completed randomized trial to test the efficacy of educational and behavioral strategies for improving adherence to regimens for PRDs. Their single-subject design studies involved monitoring adherence in a group of patients and experimentally evaluating interventions for those with the lowest levels of adherence and those identified by pediatric rheumatologists as experiencing compromised function. Case series have generally indicated positive effect for a parent-managed token reinforcement program in improving treatment adherence for children with PRD.

Rapoff and colleagues also tested the effects of less complex and labor-intensive behavioral strategies, such as self-monitoring and positive verbal feedback, combined with educational strategies (e.g., verbal and written information about medications, the importance of adherence, and strategies for improving adherence). In general, these studies have also reported positive effects.

In a new randomized trial designed to prevent problems with adherence to treatment for juvenile rheumatoid arthritis (JRA), patients and parents in the experimental group were given verbal, written, and audiovisual information from a nurse about adherence improvement strategies, including prompting, monitoring, positive reinforcement, and discipline techniques. Control group patients and parents were given verbal, written, and audiovisual information about JRA, but no specific intervention information about adherence improvement strategies. Preliminary results indicate that the experimental group demonstrated better adherence to treatment, but no differences were found between the experimental control groups on disease activity, limitations, or direct and indirect cause.

In illustrating the relevance of prevention-based models to facilitate adherence to treatment regimens for chronic pediatric diseases, Rapoff and colleagues describe the advantages of different models of primary, secondary, and tertiary prevention, including selection of candidates for intervention strategies and interventionists. Rapoff argues that all three levels of prevention are necessary, potentially cost-effective, and require input from different professionals including pediatric psychologists. Empirical validation of prevention strategies for facilitating adherence to medical treatment is necessary using multicenter, collaborative research studies.

The next two chapters described the results of family-centered interventions to promote treatment adherence among adolescents with insulin-dependent diabetes mellitus (IDDM). In chapter 15, Anderson and her colleagues report the results of an office-based intervention designed to maintain parent–adolescent teamwork in diabetes management without increasing diabetes-related conflict between parent and teen. Participants were randomly assigned to one of three groups: Teamwork Intervention, Attention Control, or Standard Care. They were then followed for a year. The teamwork intervention emphasized parent–teen responsibility sharing for diabetes tasks and ways to avoid such conflicts.

Consistent with their hypotheses, this research group found no deterioration in parental involvement in insulin administration in the Teamwork Intervention group. In contrast, significantly more parents in the comparison groups demonstrated a lessening of parental involvement in insulin administration. Similar findings were obtained for parental involvement in blood glucose monitoring, with no deterioration in parental involvement in the teamwork group compared with a trend for an increased number of parents in the comparison groups showing deterioration in parental involvement in blood glucose monitoring. Families in the teamwork group also reported decreased levels of diabetes-specific conflict in contrast to the comparison groups.

In general, parental involvement in diabetes management tasks predicted positive adherence to blood glucose monitoring. Glycemic control improved significantly as the frequency of blood glucose monitoring increased. Consistent with other research, parental involvement in diabetes-related tasks decreased in families not exposed to intervention that focused on fostering parent–adolescent teamwork at regular diabetes follow-up visits.

The results of this innovative intervention underscore the importance of interdependence between parents and teens in the management of illnesses such as diabetes. One innovation of this study was the implementation of a relatively low-cost, low-intensity intervention integrated into routine diabetes follow-up medical care. The findings support the need for diabetes management teams to encourage more positive parent–child patterns of responsibility sharing during the preadolescent and early adolescent years when such behaviors are being established. Moreover, establishing parent–adolescent teamwork early in adolescence may provide the opportunity to improve management strategies that not only support the control of blood sugar, but prevent diabetes-related conflict.

In chapter 16, Wysocki and colleagues report their work on the application of behavioral family systems therapy (BFST), which focuses on improving family communication, problem solving, and conflict resolution, adolescent adjustment IDDM, diabetes treatment adherence, and blood sugar control. This intervention was selected based on the hypothesis that reduction of parent–adolescent conflict and improvement in family communication would result in improved diabetes management and control. Wysocki and colleagues reported durable effects of BFST on parent–adolescent conflict and skill deficits, resulting in a lessening of general and diabetes-related conflict and negative communication in mothers and adolescents compared with either educational support or standard medical care. No effects were found for positive communication or self-report measures of the quality of family relationships. Contrary to hypotheses, the BFST intervention did not result in improvements in treatment adherence, nor did it improve diabetes control and health care utilization.

Wysocki and colleagues describe the lessons they learned while implementing this intervention, including strategies of recruiting and maintaining a large sample of clinically appropriate families to participate in a randomized clinical trial of intervention. They found that careful randomization did not necessarily result in equivalent groups. Wysocki and colleagues critically examine the assumptions that underlie their research program in light of their data. For example, they question their assumption that family conflict is necessarily a powerful determinant of treatment adherence and control of IDDM in light of the fact that family conflict was lessened without affecting control and management of diabetes. Moreover, the magnitude of change that was achieved in the quality of parent–adolescent relationships may have been too small to yield generalizable benefits in diabetes outcomes. The authors' cogent suggestions for future research include using BFST as a preventive intervention for younger adolescents and identifying and targeting each adolescent's specific barriers to treatment adherence.

The next two chapters described interventions that were designed to promote adherence to treatment in cystic fibrosis (CF), which involves a demanding regimen. Quittner and colleagues (chap. 17) describe family-based interventions designed to increase treatment adherence in adolescents with CF, modeled on the BFST approach described in the previous chapter. This intervention was based on evidence that adolescents' interest in greater independence may conflict with demands of their medical treatment and that the family communication and intensity of conflict may be associated with adherence problems.

Quittner and colleagues' study compares the efforts of standard medical care to two structured interventions: (a) family intervention training, which focused on providing specific information about CF and included activities that engage the teen and parents in a learning experience; and (b) BFST, which focused on enhancing problem-solving and communication skills to reduce family conflicts. Four major outcomes are being studied over an 18-month period: (a) adherence behaviors; (b) family conflict, communication, and coping skills; (c) long-term health outcomes; and (d) cost-effectiveness.

One of Quittner and colleagues' contributions is the description of the practical dilemmas that have arisen in the course of their intervention research. For example, they note that modifications of interventions were needed to tailor them to families of children with CF, the need for individualized treatment manuals include process-oriented information to facilitate conducting the intervention, and the importance of documenting the precise nature of the medical regimen. One difficulty encountered is that the clinical regimen may not always be clearly stated by physicians or reviewed at each clinic visit, let alone updated or adjusted for the child's age. A related problem is that the treatment regimen for CF has increased in complexity as new medications have been developed. Finally, the lack of national guidelines for medical treatment for CF patients also increases the variability of prescribed treatment. Quittner and colleagues underscore the need for health care providers to emphasize precisely what the patient is to do, when, and for how long with respect to their treatment.

In chapter 15, Stark and colleagues focus on interventions to enhance the management of adherence to the diet in CF, which is necessary to enhance nutritional status that is often compromised in children and adolescents with this condition. Stark and colleagues' research has indicated that mealtimes are a significant problem for parents of children with CF and that both parent and child behaviors interfere with effective nutritional intake. Children with CF demonstrate less interest in food and more behaviors that are incompatible with eating. Moreover, parents with children with CF increase the child's caloric intake by keeping children at the meal longer than parents of healthy children. Consequently, mealtimes are often experienced as stressful by these parents and unsuccessful in meeting the children's dietary requirements.

Stark and colleagues' research has focused on enhancing behavior therapy skills such as child management strategies along with shaping to enhance adherence to dietary management in CF. Findings indicate that children who participated in treatment increased their daily caloric intake and weight gain significantly and that such gains were maintained 24 months posttreatment.

Stark and colleagues' current multisite clinical trial is designed to compare behavioral intervention and nutrition education to nutrition education alone. Although preliminary analyses indicate an effect for both the behavioral intervention and nutritional education condition, the behavioral intervention has thus far demonstrated an increase in calories that was nearly double that associated with nutritional education. Stark and colleagues attribute the preliminary success of the program to the fact that child management skills taught to the parents were based on specific assessments and targeting of specific child behaviors that parents found most problematic. Behavioral intervention provides parents with strategies to manage children who are potentially resistant to dietary changes. Moreover, children are involved in the intervention through the use of reinforcement (e.g., sticker charts and group rewards for meeting caloric intake goals), which appeared to be important.

Stark and colleagues consider potentially generalizable implications of this research concerning interventions for dietary management for children with different chronic health conditions. They conclude that specific difficulties associated with diet warrant specific evaluation of adherence behaviors and barriers to adherence. Such research is especially important because the impact of dietary behaviors on the health of children with chronic health conditions is often not evident for months or years. Recommendations are made to conduct scientific, long-term evaluation of interventions to improve adherence to diet by using parent training for behavioral child management skills and should be evaluated in other illness populations.

In chapter 19, Sandberg and colleagues describe the importance of growth hormone (GH) therapy for children with GH insufficiency. Their chapter documents that large numbers of patients demonstrate either intermittent or poor adherence as indicated by the number of self-reported missed GH injections. These authors describe the costs of GH therapy noncompliance on the child and family, health care providers, and health care system.

Sandberg and colleagues consider the challenges associated with daily or almost daily injections of GH and the barriers to adherence to GH treatment, including fear of needles and injections, unrealistic parental and child expectations for improvements in relative height with GH therapy, and individual differences in patients' behavioral and emotional functioning prior to beginning GH treatment.

To address these issues, Sandberg and his colleagues have designed and are now implementing a new intervention program specifically designed to enhance adherence to GH therapy. Based on the Health Belief Model, this intervention includes relaxation training to enhance the management of GH injections and behavioral contracting and monitoring. This intervention is assessed by a comprehensive battery of measures and assesses child and family adjustment.

Sandberg and colleagues predict that adherence to treatment regimen is enhanced if the parent and child perceive the child's short stature as a problem. Better adherence is also predicted when parent and child demonstrate positive psychological adaptation at the start of GH treatment. Greater fear of medical procedures and unrealistic treatment expectations are expected to have a negative influence on adherence.

Thus far, several challenges have been experienced in delivering the intervention program such as preexisting emotional and behavior problems that precluded randomization to the intervention and difficulties with scheduling patients for sessions. However, most families have appreciated the opportunity to learn about their child's health problem and recommended treatment in a setting that is removed from the busy circumstances of the typical outpatient endocrinology clinics.

CHAPTER FOURTEEN

Facilitating Adherence to Medical Regimens for Pediatric Rheumatic Diseases: Primary, Secondary, and Tertiary Prevention

Michael A. Rapoff

University of Kansas Medical Center, Kansas City, KS

Pediatric rheumatic diseases (PRDs) are chronic multisystem disorders that involve acute and chronic tissue inflammation of the musculoskeletal system, blood vessels, and skin. Prevalence estimates are that between 160,000 and 190,000 children in the United States have a rheumatic disease. The most common PRD is juvenile rheumatoid arthritis (JRA), accounting for between 75% and 83% of children with a rheumatic disease (Cassidy & Petty, 1995).

Criteria for the diagnosis of JRA include: (a) age at onset < 16 years, (b) arthritis (defined as joint swelling or two or more of the following signs: limitation of range of motion, tenderness or pain on motion, and increased warmth) in one or more joints, (c) duration of disease 6 weeks or longer, and (d) exclusion of other forms of juvenile arthritis. There are three general subtypes of JRA, which are defined by the type of disease pattern manifested during the first 6 months: pauciarticular, polyarticular, and systemic-onset. Pauciarticular JRA involves arthritis in four or fewer joints, affects 50% of children with JRA, and has the best long-term prognosis. Polyarticular JRA involves arthritis in five or more joints, affects 40% of children with JRA, and has a guarded to moderately good prognosis. Systemic-onset JRA is characterized by arthritis in a variable number of joints accompanied by fever and a rash, affects 10% of children with JRA, and has a moderate to poor prognosis (Cassidy & Petty, 1995). Medical treatment objectives for JRA include reduction of pain and inflammation, preservation of function, and prevention of joint deformities and destruction. Comprehensive treatment of JRA includes pharmacotherapy—primarily nonsteroidal anti-inflammatory medications (NSAIDs)—physical and occupational therapy, and psychosocial support.

Children with JRA and their parents are usually asked to adhere consistently and over a long period of time to a variety of therapeutic regimens—most notably, medications, therapeutic exercises, and splinting of joints. Many of these regimens may have delayed beneficial effects and in the short term may cause negative side effects, such as gastrointestinal irritation and pain. This constellation of factors associated with JRA and its treatment (i.e., the need for consistent adherence over a long period of time, delayed beneficial effects, and negative side effects) has been predictive of greater adherence problems to medical regimens for chronic pediatric diseases (Rapoff, 1989). Although the majority of children with JRA (~70%) have a favorable long-term outcome in terms of global functional status (Levinson & Wallace, 1992), there are no data to address whether this outcome is differentially impacted by adherence to prescribed regimens.

The purpose of this chapter is to: (a) examine the prevalence and type of adherence problems to medical treatments for PRDs (primarily JRA), (b) review studies on improving adherence to regimens for PRDs (again primarily JRA) conducted by our pediatric rheumatology group at the University of Kansas Medical Center, and (c) propose a prevention model for facilitating adherence to regimens for chronic pediatric diseases such as rheumatic diseases.

PREVALENCE AND TYPES OF ADHERENCE PROBLEMS IN THE TREATMENT OF PRDs

The few studies that have specifically addressed adherence to regimens for PRDs have primarily focused on JRA. Two retrospective studies by Litt and her colleagues examined adherence to salicylate medications in the treatment of JRA. In the first study (Litt & Cuskey, 1981), adherence among 82 patients with JRA was assessed using serum salicylate assays, with patients classified as *adherent* if their mean salicylate levels over a 19-month period were above 20 mg/dl. Some 55% of adolescents ($N = 38$) and 55% of children ($N = 44$) were found to be adherent. In the second study (Litt, Cuskey, & Rosenberg, 1982), adherence among 38 adolescents with JRA was assessed using serum salicylate assays obtained over a 12-month period, with patients again classified as adherent if their salicylate levels were more than 20 mg/dl. Again, 55% of the adolescents were adherent. In these two studies, the appropriate level of adherence was determined by established therapeutic salicylate levels that fall within the range of 15 to 25 mg/dl as measured by serum assay. The anti-inflammatory effects of salicylates are generally not observed below serum levels of 15 mg/dl, and toxic effects are likely to result with levels above 30 mg/dl (Cassidy & Petty, 1995).

In three separate within-subject design studies involving five patients with JRA (ages 3–14 years) who were suspected of having adherence problems by their pediatric rheumatologist, our research group assessed baseline adherence with salicylates and other medications, including naproxen, penicillamine, prednisone, and tolmetin sodium (Rapoff, Lindsley, & Christophersen, 1984; Rapoff, Purviance, & Lindsley, 1988a, 1988b). Adherence was assessed by parental observations or pill counts with independent interobserver reliability assessments conducted by an investigator in the patients' homes or in the clinic (average interobserver agreement exceeded 90%). Mean baseline adherence levels with these medications among the five patients ranged from 38% to 59%.

Our group also assessed adherence to prednisone for three patients with PRDs; two females, 17 and 18 years with systemic lupus erythematosus, and a 11-year-old female with dermatomyositis (Pieper, Rapoff, Purviance, & Lindsley, 1989). Prednisone is a glucocorticoid agent that is a standard part of treatment for lupus and dermatoymotis, particularly during acute exacerbations to control inflammation and systemic symptoms such as fever (Cassidy & Petty, 1995). Adherence was monitored by parental or patient pill counts over the phone with independent reliability pill counts obtained by an investigator in the clinic (agreement averaged 99%). Unexpectedly, patients were found to be overmedicating as well as undermedicating. Therefore, *acceptable adherence* for this study was defined as 80% to 120% of prescribed doses taken as assessed by pill counts (which follows the convention in the literature of allowing a 20% deviation from 100% adherence). The percentage of pill counts in this acceptable range during baseline ranged from 7% to 38% across the three patients.

Children with PRDS also have to adhere to regimens other than medications, such as therapeutic exercise and wearing joint splints (to prevent contractures). Two studies have assessed parental and patient perceptions of adherence problems with these types of regimens as well as medications. In the first study (Rapoff, Lindsley, & Christophersen, 1985), an adherence questionnaire was administered to 37 parents of children with JRA (mean age of children was 12 years). The children were prescribed medications and range-of-motion exercises, splints, or both. Parents rated the degree of difficulty they had in motivating their children to adhere to the different types of regimens and noted any negative reactions their children had to the regimens. The parents reported more adherence problems with prescribed exercises as compared with medications or splint wearing. Negative reactions to medications were noted by 43% of parents, with the most common reactions being complaining about taking medications, forgetting to take them, and refusing to take them. With reference to exercises, 60% of parents reported that their children had negative reactions, with the most frequent being complaining, refusing to do the exercises, and crying. Also 43% of parents reported that their children had negative reactions to wearing splints; the most common reactions were refusing to wear splints, questioning the efficacy of splints, and being embarrassed about wearing the splints at school or around friends.

In the second study (Hayford & Ross, 1988), an adherence questionnaire was administered to 93 parents of children with JRA and to 41 of the children with JRA. As with the Rapoff et al. (1985) study, adherence was reported to be lower for exercises as compared with medications. The proportion of parents and children reporting adequate adherence with medications (95% and 89%, respectively) was significantly greater than the proportion of parents and children who reported adequate adherence for exercises (67% and 47%, respectively).

In the aggregate, these data suggest that the extent of adherence to medications for PRDs can vary widely across different patient samples and methods of assessing adherence, but is similar to adherence levels for other chronic pediatric disease regimens (Rapoff, 1999). What is not known from these studies is the *optimal* level of adherence to regimens for PRDs. The two questionnaire studies would suggest that adherence to therapeutic exercises for PRDs is more problematic than adherence to medications. Therapeutic exercises are an important part of the treatment program for JRA and help improve or maintain joint range of motion and muscle strength (Cassidy & Petty, 1995). Intervention studies that specifically target improvements in exercise adherence are rare in the literature and would be an important contribution. However, there are a few studies that have targeted improvements in adherence to regimens (primarily medications) for pediatric rheumatic diseases.

ADHERENCE INTERVENTION STUDIES IN PEDIATRIC RHEUMATOLOGY

Our pediatric rheumatology group at the University of Kansas Medical Center has published four single-subject design studies and recently completed a randomized group trial to test the efficacy of educational and behavioral strategies for improving adherence to regimens for PRDs (primarily for patients with JRA and primarily to improve medication adherence). Our research strategy for the single-subject design studies was to monitor adherence in a group of patients and then experimentally evaluate interventions for those with the lowest levels of adherence and/or those identified by the pediatric rheumatologists as experiencing compromised function possibly due to low adherence. The recently completed group trial involved a preventive approach. We recruited newly diagnosed patients with JRA or *inception cohorts* (Haynes, 1979) and randomly assigned them to an adherence intervention or attention-placebo control group. Our goal in this study was to prevent the anticipated drop-off in adherence to medications that frequently occurs among chronically ill patients as they move further from the time of initial diagnosis and treatment (Rapoff, 1999).

Single-Subject Design Studies

Two studies have examined the efficacy of parent-managed token reinforcement programs in altering adherence to regimens for JRA. The first study (Rapoff et al., 1984) focused on improving adherence to medications, splint wearing, and prone lying (to prevent hip contractures) for a 7-year-old female with severe systemic-onset JRA. Adherence was assessed by parental observations with acceptable interobserver reliability ($\emptyset$94%) obtained with an investigator conducting independent observations in the home. Mean baseline adherence was low for medications (59%) and virtually absent for splint wearing (0%) and prone lying (0%). Introduction of the token system increased adherence to 95% for medications, 77% for splint wearing, and 71% for prone lying. At 10-week follow-up (with the token system withdrawn), adherence to medications, splint wearing, and prone lying averaged 90%, 91%, and 80%, respectively. Although functioning was not formally assessed, the pediatric rheumatologist anecdotally noted concomitant improvements in function for this patient, such as greater hip extension.

The second study (Rapoff et al., 1988a) also tested the efficacy of a token system program in improving adherence to medications for a 14-year-old male with polyarticular JRA. Adherence was assessed by weekly pill counts obtained from the patient's mother over the phone with independent counts by an investigator in the clinic (agreement with the mother's count was 100%). A withdrawal (reversal), single-subject design was employed to evaluate the effects of the intervention on adherence and several clinical outcome parameters (e.g., active joint counts). Medication adherence averaged 44% during baseline, increased to an average of 59% during a simplified regimen condition (when the dosage was reduced from four to three times a day), and further increased and remained at 100% during the first token system phase. There was a decreasing trend in adherence during a token system withdrawal phase (mean = 77%), an increase during the second token system phase (mean = 99%), and an average of 92% during the maintenance phase (when the token system was not in effect but could be reinstated if adherence dropped below 80% for 2 consecutive weeks). At the 9-month follow-up (no token system in effect and no contingency for reinstatement), adherence averaged 97%. Although they were not as straightforward as the adherence results, improvements were noted in clinical outcomes during the token system and follow-up phases (e.g., ≤5 active joints) relative to baseline and the token system withdrawal phase (e.g., ∅10 active joints).

Although the previously mentioned studies show that token systems can be effective in improving adherence, they are labor-intensive for families and require well-trained personnel to implement and monitor. Therefore, we conducted two studies that evaluated less complex behavioral strategies (such as self-monitoring and positive verbal feedback) combined with educational strategies (verbal and written information about medications, the importance of adherence, and strategies for improving adherence). The first study (Rapoff et al., 1988b) included three female patients with JRA, ages 3, 10, and 13 years. Adherence was again assessed by weekly pill counts obtained from parents over the phone with independent counts by one of us in the clinic (agreement was 100%). A multiple baseline across subjects design was used to evaluate the efficacy of the intervention. Baseline medication adherence averaged 38% and 54% for two of the patients and increased during the intervention phase to an average of 97% and 92%, respectively. Adherence only increased slightly for the third patient, from an average of 44% during baseline to an average of 49% during the intervention phase. Adherence decreased for all three patients at 4-month follow-up (means ranged from 24%–89%). The patient for whom the intervention was least effective was a 13-year-old who had less parental supervision of her regimen and whose mother admitted she was nonadherent to medications prescribed to treat her arthritis. Unfortunately, clinical outcomes were not reported for these patients.

The second study (Pieper et al., 1989) evaluated less complex behavioral and educational strategies for three females with PRDs: Patient 1 was a 17-year-old with systemic lupus erythematosus (SLE), Patient 2 was an 18-year-old with SLE, and Patient 3 was an 11-year-old with dermatomyositis (DM). All three patients were prescribed alternate-day prednisone to control their diseases. Adherence to prednisone was assessed by weekly pill counts obtained from patients or parents by phone and independent counts by one of us in the clinic (agreement averaged 99%). Because patients were found to be overmedicating as well as undermedicating, we defined *acceptable adherence* as between 80% and 120% of doses taken as determined by pill counts. A multiple baseline across subjects design was used to evaluate the intervention. Baseline adherence averaged 38%, 7%, and 33%, respectively, for Patients 1, 2, and 3. Adherence improved for all three patients during the intervention phase, averaging 89%, 67%, and 88%, respectively, for

Patients 1, 2, and 3. At 6-month follow-up, adherence averaged 100% for all three patients. Twelve-month follow-up was only available for Patients 1 and 3 because Patient 2 left town to attend college. For Patients 1 and 3 at 12-month follow-up, two of their three weekly pill counts were in the acceptable range (80%–120%). Unfortunately, clinical outcomes were not monitored for these three patients.

A Randomized Medication Nonadherence Prevention Group Trial

The purpose of this study was to experimentally validate an intervention to prevent medication adherence problems among children and adolescents who were newly diagnosed with JRA (Rapoff, 1997). This study makes a significant contribution by addressing several methodological issues identified in the adherence literature (Haynes, 1979; Rapoff & Barnard, 1991; Varni & Wallander, 1984): (a) recruitment of *inception cohorts* or patients beginning their treatment regimens; (b) using a microelectronic monitor to measure adherence; (c) assessing disease activity and limitations to determine covariation with adherence; (d) assessment of direct and indirect health care costs to determine whether costs are affected by adherence interventions; (e) utilizing an attention-placebo control group to rule out extra attention as a nonspecific variable in the adherence intervention; and (f) patients and parents participated for 13 months, which allowed for repeated assessments of adherence, disease activity/limitations, and health care costs (extensive follow-up is rare in the literature).

Patients were matched by age and type of JRA and then randomly assigned to the experimental or (attention-placebo) control groups. Patients and parents in the experimental group were given verbal, written, and audiovisual information from a nurse about adherence improvement strategies, including prompting, monitoring, positive reinforcement, and discipline techniques (see Rapoff, 1998). Control group patients and parents were given verbal, written, and audiovisual information about JRA and treatments by the same nurse, but no specific information about adherence improvement strategies. Patients and parents in both groups received their respective interventions during a 1½-hour clinic visit and were then telephoned by the nurse biweekly for 2 months and then monthly for 10 months. The content of the phone calls centered around the information presented during the initial clinic visit. To maintain treatment integrity, specific protocol checklists for each group were used by the nurse, and a research assistant was present during clinic visits to prompt the nurse if she omitted any component of the interventions (this was rarely necessary).

Dependent variables included adherence, disease activity/limitations, and direct/indirect health care costs. Adherence was assessed using the Medication Event Monitoring System or MEMS (Aprex Corporation), which is a medication cap containing microelectronics that records the date and time the cap is removed. Disease activity was assessed by the pediatric rheumatologists following physical examinations, including the number of active joints (those with pain, swelling, and limitation of motion), number of minutes of morning stiffness, and a global disease severity rating (ranging from 0 = *off medication, in remission* to 4 = *severe*). When appropriate for medical follow-up, blood was drawn to obtain an erythrocyte sedimentation rate (Westergren method) as a general indicator of disease activity (normal values in our laboratory are <20 mm/hr). Activity limitations were assessed by having the parents complete the Childhood Health Assessment Questionnaire (CHAQ). The CHAQ is a functional assessment instrument designed to assess limitation due to illness over the past week in the areas of dressing and grooming, arising, eating, walking, hygiene, reach, grip, and play activities (Singh, Athreya, Fries, & Goldsmith, 1994). Direct health care costs included charges for clinic visits, laboratory and radiographic procedures, and hospitalizations, which were obtained from the patients' medical records. Indirect costs were recorded by parents, including those related to transportation to the clinic, parking, meals, lodging, employment (work missed and income lost), child care for other children in the family, and medications.

Fifty-four patients were entered in the study and had some usable data over the 13-month period required for participation ($n = 29$ in the experimental group and $n = 25$ in the control group). Mean age of the total sample was 7.8 years (range of 2–16 years) and 74% were female. The mean socioeconomic level was 45.75 (range of 15–64), corresponding to *medium business, minor professional, technical* social strata as determined by the Hollingshead Index. About half the sample (52%) had polyarticular JRA, whereas 31% had pauciarticular and 17% systemic-onset JRA. There were no significant baseline differences on demographic or disease-related variables between the two groups, with the exception of significantly more siblings, on average, for control group patients.

We hypothesized that experimental group patients would show significantly higher adherence over time and less disease activity, functional limitations, and health care costs as compared with control group patients. Adherence data (see Fig. 14.1) were aggregated by quarters following baseline (Quarter 1 = the first 3 months following baseline, etc.). Analysis of covariance (ANCOVA) for repeated measures (with baseline adherence as the covariate) showed a significant group ($p = .016$) and Group × Time interaction ($p = .047$). Follow-up multiple comparisons (using Duncan's test) showed significantly higher adherence ($p = <.01$) for the experimental

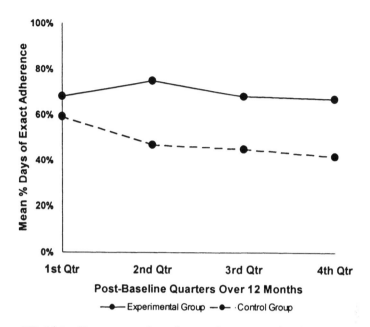

FIG. 14.1.   Mean percent days of exact adherence postbaseline over a 12-month period for patients with JRA, randomized to an adherence-enhancement (experimental) group or an attention-placebo (control) group.

group compared with the control group during Quarters 2 (75% vs. 47%), 3 (68% vs. 45%), and 4 (67% vs. 42%), but not Quarter 1 (68% vs. 59%).

Separate ANCOVA for repeated measures and follow-up multiple comparisons were also run on sedimentation rate, global disease activity, active joint counts, morning stiffness, CHAQ Disability Index, direct costs, and indirect costs. These analyses show no significant differences between the experimental and control groups on disease activity/limitations or direct and indirect costs.

The adherence data for this study supported our prediction that a nurse-administered adherence intervention can significantly enhance adherence to medications for newly diagnosed patients with JRA relative to an attention-placebo control condition. This finding was encouraging because most pediatric rheumatology treatment centers have a nurse clinician as a central member of the medical team, and nurses are in a unique position to offer patients and their families guidance about maintaining adherence to prescribed treatments.

The disease activity/limitations and health care cost results were unexpected and disappointing, and thus need to be explained. The lack of significant differences in disease-related outcomes found in this study is consistent with the available literature that raises doubts about the relationship between treatment adherence and outcomes of chronic health conditions. In addition, several other issues should be considered in interpreting these findings (Rapoff & Barnard, 1991). Patients in this study had relatively mild disease (e.g., baseline global disease severity averaged 2.21 for the experimental group and 1.96 for the control group or generally *mild* disease severity). Thus, "floor effects" (or low disease activity levels) may have prevented detection of improvements that could be differentially attributed to the adherence intervention. Also, the level of adherence for control patients may have been sufficient (given the wide therapeutic range for some NSAIDs) to control their disease symptoms. Nevertheless, these results remain disappointing because the optimal outcomes of adherence interventions is that patients get better, feel better, and do better (Rapoff, 1999).

Regarding the health care cost results, facilitating adherence to chronic illness treatment may increase rather than decrease costs (especially in the short term) because patients and families may be more consistent in pursuing medical follow-up and purchasing medications. Also, disease severity is generally the most powerful predictor of health care costs because those patients with more severe disease may require more follow-up visits, procedures, medications, or other treatments. Distinguishing potentially unnecessary or preventable health care costs (the costs of diagnostic and treatment services because of poor adherence) from necessary or inevitable costs is needed to determine whether improved adherence to treatment reduces unnecessary costs. Finally, patients may need to be monitored over more extended periods of time (such as 3–5 years) than was done in this study to allow the health and economic benefits of adherence interventions to accrue (we are currently doing this for patients in this study).

Implications of Intervention Studies

In taking stock of the adherence intervention studies our group has completed over the past 13 years, we have taken two different approaches to addressing nonadherence to medical regimens for PRDs. In the single-subject design studies, we attempted to evaluate adherence interventions for patients who were suspected of having low adherence and compromised health presumably due to low adherence. This approach might be considered a *tertiary* prevention strategy in that we attempted to prevent further negative effects on health and well-being that might be attributable to nonadherence. Although there were substantial improvements in adherence for most patients, health or disease outcomes were rarely assessed; when they were assessed, the results did not clearly indicate improvements in outcomes that could be attributed to the adherence interventions.

Our recent group intervention trial may represent a *secondary* or *primary* prevention strategy in that we tried to detect and reduce nonadherence early in the course of treatment or prevent nonadherence from occurring to preserve the health and well-being of patients. Again, significant improvements in adherence could be attributed to the intervention, but preliminary analyses failed to show improvements in outcomes or reduced health care costs.

A PREVENTION MODEL FOR FACILITATING ADHERENCE TO REGIMENS FOR CHRONIC PEDIATRIC DISEASES

To conclude this chapter, I describe a prevention model that can be applied to nonadherence to medical regimens for pediatric chronic illnesses and has potential implications for health care delivery. The word *prevent* means to *hinder, obviate*, or, in the older sense, *go before, anticipate* (Skeat, 1953). From a clinical, epidemiological perspective, what is being anticipated or obviated are threats to the health and well-being of people, such as life-altering and/or life-threatening diseases. In medicine, there are three general levels of prevention: primary, secondary, and tertiary (Fletcher, Fletcher, & Wagner, 1988). *Primary prevention* involves clinical activities that seek to remove identified risk factors so as to prevent diseases from occurring (e.g., immunizations to prevent communicable diseases). *Secondary prevention* involves clinical activities that attempt to detect diseases early (possibly during asymptomatic stages) and initiate treatment to stop diseases from progressing (e.g., screening for hypertension to identify those who have high-blood pressure and initiate anti-hypertensive drug, dietary, and exercise regimens). *Tertiary prevention* involves clinical activities that prevent further decrements in health and well-being for those persons who are already affected by disease (e.g., beta-blocker drugs to reduce mortality following a myocardial infarction). Each of these levels of prevention may be applicable to nonadherence to treatment regimens for pediatric chronic illness, which is a potential threat to the health and well-being of children and adolescents.

Before considering primary, secondary, and tertiary prevention approaches to addressing medical nonadherence, several caveats are in order. First, prevention efforts require that we have a valid, reliable, and clinically feasible way to detect or assess nonadherence. Although no such *ideal* measure exists, 24-hour recall interviews (in clinics or by phone) seem to represent our best option to date: They are reliable, valid, and feasible for routine and serial assessments of adherence. Second, information obtained from routine and serial assessments of adherence should allow us to identify the presence of *clinically significant nonadherence*, which can be defined as inconsistencies in following a particular regimen that may result in compromised health and well-being for particular patients with particular diseases. Previous attempts at determining levels of adherence that are necessary to prevent potentially deleterious health outcomes have been arbitrary and not biologically based (e.g., *adequate adherence* defined as taking ∅80% of prescribed medication doses). Third, because the desired outcome of adherence interventions is that patients get better, feel better, and do better, we need both traditional (e.g., clinical signs and symptoms) and quality-of-life measures of disease and health status that are valid, reliable, and clinically feasible (Rapoff, 1999). Clearly further research is needed to address these important issues before a comprehensive approach to preventing medical nonadherence can be realized.

Figure 14.2 is a schematic diagram of a preventive approach to addressing medical nonadherence to chronic disease regimens. At each level of prevention, there is a brief description of those patients who might benefit from the various approaches, examples of strategies that could be employed to facilitate adherence, and the person(s) who would be responsible for implementing the strategies.

Primary Prevention

Primary prevention efforts would seem to be most relevant for those patients who have not yet exhibited clinically significant nonadherence— possibly those who are recently diagnosed with a chronic illness or those who are able to sustain adequate adherence over time with basic levels of

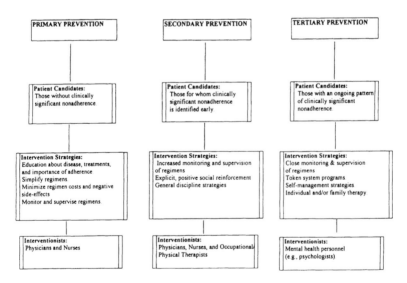

FIG. 14.2. Primary, secondary, and tertiary prevention approaches to medical nonadherence.

support and education. Interventions at this level would involve primarily educational and organizational strategies and less complicated behavioral strategies, such as:

⟨ Ongoing and comprehensive education about the chronic disease (including etiology, course, and prognosis), the treatment regimen (including the nature, purpose, and possible outcomes of treatments, as well as possible negative side effects of treatment), and the benefits of consistent adherence (such as improved regimen efficacy).

⟨ Modeling and rehearsing regimen tasks when first prescribed and in an ongoing fashion as needed (such as modeling correct use of a metered dose inhaler for children with asthma).

⟨ Presentation of information in effective verbal, written, and multimedia formats to enhance learning and retention of information (such as detailed treatment manuals or pamphlets that are readable and attractive to patients and families).

⟨ Making health care more accessible and attractive to patients and families (such as outreach clinics and consumer-friendly settings).

⟨ Increasing health care provider supervision of treatment regimens (such as inquiring about adherence problems during routine follow-up visits and tracking changes providers make in regimens over time).

⟨ Simplifying and minimizing the negative side effects of regimens (such as reducing the number of medications and taking medications that irritate the gastrointestinal tract with food or antacids).

⟨ Teaching patients and families to monitor adherence (such as charts or graphs posted on the refrigerator at home).

Primary health care providers, particularly nurses, could implement these strategies as part of routine follow-up care for patients with chronic diseases. The role of pediatric psychologists and other specialists would be to develop, conduct, and evaluate continuing education programs for physicians and nurses that focus on these types of strategies for facilitating adherence (e.g., Maiman, Becker, Liptak, Nazarian, & Rounds, 1988).

Secondary Prevention

Secondary prevention might be most applicable to those patients for whom clinically significant nonadherence has been identified early on, when nonadherence is *asymptomatic* or has yet to (but eventually would) compromise their health and well-being. Interventions at this level would be more complex and time-consuming than those at the previous level and might include the following:

- ⟨ Re-education as needed about the disease, treatment regimen, and the importance of consistent adherence.
- ⟨ More extensive monitoring of regimen adherence by parents and patients.
- ⟨ More explicit and consistent positive social reinforcement programs (e.g., praise) to promote adherence to treatment.
- ⟨ General parenting instruction including discipline strategies (such as time-out for younger children and time-limited *grounding* or withdrawing of privileges for older children).

Primary (physicians and nurses) and allied (e.g., occupational therapists) health care providers could be trained to implement these strategies. Again, the role of pediatric psychologists and other specialists would be to develop, conduct, and evaluate programs to train primary and allied health care providers how to implement these strategies.

Tertiary Prevention

Tertiary prevention efforts would be reserved for those patients with a chronic pattern of clinically significant nonadherence that is presumed to have deleterious effects on their health and well-being. Strategies at this level are the most complex and time-consuming and might include the following:

- ⟨ Token system programs (such as point systems, where patients earn tokens for adherence, lose tokens for nonadherence, and purchase privileges with tokens).
- ⟨ Contingency contracting (explicit written contracts that specify regimen tasks to be performed and consequences for adherence and nonadherence).
- ⟨ Self-management training (such as problem-solving training to anticipate and manage obstacles to adherence).
- ⟨ Individual and/or family therapy to address more serious patient or family problems that impact medical adherence (such as depression or dysfunctional family interactions).

Because of the demanding and technical nature of these strategies, mental health practitioners, who have extensive training and experience with chronically ill patients and their families, would be responsible for implementing strategies at this level. By virtue of their specialized training in providing services to children with chronic illness and their families, pediatric psychologists are particularly well suited to assist patients and families and evaluate interventions for improving adherence.

Recommendations for Research

Empirical efforts to validate strategies for improving adherence are predicated on having adequate measures of adherence and disease or health outcomes. Because all measures of adherence have costs and benefits (see Riekert & Drotar, chap. 1, this volume), a prudent strategy would be to use multiple measures of adherence. For medication adherence, this might involve a combination of assays and electronic monitors. Periodic assays would confirm actual ingestion of medications, and electronic monitors would provide continuous and precise data on dose frequency and timing. For nonmedication regimens, a promising combination might be structured telephone interviews to obtain periodic and precise information on the frequency of timing of regimen tasks (e.g., the frequency and timing of insulin injections for children with diabetes) combined with occasional direct observations by parents to confirm interview-derived reports. Assessments of disease or health outcomes are also needed to demonstrate the clinical utility of adherence interventions and should include traditional disease activity measures (e.g., clinical signs and symptoms and laboratory tests) and quality of life measures (both generic and disease specific).

In reviewing the intervention studies by our group and others (see Rapoff, 1999, for a recent review), it seems that most adherence interventions employ a tertiary prevention approach. Across these studies, small numbers of patients are exposed to fairly complex educational and behavioral strategies implemented by highly trained mental health practitioners. Few studies have approached the problem of medical nonadherence from a primary or even secondary prevention perspective. All three levels of prevention may be necessary, cost-effective, and require input from pediatric psychologists. Primary and secondary preventive approaches have the potential to prevent or minimize the deleterious effects of medical nonadherence and may be cost-effective for newly diagnosed patients. Tertiary prevention efforts would be reserved for those patients and families who, for a variety of reasons, do not maintain adequate levels of adherence to prescribed medical regimens (some justifiable reasons too, like the regimen does not help). Tertiary prevention could also be cost-effective if it reduces overutilization of health care resources attributable to medical nonadherence.

There is a need to move beyond correlational studies to experimental manipulations of variables to improve adherence. The choice of experimental designs is critical. Single-subject designs are particularly well suited for tertiary prevention studies because they accommodate small sample sizes and allow for changes in intervention protocols to address variables that uniquely affect the adherence of individual patients. Randomized, between-group designs that include an attention-placebo control group comparison would be best suited for validating primary or secondary level adherence interventions.

Because chronic diseases affect relatively small numbers of children and adolescents, empirical validation of primary, secondary, and tertiary prevention strategies for facilitating adherence to medical regimens will require multicenter collaborative research studies. Our medical colleagues have long recognized the value of multisite investigations when evaluating promising medical treatments for chronic diseases. We should follow their lead. This should improve our chances of obtaining funding and demonstrating the value of our efforts to facilitate adherence.

ACKNOWLEDGMENT

The research reported in this chapter was supported in part by Allied Health Professional Grants from the Arthritis Foundation and by a grant from the Maternal and Child Health Research Program (MCJ-200617). I would like to thank past and present colleagues at the University of Kansas Medical Center, Department of Pediatrics: Carol Lindsley, MD, Judy Morris, RN, Nancy Olson, MD, Joni Padur, PhD, Kathryn Pieper, PhD, Mark Purviance, PhD, and Susan Wright, OTR, who tolerated me and taught me about the value of teamwork.

REFERENCES

Cassidy, J. T., & Petty, R. E. (1995). *Textbook of pediatric rheumatology* (3rd ed.). Philadelphia: W. B. Saunders.

Fletcher, R. H., Fletcher, S. W., & Wagner, E. H. (1988). *Clinical epidemiology: The essentials* (2nd ed.). Baltimore: Williams & Wilkins.

Hayford, J. R., & Ross, C. K. (1988). Medical compliance in juvenile rheumatoid arthritis: Problems and perspectives. *Arthritis Care and Research, 1*, 190–197.

Haynes, R. B. (1979). Determinants of compliance: The disease and the mechanics of treatment. In R. B. Haynes, D. W. Taylor, & D. C. Sackett (Eds.), *Compliance in health care* (pp. 49–62). Baltimore: Johns Hopkins University Press.

Levinson, J. E., & Wallace, C. A. (1992). Dismantling the pyramid. *Journal of Rheumatology, 19*, 6–10.

Litt, I. F., & Cuskey, W. R. (1981). Compliance with salicylate therapy in adolescents with juvenile rheumatoid arthritis. *American Journal of Diseases of Children, 135*, 434–436.

Litt, I. F., Cuskey, W. R., & Rosenberg, A. (1982). Role of self-esteem and autonomy in determining medication compliance among adolescents with juvenile rheumatoid arthritis. *Pediatrics, 69*, 15–17.

Maiman, L. A., Becker, M. H., Liptak, G. S., Nazarian, L. F., & Rounds, K. A. (1988). Improving pediatricians' compliance-enhancing practices: A randomized trial. *American Journal of Diseases of Children, 142,* 773–779.

Pieper, K. B., Rapoff, M. A., Purviance, M. R., & Lindsley, C. B. (1989). Improving compliance with prednisone therapy in pediatric patients with rheumatic disease. *Arthritis Care and Research, 2,* 132–135.

Rapoff, M. A. (1989). Compliance with treatment regimens for pediatric rheumatic diseases. *Arthritis Care and Research, 2*(Suppl.), 40–47.

Rapoff, M. A. (1997). *Prevention of medication compliance problems.* Kansas City, KS: University of Kansas Medical Center.

Rapoff, M. A. (1998). *Helping children follow their medical treatment program: Guidelines for parents of children with rheumatic diseases.* (Available from the author, University of Kansas Medical Center, Department of Pediatrics, 3901 Rainbow Blvd., Kansas City, KS 66160-7330.)

Rapoff, M. A. (1999). *Adherence to pediatric medical regimens.* New York: Plenum.

Rapoff, M. A., & Barnard, M. U. (1991). Compliance with pediatric medical regimens. In J. A. Cramer & B. Spilker (Eds.), *Patient compliance in medical practice and clinical trials* (pp. 73–98). New York: Raven.

Rapoff, M. A., Lindsley, C. B., & Christophersen, E. R. (1984). Improving compliance with medical regimens: Case study with juvenile rheumatoid arthritis. *Archives of Physical Medicine & Rehabilitation, 65,* 267–269.

Rapoff, M. A., Lindsley, C. B., & Christophersen, E. R. (1985). Parent perceptions of problems experienced by their children in complying with treatments for juvenile rheumatoid arthritis. *Archives of Physical Medicine & Rehabilitation, 66,* 427–430.

Rapoff, M. A., Lindsley, C. B., & Purviance, M. R. (1991). The validity and reliability of parental ratings of disease activity in juvenile rheumatoid arthritis. *Arthritis Care & Research, 4,* 136–139.

Rapoff, M. A., Purviance, M. R., & Lindsley, C. B. (1988a). Improving medication compliance for juvenile rheumatoid arthritis and its effect on clinical outcome: A single-subject analysis. *Arthritis Care and Research, 1,* 12–16.

Rapoff, M. A., Purviance, M. R., & Lindsley, C. B. (1988b). Educational and behavioral strategies for improving medication compliance in juvenile rheumatoid arthritis. *Archives of Physical Medicine and Rehabilitation, 69,* 439–441.

Singh, G., Athreya, B. H., Fries, J. F., & Goldsmith, D. P. (1994). Measurement of health status in children with juvenile rheumatoid arthritis. *Arthritis & Rheumatism, 37,* 1761–1769.

Skeat, W. W. (1953). *An etymological dictionary of the English language* (rev. ed.). New York: Oxford University Press.

Varni, J. W., & Wallander, J. L. (1984). Adherence to health-related regimens in pediatric chronic disorders. *Clinical Psychology Review, 4,* 585–596.

CHAPTER FIFTEEN

An Intervention to Promote Family Teamwork in Diabetes Management Tasks: Relationships Among Parental Involvement, Adherence to Blood Glucose Monitoring, and Glycemic Control in Young Adolescents With Type 1 Diabetes

Barbara J. Anderson
Julienne Brackett
Joyce Ho
Lori M. B. Laffel
Joslin Diabetes Center, Boston, MA

The Diabetes Control and Complications Trial (DCCT) focused the diabetes community on the primary importance of glycemic outcomes for the prevention or delay of diabetes complications. In the DCCT, adherence to a demanding regimen that included multiple insulin injections (or pump therapy) and monitoring blood glucose concentrations four or more times daily was required of the intensively treated participants, including the adolescents. Because the DCCT demonstrated that improved glycemic control reduced the rate of diabetes complications (Diabetes Control and Complications Trial, 1994), it is important to identify supports for and barriers to adherence in all patients with Type 1 diabetes, especially adolescent patients. There is a consensus among empirical studies (Anderson & Laffel, 1996; Daneman, Wolfson, Becker, & Drash, 1981; U.S. Department of Health, Education, and Welfare, 1976; White, Waltman, Krupin, & Santiago, 1981) that glycemic control and adherence to diabetes management tasks deteriorate significantly during the adolescent years in patients with Type 1 diabetes. In particular, adherence to blood glucose monitoring has been identified as challenging for many children and adolescents with Type 1 diabetes (Belmonte et al., 1988; Wysocki, 1994).

The early adolescent years are consistently identified as a period of deteriorating blood glucose control (Blethen, Sargeant, Whitlow, & Santiago, 1981; Cerreto & Travis, 1984; Daneman et al., 1981) and heightened family conflict over adherence to diabetes management tasks (Anderson, 1984; Johnson, 1982). Moreover, cross-sectional and prospective studies (Anderson, Miller, Auslander, & Santiago, 1981; Hanson, Henggeler, & Burghen, 1987; Hauser et al., 1990; Jacobson et al., 1987, 1990) reveal that both diabetes-specific family conflict and general family conflict are associated with lower adherence rates in adolescents. Unfortunately, these struggles occur within the broader context of increased expectations by parents and health care providers for the young adolescent to assume more independence in responsibility for diabetes management tasks like blood glucose monitoring (Anderson, Auslander, Jung, Miller, & Santiago, 1990; Follansbee, 1989). Furthermore, in the post-DCCT era, parents as well as health care providers have increased expectations for good glycemic control in adolescents with diabetes (Grey et al., 1998).

In recent family studies (Anderson et al., 1990; Wysocki et al., 1996), it has been documented that there is an erosion of parental involvement in and support for diabetes management tasks over the early adolescent years. Furthermore, there is consistent agreement among empirical studies (Anderson et al., 1990; Burns, Green, & Chase, 1986; Ingersol, Orr, Herrold, & Golden, 1986; Weissberg-Benchell et al., 1995; Wysocki et al., 1996) that children and adolescents who assume early sole responsibility for their diabetes management are less adherent, have more mistakes in their self-care (e.g., incorrect insulin dose adjustment), and are in poorer glycemic control than those whose parents remain involved.

From the perspective of general adolescent development, a consensus appears to be developing among investigators (Irwin, 1987; Laursen, Coy, & Collins, 1998) that separation from parents during early adolescence increases young teens' vulnerability to negative peer influence. Engagement or teamwork between parent and young teen has been shown to enhance ego development and individuation and to have a positive impact on health, academic, and socioemotional outcomes (Grolnick & Slowiaczek, 1994; Resnick et al., 1997). Current research (Resnick et al., 1997) also supports the corollary that early distancing from parents puts the young adolescent at risk for health-compromising behaviors.

However, parental involvement can also lead to conflict and stress in the parent–adolescent relationship. It is clear that supportive behaviors must be individualized depending on the adolescent's developmental level and temperament, as well as the circumstances of each family (Holmbeck, 1993). Parent involvement can at times undermine healthy adolescent self-care behavior, as in the behavioral interaction cycle of *miscarried helping* (Coyne & Anderson, 1988) that occurs when the offered help shames, blames, or humiliates the patient. In the context of a chronic illness like diabetes, miscarried helping can escalate parent–adolescent conflict and undermine adolescent adherence and positive medical outcomes (Anderson & Coyne, 1993; Miller-Johnson et al., 1994).

Two priorities stand out from the recent research literature on adolescents with diabetes and their families: Sustaining parent involvement and minimizing parent–adolescent conflict are both important for adherence to the diabetes regimen and positive health outcomes over the early adolescent years. In addition, there is a need for interventions that focus on optimizing family behaviors as well as glycemic control (Drotar, 1997).

The purpose of this study was to design and evaluate an office-based intervention aimed at maintaining parent–adolescent teamwork in diabetes management tasks without increasing diabetes-related conflict between parent and teen. Priority was given to the development of a family-focused and low-cost intervention that could be integrated into the regular follow-up appointments of youth with diabetes. In this era of health care reform and cost containment, our focus was also to design an intervention that would provide recommendations for health care providers that realistically could be translated into office-based care on a wide-scale basis. Specific hypotheses included the following: (a) families participating in an intervention focused on maintaining parent–adolescent teamwork in the tasks of diabetes management will demonstrate significantly less deterioration in parental involvement in diabetes tasks (insulin administration and blood glucose monitoring) as compared with families receiving traditional didactic diabetes education or routine medical care; (b) families participating in an intervention focused on maintaining parent–adolescent teamwork in the tasks of diabetes management will not show a significant increase in diabetes-related family conflict despite increased parental involvement in diabetes tasks as compared with families receiving traditional didactic diabetes education or routine medical care; (c) across all study families, higher levels of parental involvement in the tasks of diabetes management are significantly related to increased adherence to daily blood glucose monitoring; and (d) across all study families, increased adherence to daily blood glucose monitoring is significantly related to better glycemic control (lower HbA_{1c}) over the 24-month duration of the study.

RESEARCH DESIGN AND METHODS

Participants

Study participants were pre- and young adolescents with insulin-dependent diabetes mellitus (IDDM), ages 10 to 15 years, who were patients in the Pediatric Unit of the Joslin Diabetes Center and their parents. Patient records were reviewed for the following eligibility criteria: duration of

IDDM greater than 1 year, reasonable glycemic control, similar to eligibility criteria for adolescents in the DCCT (Diabetes Control and Complications Trial, 1994; glycosylated hemoglobin, HbA_{1c} from 6.6% to 10.4% [reference range 4.0%–6.0%]), no documented serious medical or psychiatric condition in the patient or their parents (as defined by a medical diagnosis recorded in the patient's chart by the patient's physician), residence in New England or New York, at least one outpatient medical visit in the previous year, and ability to come to Joslin for medical visits three to four times over the next calendar year.

Letters of introduction were mailed to each eligible family followed by telephone contact. Of the 140 eligible families, 89 (or 64% of eligible families) agreed to participate. Most families who refused participation were not able to make the time commitment for three to four outpatient visits over the 1-year study period. There were no significant differences between study families and those who declined study participation with respect to attained age, disease duration, frequency of injections per day, or glycemic control measured as HbA_{1c}. Joslin's Committee on Human Subjects approved this study and written informed consent was obtained from all families prior to entry.

Procedure

Subjects were randomly assigned to one of three study groups (Teamwork Intervention, Attention Control, or Standard Care) stratified according to age and gender to ensure equal representation of younger (10–12 years) and older (13–15 years) male and female patients in each group. Two families (one in Standard Care and one in Attention Control) were lost to follow-up due to changes in residence and health insurance coverage after the first study visit and were excluded. Two additional families from Teamwork Intervention were excluded due to the identification of serious maternal psychiatric conditions (exclusion criteria). Thus, the final sample included 85 families: 28 in Teamwork, 30 in Attention Control, and 27 in Standard Care.

Design

During the 12-month study period, subjects in all three study groups had routine ambulatory appointments for their diabetes care at 3- to 4-month intervals from members of the pediatric diabetes team. Families randomly assigned to the Teamwork Intervention and Attention Control conditions also met individually with a research assistant for 20- to 30-minute intervention sessions immediately before or after the routine medical appointment during the 12-month study period. Families in all three groups were followed up for an additional 12-month period with ascertainment of glycemic control at each visit during the entire 24-hour period.

For all patients, the health care team gathered adherence assessments and clinical data at each visit. During the medical visit, interval history and physical examination, including staging of sexual development by the method of Tanner (Marshall & Tanner, 1969, 1970), were completed. In addition, at each visit, a research assistant conducted a brief joint patient and parent interview to update demographic information and assess the division of responsibility for diabetes management tasks in the family over the preceding 3 months. Self-reported questionnaire data were gathered from all families at the beginning and end of the 12-month study period.

Teamwork Intervention Condition.   The intervention for families in the Teamwork condition focused on the importance of parent–teen responsibility sharing for diabetes tasks and ways to avoid conflicts that undermine family teamwork. The modules focused on common conflicts or issues that may interfere with parent–adolescent teamwork around diabetes management (see Table 15.1). The modules were delivered to families by research assistants who were college graduates with no prior training in diabetes. The research assistants received diabetes training by observing a multidisciplinary pediatric team for 2 months prior to study onset. At each visit, the research assistant met with each family for approximately 20 to 30 minutes, encouraged active family discussion, and provided brief written materials designed to reinforce the module topic. The current Teamwork intervention was based on written materials that can be transported to any office-based practice and can guide and support recommendations for encouraging parent–adolescent teamwork from diagnosis through various stages of development. These written materials were designed to foster greater understanding and cooperation between the patient and family members and between family members and the health care team. The modules emphasized these

TABLE 15.1
Intervention Module Topics

Session	Time in 12-month Study	Study Condition	
		Teamwork Intervention	*Attention Control*
1	Baseline	Effects of growth and puberty on diabetes management. Need for parental involvement during this period	Telling others about your diabetes
2	3–4 months	Coping with common conflicts around blood glucose monitoring	Effects of stress on diabetes
3	6–8 months	Preventing conflicts around food	Making healthy choices from the meal plan
4	9–12 months	Parental support for exercise	Effects of exercise on diabetes

key points: (a) multiple causes of high and low blood glucose levels during early adolescence, (b) realistic expectations for blood glucose levels and behaviors during early adolescence, and (c) importance of parents maintaining involvement with insulin injections and blood glucose monitoring without shaming and blaming the young teen.

At the conclusion of the first session, the young adolescent and parent negotiated a responsibility sharing plan for insulin administration and blood glucose monitoring. This plan outlined who would be responsible for the different tasks involved in insulin injections, such as deciding the insulin dose, drawing up insulin, and doing the injection, as well as for the tasks of blood glucose monitoring. The plan also indicated whether a parent would supervise the injection and/or know the blood sugar value. The plan emphasized the need for the family to work as a team to manage diabetes, with the parents offering hands-on as well as emotional support to the adolescent. This plan was reviewed, reinforced, and/or renegotiated at each subsequent visit during the 12-month study period. Adolescents and parents accepted the Teamwork intervention enthusiastically and actively engaged in negotiating a family teamwork plan.

Attention Control Condition. The Attention Control group received the equivalent time (20–30 minutes per medical visit) and attention from the research assistant as provided to families in the Teamwork group. The Attention Control sessions provided didactic, traditional diabetes education with no focus on parental involvement (see Table 15.1). No plan for parent–adolescent teamwork was negotiated.

Standard Care Condition. Families randomly assigned to the Standard Care condition received routine clinical care from the diabetes team every 3 to 4 months over the 12-month study period. Families in this group had no intervention sessions with a research assistant.

Outcomes

Four levels of data are reported in this chapter: parent involvement in diabetes management, diabetes-related family conflict, adherence to blood glucose monitoring, and glycemic control (HbA$_{1c}$).

Measures of Parental Involvement in Diabetes Management Tasks. To assess the division of responsibility within families during a typical day for two major tasks of diabetes management (insulin injections and blood glucose monitoring), the investigators developed an interview to ascertain the current insulin injection and blood glucose monitoring routines in the family. The specific coding details for these two measures have been reported previously (Anderson, Ho, Brackett, Finkelstein, & Laffel, 1997). Briefly, families were asked who was usually (in the past month) responsible for five components of injecting insulin and for four components of monitoring blood sugars. Because there is no single set of parent behaviors that constitutes an involved parent, the components of parent involvement in insulin injections or blood sugar monitoring were combined to create the Insulin Routine Score and Blood Glucose Monitoring (BGM) Score. Component behaviors for insulin administration and blood glucose monitoring were coded with the creation of two composite scores ranging from 1 to 4: with: 1 = *no parental involvement* (adolescent has total responsibility), 2 = *minimal parental involvement*, 3 = *moderate parental involvement*, and 4 = *maximum parental involvement* (adolescent has no responsibility). Because the coding systems involved combining component behaviors into the higher order combinations of parent involvement, reliability of this coding system was checked independently by two trained research assistants. Comparison of the coding by each research assistant revealed 94% interrater reliability. Reliability checks were maintained throughout the study period.

Measure of Diabetes-Related Conflict. At baseline and 12 months, parents completed the Diabetes Family Conflict Scale to assess the degree of family conflict in 17 diabetes management tasks (Rubin, Young-Hyman, & Peyrot, 1989). The level of conflict in the family over diabetes-specific tasks was rated on a 3-point scale (1 = *always hassle* and 3 = *never hassle*). To score this measure, we summed the number of items in which any level of conflict was acknowledged. Therefore, scores could range from 0 to 17, with a 17 indicating conflict on all items.

Measure of Adherence to Blood Glucose Monitoring. For an assessment of the adolescent's adherence to blood glucose monitoring, a rating scale was completed independently by the adolescent's care provider during the medical visit. The Adherence Scale used in this study was a modified version of the scale developed by Jacobson et al. (1990) for use in a longitudinal study of adolescents with Type 1 diabetes. To assess adherence to blood glucose monitoring, the physician was asked to rate the daily frequency of glucose monitoring in the 3 to 4 months preceding the medical office visit according to the following scale: 0 to 1, 2, 3, or 4 or more blood glucose checks per day.

Measure of Glycemic Control. Blood sampling to assess glycemic control occurred at each visit. Initially, total glycosylated hemoglobin (HbA$_1$) was measured by electrophoresis (reference range 5.4%–7.4%, Corning Medical and Scientific, Corning, NY). However, during the study, lab methodology changed to a method measuring HbA_{1c} (reference range 4.0%–6.0%) employing high-performance liquid chromatography (Bio-Rad Variant, Hercules, CA). To allow for comparison between HbA_1 and HbA_{1c} values, a conversion formula derived from a regression analysis of 700 samples analyzed by both methods was used (HbA_{1c} = .77HbA_1 + .44). All glycemic control data are reported as HbA_{1c} values.

Statistical Analysis.   Statistical analysis of the data was performed using SAS for Windows (Release Version 6.12). Means and standard deviations are presented unless otherwise indicated. The analyses include unpaired t tests, analysis of variance (ANOVA), Pearson bivariate correlations, chi-square, and multivariate analysis. In general, univariate analyses were examined first. The complex relationships among the developmental, behavioral, and biological variables called for multivariate analyses to control for potentially confounding covariates. P values of less than .05 were considered significant.

Results

Baseline.   Baseline values were examined to ensure comparability of study groups at entry. There were no significant differences in demographic or clinical characteristics across the three study groups as presented in Table 15.2. Patients were about 12.5 years of age with duration of diabetes of approximately 5.5 years. More than 50% of patients in each group were receiving three injections per day and were checking blood sugars three or more times per day. It is important to note the striking homogeneity and relative intensity in home-care behaviors among the patients across the three study groups. This intensity is due, in part, to the eligibility criteria established for this longitudinal research sample, and the homogeneity reflects adequate randomization.

Table 15.3 presents baseline values for measures of parent involvement in insulin injections and blood glucose monitoring for the three study groups. There were no significant differences between the three study groups at baseline with respect to level of parental involvement in insulin administration or blood glucose monitoring (BGM) tasks. More than 50% of parents in each of the study groups demonstrated moderate or maximum involvement in insulin administration, and more than 40% of parents in each group demonstrated moderate or maximum involvement in BGM at Baseline.

Table 15.3 also presents baseline values for the three study groups with respect to Rubin's Diabetes Conflict Scale. On this Conflict Scale, parents, on average, endorsed approximately 4 out of 17 conflict items. For this measure of parent-reported diabetes-related family conflict, there were no statistically significant differences across the three study groups at baseline.

TABLE 15.2
Baseline Patient Characteristics by Study Condition

Characteristic	Teamwork Intervention (n = 28)	Attention Control Intervention (n = 30)	Standard Care (n = 27)
Age (yrs) $\bar{x} \pm SD$	12.7 ± 1.40	12.7 ± 1.40	12.5 ± 1.40
Duration (yrs) $\bar{x} \pm SD$	5.3 ± 2.56	6.1 ± 2.78	5.2 ± 2.17
HbA$_{1c}$ $\bar{x} \pm SD$	8.3 ± 1.10%	8.7 ± 1.19%	8.6 ± 0.97%
Insulin U/kg/day $\bar{x} \pm SD$	0.97 ± 0.270	0.94 ± 0.200	0.93 ± 0.179
Injections per day			
% on 2	39%	33%	19%
% on 3	61%	67%	81%
Frequency of BGM/day			
0–1/day	7%	7%	0%
2–3/day	61%	63%	78%
4+/day	32%	30%	22%
Gender (% Male)	50%	50%	52%
Developmental stage			
Prepubertal (Tanner Stage I)	22%	13%	26%
Pubertal (Tanner Stages II–IV)	64%	63%	59%
Postpubertal (Tanner Stage V)	14%	23%	15%
Family structure			
% single parent	21%	20%	15%
% two parent	79%	80%	85%

Outcomes of the 12-Month Study Period: Impact on Teamwork and Conflict. Table 15.3 also displays the 12-month study data for parent involvement in insulin administration and blood glucose monitoring, family conflict, and glycemic control. A series of chi-square analyses and repeated measures ANOVA was carried out examining changes in parent involvement, family conflict, and glycemic control over the 12-month study period. Because we found no statistically significant differences between families in the Attention Control and Standard Care groups after the 12-month study period on these key outcome variables, for additional longitudinal data analyses and presentation of results we combined these two study groups to form a single Comparison group ($N = 57$).

The primary goal of this intervention was to prevent deterioration in parental involvement with diabetes management tasks, which often occurs during early adolescence. With respect to involvement in both insulin administration and blood glucose monitoring, we defined *deterioration* in parental involvement as decreasing involvement by one or more categories, as defined earlier, in measures of parental involvement. Figure 15.1 presents the percentage of parents demonstrating increased involvement, no change, and deterioration of parent involvement in insulin administration and blood

TABLE 15.3
Baseline and 12-Month Values for Parent Involvement, Family Conflict, and Metabolic Control by Study Condition

Characteristic	Teamwork Intervention (n = 28)		Attention Control Intervention (n = 30)		Standard Care (n = 27)	
	Baseline	12 Months	Baseline	12 Months	Baseline	12 Months
Insulin involvement (% of families)						
None	10.7	3.6	6.7	6.7	0.0	7.4
Minimal	28.6	25.0	33.3	36.7	37.0	25.9
Moderate	42.9	67.9	43.3	40.0	48.2	51.8
Maximum	17.9	3.6	16.7	16.7	14.8	14.8
BGM involvement (% of families)						
None	10.7	10.7	10.0	16.7	7.4	3.7
Minimal	50.0	28.6	33.3	40.0	51.9	66.7
Moderate	25.0	50.0	40.0	30.0	40.7	29.6
Maximum	14.3	10.7	16.7	13.3	0.0	0.0
Family conflict (Rubin) $\bar{x} \pm SD$ 2.06	4.8 ± 3.09	3.8 ± 2.75	3.6 ± 2.77	3.9 ± 3.02	3.5 ± 2.34	3.9 ±
Unsupportive parent behavior (DFBC) $\bar{x} \pm SD$	13.8 ± 4.5	11.1 ± 3.8	11.7 ± 3.62	11.1 ± 3.53	13.8 ± 3.8	13.1 ± 3.9
HbA$_{1c}$ (%) $\bar{x} \pm SD$ 0.63	8.3 ± 1.10	8.9 ± 1.05	8.7 ± 1.19	8.7 ± 0.94	8.6 ± 0.97	8.7 ±

glucose monitoring from baseline to the end of the 12-month intervention period for the Teamwork group contrasted with the Comparison group.

There was no deterioration in parental involvement in insulin administration in any family in the Teamwork group (Fig. 15.1, Panel A). Significantly more parents in the Comparison group (16%) showed deterioration in parental involvement in insulin administration ($\chi^2 = 4.95$, $df = 1$, $p < .03$).

A

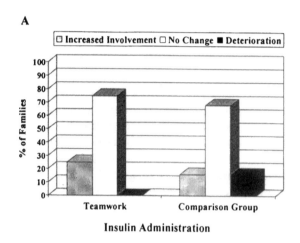

Insulin Administration

B

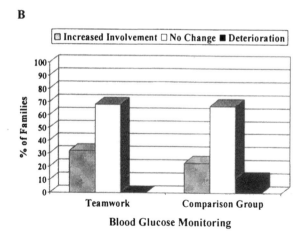

Blood Glucose Monitoring

FIG. 15.1. Changes in the level of parental involvement according to study group. (A) Comparison of insulin administration involvement. Significant difference between the two groups in number of families showing deterioration in involvement in insulin administration ($\chi^2 = 4.95$, $df = 1$, $p < .03$). (B) Comparison of blood glucose monitoring involvement. A trend ($p = .075$) was noted between the groups in number of families showing deterioration in involvement in blood glucose monitoring.

Figure 15.1, Panel B presents the percentage of parents demonstrating increased involvement, no change, or deterioration of parent involvement in blood glucose monitoring over the 12-month study period for the two groups. Again there was no deterioration in parental involvement in any family in the Teamwork group compared with 11% of parents in the Comparison group who showed deterioration in parental involvement in blood glucose monitoring. There was a trend for this change in parental involvement to reach statistical significance ($\chi^2 = 3.17$, $df = 1$, $p < .075$).

We also investigated the impact of the Teamwork Intervention on the level of diabetes-related conflict in the family. Because the Teamwork parents were more engaged with their adolescents around diabetes tasks, they had more potential for family conflict over diabetes-related tasks than did families in the Comparison group. Figure 15.2 presents the mean level of diabetes-related family conflict from the Diabetes Conflict Scale by the two groups at baseline and at the end of the 12-month study period. ANOVA revealed that Teamwork families reported decreased levels of diabetes-specific conflict at the end of the study period, as shown by a significant Group by Time Interaction ($F = 4.97$, $df = 1$, $p < .02$). No significant change in the level of conflict was reported in the Comparison group.

Follow-Up Period 12 to 24 Months: Relationships Among Family Teamwork, Adherence, and Glycemic Control. We did not hypothesize changes in HbA$_{1c}$ during the 12-month intervention period because

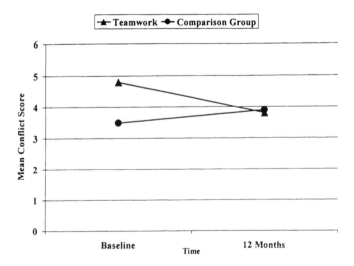

FIG. 15.2. Mean scores on Diabetes Family Conflict Scale (Rubin et al., 1989) at baseline and 12 months according to study condition. A significant group by time interaction was found ($F = 4.96$, $df = 1$, $p < .03$).

the focus of this intervention was on changing family behavior patterns and not directly on factors more likely to impact immediately on glycemia, such as intensity of the diabetes treatment regimen. However, once family behavior patterns around teamwork and conflict were changed, we explored the linkages between family teamwork and adherence as well as adherence and glycemic control over the subsequent 12-month period—from 12 to 24 months. Therefore, in the next analyses, we no longer looked at families with respect to group assignment, but at predictors of these important outcomes.

First, we summed the results of the Adherence Rating Scale for every office visit over Months 3 to 24 of the study period to derive a Cumulative BGM index ($M = 11.6 \pm 2.96$), which ranged between 5 and 16. In a multivariate analysis, we examined predictors (age, diabetes duration, gender, and parental involvement) of Cumulative BGM adherence over the 24-month study period. The level of parent involvement in diabetes management tasks at 24 months significantly predicted cumulative BGM adherence ($R^2 = .25; p < .003$). With respect to diabetes management tasks, the family patterns that reflected no family teamwork—Adolescent Only and Parent Only—were related to the lowest levels of BGM adherence over the 24-month study period.

Finally, we examined the relationship between adherence to BGM at 24 months and a cumulative index of HbA_{1c} over the 24-month study period with a multivariate analysis predicting cumulative glycemic control (HbA_{1c}) over the 24-month study period by averaging the HbA_{1c} values from every office visit at Months 3 to 24 for each patient in the study. After controlling for gender, duration of diabetes, and Tanner stage, we found that adherence to BGM at 24 months was the single significant predictor of glycemic control ($R^2 = .23; p < .02$). As indicated in Fig. 15.3, glycemic control improved significantly as the frequency of BGM increased—from an HbA_{1c} value of 9.1% when the blood glucose was checked zero to one times per day to 8.4% when the blood glucose level was checked four or more times daily.

DISCUSSION

Over the course of this study, an erosion in parental involvement in diabetes tasks occurred in the families not exposed to the intervention focused on fostering parent–adolescent teamwork at their regular diabetes follow-up visits. These results are consistent with other reports (Anderson et al., 1990; Weissberg-Benchell, 1995; Wysocki et al., 1996) that parent involvement in the tasks of diabetes management deteriorates in young adolescents over time with increasing age and disease duration.

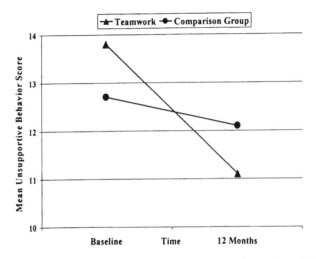

FIG. 15.3.   Relationship between mean HbA$_{1c}$ over 24 months and BGM adherence at 24 months.

However, clinicians who work with adolescents with diabetes are only beginning to recognize the importance of continued parent involvement on glycemic and behavioral outcomes in this group of patients. This recent focus on the family among clinicians and researchers is consistent with developmental theories that conceptualize the major task of the adolescent period as movement away from dependence on the family, not toward independence, but rather toward interdependence. Interdependence does not require adolescents to distance themselves emotionally from parents, but rather requires a reorganization in which family members renegotiate and redistribute responsibilities and obligations (Baumrind, 1987). A large empirical study, The National Longitudinal Study of Adolescent Health (Resnick et al., 1997), investigated a representative sample of 12,000 adolescents and concluded that parental involvement was the single most important predictor of positive adolescent outcomes, such as school success and avoidance of drug use and teen pregnancy.

The current study was carried out within the context of this recent recognition of the value of parental involvement in adolescent development. We designed a relatively low-cost, low-intensity intervention that was integrated into the routine diabetes follow-up medical care of young adolescent patients. This Teamwork intervention was focused on preventing the normative erosion in parental involvement in diabetes management. Consistent with this focus, we found that, within the Teamwork Intervention condition, parents and teens were able to sustain shared responsibility for insulin administration significantly more than families in the Attention Control and Standard Care conditions. In addition, there was a trend for parents and teens in the Teamwork condition, as compared with families in the Comparison groups, to sustain and even increase involvement with blood glucose monitoring tasks.

One of the most important findings in this study is that families in the Teamwork group with sustained parental involvement in both insulin tasks and blood glucose monitoring did not experience an increase in diabetes-related family conflict. In fact, families in the Teamwork condition, who were more engaged around diabetes tasks and thus had more potential for conflict, reported less conflict than families in the Comparison group. This is important given new research on adolescent development (Laursen et al., 1998) that the affective intensity (i.e., the level of hurt and pain) of parent–adolescent conflicts typically increases between the early adolescent period and the mid- to late-adolescent period. This suggests that pediatric diabetes comprehensive care teams can provide families with anticipatory guidance to encourage more positive parent–child patterns of responsibility sharing during the preadolescent and early adolescent years when family behaviors are being established. With this intervention approach, some of the entrenched and intense diabetes-related conflicts that are frequently encountered between older adolescents and their parents can possibly be prevented.

In this post-DCCT era, it is not family conflict, but improvements in adherence to diabetes management tasks and glycemic control that are receiving the most attention. This is based on the clear demonstration from the DCCT that improved glycemic control during adolescence has the potential to prevent and/or delay early physiological complications (Diabetes Control and Complications Trial, 1994; Drash, 1993). Thus, there is a need for practical interventions that focus on enhancing adherence and glycemic control in this high-risk group.

It is important to recall that the immediate targets of the Teamwork Intervention were not glycemic parameters or adherence behaviors, but rather family behavior patterns. Therefore, it is not surprising that the Teamwork Intervention did not lead to immediate or dramatic improvements in glycemic control in the participating adolescent patients. However, our data suggest that after changes in family interaction patterns have been demonstrated, parental involvement in diabetes care and lower levels of family conflict are related to higher levels of BGM adherence over the 24-month study period. This suggests that the establishment of parent–adolescent teamwork early in adolescence may provide the opportunity to intensify management strategies because they can be supported within the family to improve glycemic control. Similarly, reporting on results of a pioneering family-based group intervention with adolescents with diabetes, Delamater and colleagues (1991) also suggested that decreasing family conflict may have positive effects on the glycemic and behavioral outcomes of adolescents with Type 1 diabetes. One valuable application of this Teamwork intervention strategy may be in combining it with more medically based approaches that intensify insulin therapy to improve glycemic control, such as the approach reported by Grey and colleagues (1998) with medical treatment intensification with adolescent patients. For adolescents, who are our most metabolically at-risk group of patients with Type 1 diabetes, new pediatric diabetes intervention models to improve adherence and medical outcomes may be most effectively built from a synthesis of several current approaches that must target not only insulin regimens, but also family interaction patterns.

It is crucial for present-day intervention approaches in chronic disease to be generalizable across broad groups of patients and health care delivery systems (Glasgow et al., 1999). From a public health perspective, a low-cost intervention, such as the Teamwork Intervention integrated into routine diabetes medical care, may be appropriate for families for whom group-based interventions or therapy approaches are neither acceptable nor affordable (Glasgow et al., in press).

However, several cautions must be emphasized in discussing the results of this study. First, these findings are based on a small sample size of 85 families. One consequence of the eligibility criteria set for this longitudinal intervention research was a homogeneous group of participating families. To minimize subject attrition over the 24-month study period, more at-risk families were not included in this initial study. This intervention needs to be replicated with a larger, more heterogeneous and higher risk sample of families. In fact, the clinical benefits may be greater if more at-risk patients were included in the study. Second, because the intervention period of this study was relatively brief, this approach should be replicated over longer intervention and follow-up time periods.

Recently investigators and clinicians have recognized the complexity of measuring adherence to the diabetes regimen (Johnson, 1992; McNabb, 1997). Our data suggest that the frequency of BGM provides an important marker of "engagement with the treatment regimen" that can be reliably and realistically measured. However, our research questions were focused on the fundamental aspect of whether blood glucose data were available to the family and health care team, rather than how the results were interpreted (Anderson et al., 1997). The results of BGM provide important information for the health care team as well as for the patient–family unit. This information permits the health care team to prescribe appropriate insulin dosages and make other adjustments in the meal plan or exercise program as needed. It also provides patients and families with immediate information on which to adjust the diabetes management plan. Understanding how to react to blood glucose results is important for families of youth with Type 1 diabetes trying to achieve optimal glycemic control.

Therefore, future studies should assess both the availability and use of BGM results by families.

To conclude, contemporary theories of adolescent development focus on the transformation of the parent–adolescent relationship and the processes that foster continuity of parental influences and minimize the disruption of these influences. The recently published report *Great Transitions* by the Carnegie Council on Adolescent Development (1995) emphasized the importance of reengaging parents with their young adolescents to promote educational achievement and good health outcomes. Interventions focused on adolescents with diabetes will benefit from this broader cultural awareness that continued parent involvement during adolescence protects youth from many high-risk behaviors and negative developmental outcomes. The model of pediatric diabetes care for the new millennium needs to incorporate a public health approach and be built on new developmental constructs of the adolescent–parent relationship, which educate both health care teams and families about the value of a partnership between the parent and the young adolescent when adherence to complex regimen is critical, as it is in Type 1 diabetes.

ACKNOWLEDGMENT

This study was financially supported by a grant (DK-46887) from NIDDK to Barbara Anderson. Portions of this chapter were presented in oral form at the 57th annual meeting of the American Diabetes Association in June 1997 in Boston, MA. We wish to acknowledge contributions of the clinical team in the Pediatric Unit of the Joslin Diabetes Center: Dr. Joan Mansfield, Dr. Alyne Ricker, Dr. Joseph Wolfsdorf, as well as Louise Crescenzi, Paula Michel Fanizzi, Cindy Pasquarello, and Kristen Rice.

REFERENCES

Anderson, B. J. (1984). The impact of diabetes on the developmental tasks of childhood and adolescence: A research perspective. In M. Nattrass & J. V. Santiago (Eds.), *Recent advances in diabetes* (pp. 165–171). London: Churchill Livingston.

Anderson, B. J., Auslander, W. F., Jung, K. C., Miller, J. P., & Santiago, J. V. (1990). Assessing family sharing of diabetes responsibilities. *Journal of Pediatric Psychology, 15,* 477–492.

Anderson, B. J., & Coyne, J. C. (1993). Family context and compliance behavior in chronically ill children. In N. Krasnegor, L. Epstein, S. B. Johnson, & S. J. Yaffe (Eds.), *Developmental aspects of health compliance behavior* (pp. 77–89). Hillsdale, NJ: Lawrence Erlbaum Associates.

Anderson, B. J., Ho, J., Brackett, J., Finkelstein, D., & Laffel, L. (1997). Parental involvement in diabetes management tasks: Relationships to blood glucose monitoring adherence and metabolic control in young adolescents with IDDM. *Journal of Pediatrics, 130,* 257–265.

Anderson, B. J., & Laffel, L. (1996). Behavioral and family aspects of the treatment of children and adolescents with IDDM. In D. Porte, R. Sherwin, & H. Rifkin (Eds.), *Ellenberg and Rifkin's diabetes mellitus* (5th ed., pp. 811–825). Stamford, CT: Appleton & Lange.

Anderson, B. J., Miller, J. P., Auslander, W. F., & Santiago, J. V. (1981). Family characteristics of diabetic adolescents: Relationship to metabolic control. *Diabetes Care, 4*, 586–594.

Baumrind, D. (1987). A developmental perspective on adolescent risk taking in contemporary America. In C. E. Irwin (Ed.), *Adolescent social behavior and health* (pp. 93–126). San Francisco: Jossey-Bass.

Belmonte, M. M., Schiffrin, A., Dufresne, J., Suissa, S., Goldman, H., & Polychronakos, C. (1988). Impact of SBGM on control of diabetes as measured by HbA_1: 3-year survey of a juvenile IDDM clinic. *Diabetes Care, 11*, 484–488.

Blethen, S. L., Sargeant, D. T., Whitlow, M. G., & Santiago, J. V. (1981). Effect of pubertal stage and recent blood glucose control on plasma somatomedin C in children with insulin-dependent diabetes mellitus. *Diabetes, 30*, 868–872.

Burns, K. L., Green, P., & Chase, H. P. (1986). Psychosocial correlates of glycemic control as a function of age in youth with IDDM. *Journal of Adolescent Health, 7*, 311–319.

Carnegie Council on Adolescent Development. (1995). *Great transitions: Preparing adolescents for a new century.* New York: Author.

Cerreto, M. C., & Travis, L. B. (1984). Implications of psychological and family factors in the treatment of diabetes. *Pediatric Clinics of North America, 31*, 689–710.

Coyne, J. C., & Anderson, B. J. (1988). The "Psychosomatic Family" reconsidered: Diabetes in context. *Journal of Marital and Family Therapy, 14*, 113–123.

Daneman, D., Wolfson, D. H., Becker, D. J., & Drash, A. L. (1981). Factors affecting glycosylated hemoglobin values in children with insulin-dependent diabetes. *Journal of Pediatrics, 99*, 847–853.

Delamater, A. M., Smith, J. A., Bubb, J., Green-Davis, S., Gamble, T., White, N. H., & Santiago, J. V. (1991). Family-based behavior therapy for diabetic adolescents. In J. H. Johnson & S. B. Johnson (Eds.), *Advances in child health psychology* (pp. 293–306). Gainsville, FL: University of Florida Press.

Diabetes Control and Complications Trial Research Group. (1994). Effect of intensive diabetes treatment on the development and progression of long-term complications in adolescents with insulin-dependent diabetes mellitus: Diabetes Control and Complications Trial. *Journal of Pediatrics, 125*, 177–188.

Drash, A. L. (1993). The child, the adolescent, and the Diabetes Control and Complications Trial. *Diabetes Care, 16*, 1515–1516.

Drotar, D. (1997). Intervention research: Pushing back the frontiers of pediatric psychology. *Journal of Pediatric Psychology, 22*, 593–606.

Follansbee, D. S. (1989). Assuming responsibility for diabetes management: What age? What price? *Diabetes Educator, 15*, 347–352.

Glasgow, R. E., Kaplan, R. M., Smith, L., Wagner, E. H., Vinicor, F., & Norman, J. (1999). If diabetes is a public health problem, why not treat it as one? A population-based approach to chronic illness. *Annals of Behavioral Medicine, 21*, 159–170.

Grey, M., Goland, E. A., Davidson, M., Yu, C., Sullivan-Bolyai, S., & Tamborlane, W. V. (1998). Short-term effects of coping skills training as adjunct to intensive therapy in adolescents. *Diabetes Care, 21*, 902–908.

Grolnick, W. S., & Slowiaczek, M. L. (1994). Parents' involvement in children's schooling: A multidimensional conceptualization and motivational model. *Child Development, 65*, 237–252.

Hanson, C. L., Henggeler, S. W., & Burghen, G. A. (1987). Model of associations between psychosocial variables and health outcome measures of adolescents with IDDM. *Diabetes Care, 10*, 752–756.

Hauser, S. T., Jacobson, A. M., Lavori, P., Wolfsdorf, J. I., Herskowitz, R. D., Milley, J. E., Bliss, R., Wertlieb, D., & Stein, J. (1990). Adherence among children and adolescents with insulin-dependent diabetes mellitus over a four-year longitudinal follow-up: II. Immediate and long-term linkages with the family milieu. *Journal of Pediatric Psychology, 15*, 527–542.

Holmbeck, G. N. (1993). A model of family relational transformations during the transition to adolescence: Parent-adolescent conflict and adaptation. In J. A. Graber, J. Brooks-Gunn, & A. C. Petersen (Eds.), *Transitions through adolescence: Interpersonal domains and context* (pp. 167–199). Mahwah, NJ: Lawrence Erlbaum Associates.

Ingersoll, G. M., Orr, D. P., Herrold, A. J., & Golden, M. P. (1986). Cognitive maturity and self-management among adolescents with insulin-dependent diabetes mellitus. *Journal of Pediatrics, 108*, 620–623.

Irwin, C. E. (Ed.). (1987). *Adolescent social behavior and health.* San Francisco: Jossey-Bass.

Jacobson, A. M., Hauser, S. T., Lavori, P., Wolfsdorf, J. I., Herskowitz, R. D., Milley, J. E., Bliss, R., Gelfand, E., Wertlieb, D., & Stein, J. (1990). Adherence among children and adolescents with insulin-dependent diabetes mellitus over a four-year longitudinal follow-up: I. The influence of patient coping and adjustment. *Journal of Pediatric Psychology, 15*, 511–526.

Jacobson, A. M., Hauser, S. T., Wolfsdorf, J. I., Houlihan, J., Milley, J. E., Herskowitz, R. D., Wertlieb, D., & Watt, B. A. (1987). Psychologic predictors of compliance in children with recent onset of diabetes mellitus. *Journal of Pediatrics, 110*, 805–811.

Johnson, S. B. (1982). Behavioral management of childhood diabetes. *New Directions for Mental Health Services, 18*, 5–18.

Johnson, S. B. (1992). Methodological issues in diabetes research: Measuring adherence. *Diabetes Care, 15*, 1658–1667.

Laursen, B., Coy, K. C., & Collins, W. A. (1998). Reconsidering changes in parent–child conflict across adolescence: A meta-analysis. *Child Development, 69*, 817–832.

Marshall, W. A., & Tanner, J. M. (1969). Variations in pattern of pubertal changes in girls. *Archives of Diseases of Childhood, 44*, 291–303.

Marshall, W. A., & Tanner, J. M. (1970). Variations in pattern of pubertal changes in boys. *Archives of Diseases of Childhood, 45*, 13–23.

McNabb, W. L. (1997). Adherence in diabetes: Can we define it and can we measure it? *Diabetes Care, 20*, 215–218.

Miller-Johnson, S., Emery, R. E., Marvin, R. S., Clarke, W., Lovinger, R., & Martin, M. (1994). Parent–child relationships and the management of insulin-dependent diabetes mellitus. *Journal of Consulting and Clinical Psychology, 62*, 603–610.

Resnick, M. D., Bearman, P. S., Blum, R. W., Bauman, K. E., Harris, K. M., Jones, J., Tabor, J., Beuhring, T., Sieving, R. E., Shew, M., Ireland, M., Bearinger, L. H., & Udry, J. R. (1997). Protecting adolescents from harm: Finding for the National Longitudinal Study on Adolescent Health. *Journal of the American Medical Association, 278*, 823–832.

Rubin, R. R., Young-Hyman, D. L., & Peyrot, M. (1989). Parent–child responsibility and conflict in diabetes care [Abstract]. *Diabetes, 38*(Suppl. 2), 28.

U.S. Department of Health, Education, and Welfare. (1976). *Report of the National Commission on Diabetes, Vol. III* (DHEW Publication No. NIH 76-1022). Washington, DC: Author.

Weissberg-Benchell, J., Glasgow, A. M., Tynan, W. D., Wirtz, P., Turek, J., & Ward, J. (1995). Adolescent diabetes management and mismanagement. *Diabetes Care, 18*, 77–82.

White, N. H., Waltman, S. R., Krupin, E., & Santiago, J. V. (1981). Reversal of neuropathic and gastrointestinal complications related to diabetes mellitus in adolescents with improved metabolic control. *Journal of Pediatrics, 99*, 41–45.

Wysocki, T. (1994). The psychological context of SBGM. *Diabetes Spectrum, 7*, 266–270.

Wysocki, T., Taylor, A., Hough, B. S., Linscheid, T. R., Yeates, K. O., & Naglieri, J. A. (1996). Deviation from developmentally appropriate self-care autonomy. *Diabetes Care, 19*, 119–125.

CHAPTER SIXTEEN

Behavioral Family Systems Therapy for Adolescents With Diabetes

Tim Wysocki
Peggy Greco
Nemours Children's Clinic, Jacksonville, FL

Michael A. Harris
Neil H. White
Washington University School of Medicine, St. Louis, MO

To keep Type 1 diabetes under adequate control and avoid long-term complications of the disease, patients and families must implement a complex treatment regimen including multiple daily insulin injections and blood glucose tests, a prescribed meal plan, regular physical exercise, and problem solving based on blood glucose test results. Not surprisingly, the management of diabetes presents quite a challenge during adolescence. Numerous studies have shown that diabetes treatment adherence and diabetic control decline during adolescence (see Johnson, 1995; Wysocki & Greco, 1997, for reviews). Other studies have shown that parent–adolescent communication and conflict resolution skills may be important mediators of the efficacy of family management of diabetes (Bobrow, AvRuskin, & Siller, 1985; Miller-Johnson et al., 1994; Wysocki, 1993). The magnitude of this challenge stimulated our interest in evaluating psychological and behavioral interventions that might help adolescents and their families cope more effectively with diabetes and its treatment. About 4 years ago, in a similar chapter we described the research methods that comprised our randomized controlled trial of behaviorally oriented family therapy for adolescents with Type 1 diabetes (Wysocki, White, Bubb, Harris, & Greco, 1995). In the present chapter, we report the results of our investigation and offer suggestions for future research based on our findings.

There are several cross-sectional and longitudinal studies indicating that family conflict, in particular parent–adolescent conflict, is a key predictor of diabetes outcomes such as psychological adjustment to diabetes, adherence to the diabetes treatment regimen, and diabetic control (Bobrow et al., 1985; Lorenz & Wysocki, 1991; Miller-Johnson et al., 1994; Wysocki, 1993; Wysocki & Greco 1995; Wysocki, White, Bubb, Harris, & Greco, 1995). Therefore, families that could improve their problem-solving and communication skills might be better equipped to detect, prevent, and remedy nonadherence with diabetes treatment and manage family stress that might interfere with diabetes control. We reasoned that an intervention targeting parent–adolescent conflict could yield multiple benefits in terms of improving family communication and problem solving, encouraging better treatment adherence, and optimizing diabetic control.

Robin and Foster's (1989) Behavioral Family Systems Therapy (BFST) is a behaviorally oriented family therapy approach that seems well suited for targeting parent–adolescent conflict. BFST incorporates elements of behavior therapy with elements of systemic family therapy to improve family communication, problem solving, and conflict resolution. Although this approach had been shown effective with several clinical populations (e.g., girls with eating disorders, predelinquent youths, and adolescents with attention deficit hyperactivity disorder [ADHD]), it had never been evaluated with families of adolescents with a chronic disease such as diabetes (Wysocki et al., 1995, 1997, 1999, 2000).

We conducted a careful, randomized controlled trial of Robin and Foster's (1989) BFST with a fairly large sample of conflictual families of adolescents with diabetes. In this chapter, we provide a summary of our investigation and its results and we discuss prospects for further research in this area.

Study Design

Specific aims of the project were to: (a) conduct a randomized, controlled trial of the effects of standard medical care for IDDM either alone or augmented by 10 sessions of participation in either an Educational Support Group (ES) or BFST; (b) compare the interventions' effects on parent–adolescent relationships, adolescent adjustment to IDDM, diabetes treatment adherence, and diabetic control; and (c) assess generalization and maintenance of treatment effects.

Figure 16.1 illustrates the repeated measures, randomized treatments design that was used for this study. Families were enrolled in St. Louis, Missouri, or Jacksonville, Florida. Participants were 119 families of adolescents with IDDM who meet the following criteria: ages 12 to 17 years; IDDM for at least 1 year; living in a family situation; no other chronic diseases or major cognitive impairments; no history of treatment for a major psychiatric

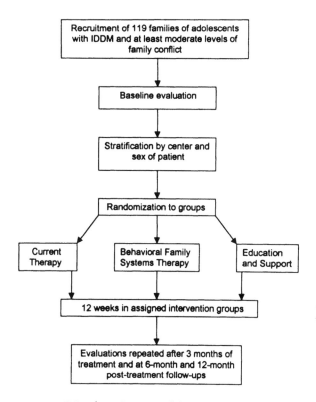

FIG. 16.1.   Diagram of the study design.

disorder in either parent or adolescent within the prior 6 months; and not incarcerated, in foster care, or in residential treatment. We only enrolled families reporting at least moderately elevated scores on each of two screening questionnaires that measure general teen–parent conflict (Prinz, 1977) and IDDM-specific conflict (Rubin, Peyrot, & Young-Hyman, 1989).

After a comprehensive baseline evaluation, described later, families were randomized to 3 months of treatment in one of three groups: Current Therapy, Education and Support, or Behavioral Family Systems Therapy, which differ as described next. Patients who were assigned to the latter two groups reverted to current therapy after completing their respective treatments for this study. Randomization was conducted by the project coordinator at the opposing site using a previously developed randomization sequence to eliminate the possibility of bias in treatment assignments.

Current Therapy (CT).   Patients in this group ($n = 41$) continued in standard medical care for diabetes by a multidisciplinary health care team. No family was seen for psychological services by any of the project staff.

On request, families were assisted in obtaining psychological services elsewhere.

Education and Support (ES).   These 40 families attended 10 sessions of a diabetes support group that was conceptualized as the best alternative therapy and as the most commonly used mental health intervention for the targeted population. The intervention was designed to provide advanced diabetes education, cultivate social support networks among adolescents and parents, and encourage proactive self-management of IDDM through training in responding appropriately to blood glucose test results. Groups consisting of two to five families each experienced all 10 ES sessions together. The ES group was also a control for the extra professional attention received by the BFT families. Group facilitators were master's level counselors. A leading expert on facilitation of support groups trained the two group leaders and ensured consistency in this intervention across the two sites. Content of group sessions was guided by the American Diabetes Association's (1990) *Diabetes support groups for young adults: A facilitator's manual.*

Behavioral Family Systems Therapy (BFST).   The 38 families in this condition received 10 sessions of BFST (Robin & Foster, 1989) consisting of three components: (a) Families were trained in communication and problem solving using conventional behavior therapy techniques of instructions, feedback, modeling, rehearsal, and behavioral homework assignments. (b) Cognitive restructuring was used to address extreme, counterproductive, or irrational beliefs held by family members. Commonly targeted beliefs among parents were that the adolescent's noncompliance indicated malicious or hostile intent toward the parents or was certainly predictive of the adolescent's ruination in the future. Common beliefs held by adolescents were that parents expected perfection of them in diabetes management and that it was worthless to strive for modest improvement. (c) Systemic family therapy techniques were used to target pathogenic family structural problems such as unclear psychological boundaries between parents and adolescents, situations in which one parent and the adolescent teamed up against the other parent, and adolescents' involvement in marital discord.

To emulate actual clinical application of BFST, each family received an individualized treatment plan tailored to the results of the baseline assessment. Results of questionnaires described next and direct observation of family communication were used by the project psychologists to select appropriate treatment targets for each family. The BFST intervention was implemented by two pediatric psychologists (MH and PG), both of whom received extensive training by Arthur Robin, PhD, one of the developers of the approach. Integrity of the intervention was ensured through critiques of audiotaped sessions by either Dr. Robin or three of the authors (TW, PG, MH). Dr. Robin also provided periodic consultation regarding intervention design for selected families.

Assessment Procedures

An evaluation protocol was completed at baseline, at the end of intervention (3 months after baseline), and again 6 and 12 months after the end of intervention. Each of these four evaluations included collection of multiple general and diabetes-specific measures.

Each evaluation began with assessment of diabetes treatment adherence using a 24-hour recall interview method (Johnson, Silverstein, Rosenbloom, Carter, & Cunningham, 1986; Johnson, Tomer, Cunningham, & Henretta, 1990). Parents and adolescents were interviewed separately by telephone three times over 2 weeks. We incorporated into this interview a similar procedure (Montemayor & Hanson, 1985) for the assessment of parent–adolescent conflict. The latter items were appended to the diabetes adherence interviews to measure the frequency, intensity, duration, topic, and manner of resolution of parent–adolescent conflict. After the series of three telephone interviews was complete, families completed the rest of the evaluation at the respective medical centers, at which time several additional general and diabetes-specific measures were collected from adolescents and their parents:

> The Parent Adolescent Relationship Questionnaire (PARQ; Robin, Koepke, & Moye, 1990) consists of parallel parent (314 items) and adolescent (280 items) forms that yield standard scores for three primary factors: Overt Conflict/Skill Deficits, Extreme Beliefs, and Family Structure, with alpha coefficients ranging from .73 to .89.

> The Issues Checklist (IC; Prinz, 1977) obtains parent and adolescent ratings of recent conflict surrounding 44 common family issues. The IC yields scores for number of conflict items endorsed and conflict frequency and intensity. Internal consistency was .74 for adolescents, .72 for mothers, and .79 for fathers.

> The Diabetes Responsibility and Conflict Scale (Rubin et al., 1989) assesses parent–adolescent conflict surrounding 15 diabetes tasks. Internal consistency for this sample was .92 for adolescents, .86 for mothers, and .89 for fathers.

> The Teen Adjustment to Diabetes Scale (TADS; Wysocki, Hough, Ward, & Green, 1992) is a 21-item Likert-type scale with parallel adolescent and parent forms that measures adolescents' behavioral, affective, and

attitudinal adjustment to diabetes. Internal consistency was .92 for adolescents, .86 for mothers, and .89 for fathers.

The Self-Care Inventory (SCI; Greco et al., 1990) is a 14-item self-report measure of diabetes treatment adherence over a 1-month interval. Internal consistency was .76 for adolescents, .81 for mothers, and .82 for fathers.

We tape-recorded two 10-minute family problem-solving discussions regarding one general and one IDDM-related issue that were identified by the family as concerns. The audiotaped interactions were coded using the Interaction Behavior Code (Prinz, 1977) by three or more independent raters. Kappa coefficients ranged from .77 to .84 for the various scores generated by this method. A blood sample was collected from the adolescents for a glycated hemoglobin (GHb) assay to measure recent diabetic control. Each family was paid $100 after each evaluation (divided between adolescents and parents), resulting in $400 during the study. Families assigned to the ES and BFT groups could earn another $100 by attending all 10 intervention sessions scheduled for their groups. These incentives were designed to enhance recruitment and retention of families.

RESULTS

Recruitment, Retention, and Treatment Integrity

Three hundred and sixty families were contacted about study participation at the two sites. Of those, 228 either denied interest in enrolling or were ineligible. Of the 132 eligible families that expressed an interest, 90% (119) enrolled in the study. Characteristics of the adolescents and their parents who were enrolled are shown in Table 16.1. Of the enrolled families, 96% (115) completed the 3-month (immediate posttreatment) evaluation. The follow-up evaluations scheduled 6 and 12 months after the conclusion of treatment were completed by 95% (113) and 91% (108) of the families, respectively. Attrition did not differ significantly among the three groups. Families in the BFST group completed 89% of scheduled therapy sessions, whereas families in the ES group attended 91% of scheduled support group sessions. Psychological services outside of the study were received by five CT families (22 sessions), three ES families (21 sessions), and no BFST families. The study results are unaffected by involvement in such services.

Unfortunately, the randomization procedure failed to yield equivalent groups at baseline on many demographic dimensions. The BFST group included significantly more single-parent families, significantly more

TABLE 16.1
Characteristics of Study Participants at Baseline

Characteristic	CT	BFST	ES
Age (mean yrs ± 1 SD)	14.3 ± 1.4	14.5 ± 1.2	14.1 ± 1.4
Duration of IDDM			
(mean yrs ± 1 SD)	5.2 ± 3.8	5.4 ± 3.8	4.5 ± 3.7
Hollingshead Index Raw Score			
(mean ± 1 SD)	43.9 ± 12.9	41.3 ± 11.8	44.3 ± 11.1
Family size			
(mean # persons ± 1 SD)	4.2 ± 1.5	4.2 ± 1.8	4.2 ± 1.4
Glycated hemoglobin			
(mean % ± 1 SD)	11.8 ± 3.1	11.9 ± 3.3	11.8 ± 2.9
Gender			
Male	20 (49%)	15 (39%)	15 (38%)
Female	21 (51%)	23 (61%)	25 (62%)
Race			
White	32 (78%)	29 (79%)	32 (80%)
African American	9 (22%)	9 (21%)	7 (17%)
Hispanic	0 (0%)	0 (0%)	1 (3%)
Tanner stage			
Prepubertal (Stage I)	0 (0%)	1 (3%)	2 (5%)
Midpubertal (Stages II–IV)	21 (51%)	17 (45%)	23 (58%)
Pubertal (Stage V)	20 (46%)	20 (52%)	15 (37%)
Family composition			
Living with both biological parents	23 (56%)	15 (39%)	27 (68%)
Living with one biological parent	14 (34%)	17 (45%)	5 (12%)
Living with one biological and			
one stepparent	3 (7%)	5 (13%)	7 (17%)
Other	1 (3%)	1 (3%)	1 (3%)

divorced parents, and significantly lower socioeconomic status (SES) than did one or both of the other groups. In addition to these demographic differences, the BFST group also manifested significantly worse status before treatment on several of the measures that served as key outcomes for the study. The Baseline scores of the three groups are shown in Table 16.2, along with an indication of significant group differences. In each instance, the BFST group had significantly worse pretreatment status than one or both of the other groups. Because of these differences, we employed repeated measures analyses of covariance (ANCOVA) as the primary data analysis technique. For each of the analyses that follow, the baseline value of the respective outcome measure was treated as the covariate, whereas the dependent variable in each analysis was a baseline to posttreatment change score in that measure. Because many of our findings are reported elsewhere in greater detail (Wysocki et al., 1997, 1999, 2000), we have presented only certain illustrative findings in this chapter so that greater attention could be given to a discussion of our findings.

TABLE 16.2
Baseline Scores (Mean ± 1 *SD*) for Each Group

Measures	CT (n = 41)	ES (n = 40)	BFST (n = 38)
Parent–Adolescent			
Relationship Questionnaire			
Overt Conflict/Skill Deficits[a]	51.2 ± 3.9	52.8 ± 5.4	53.3 ± 5.7
Extreme beliefs	49.6 ± 3.4	51.2 ± 5.1	51.1 ± 4.4
Family structure	51.7 ± 6.6	52.3 ± 6.4	51.7 ± 5.6
Issues Checklist[a]			
Number of items endorsed	15.4 ± 4.5	16.9 ± 6.0	17.4 ± 6.8
Total frequency of conflict	58.7 ± 42.3	70.8 ± 47.7	94.0 ± 133.1
Total intensity of conflict	31.0 ± 13.1	36.5 ± 13.9	40.8 ± 20.2
Recall Interview Conflict Scores			
Frequency	2.1 ± 1.9	2.1 ± 1.3	2.3 ± 1.3
Intensity	1.7 ± 1.3	1.7 ± 0.7	1.9 ± 1.2
Duration[a]	8.5 ± 9.1	11.0 ± 19.3	10.7 ± 15.5
Interaction Behavior Code			
Adolescent negative communication[a]	3.5 ± 2.1	4.3 ± 2.6	4.8 ± 2.5
Adolescent positive communication[b]	1.0 ± 0.7	0.9 ± 0.6	0.8 ± 0.6
Mother negative communication[a]	3.1 ± 1.4	4.0 ± 2.0	4.5 ± 1.9
Mother positive communication[b]	2.0 ± 0.9	2.0 ± 1.1	2.2 ± 0.9
Father negative communication	3.1 ± 1.2	3.1 ± 1.7	3.3 ± 1.3
Father positive communication[b]	1.8 ± 0.9	1.9 ± 1.1	1.5 ± 0.8
Negative reciprocity	1.7 ± 0.5	1.7 ± 0.6	1.9 ± 0.6
Positive reciprocity[b]	1.8 ± 0.5	1.9 ± 0.6	1.6 ± 0.5
Problem-solving process	2.4 ± 0.5	2.4 ± 0.4	2.4 ± 0.5
Problem resolution	2.6 ± 0.5	2.5 ± 0.5	2.6 ± 0.5
Diabetes Responsibility and Conflict Scale[a]	28.6 ± 8.3	29.5 ± 8.1	32.5 ± 9.4
Teen Adjustment to Diabetes Scale[a]	72.8 ± 10.5	77.0 ± 10.2	78.2 ± 9.7
Recall Interview Adherence Factors			
Insulin	−.11 ± .39	.09 ± .51	.02 ± .49
Testing/eating frequency[a]	−.17 ± .78	−.31 ± .58	.52 ± .75
Diet composition	−.14 ± .37	.10 ± .89	.04 ± .46
Diet amount[a]	−.22 ± .91	−.09 ± .97	.32 ± .87
Exercise	.15 ± .83	.12 ± .78	−.29 ± .58
Self-Care Inventory[a,b]	51.1 ± 6.6	49.4 ± 7.7	46.7 ± 9.3
Glycated Hemoglobin (%)	11.8 ± 3.1	11.8 ± 2.9	11.9 ± 3.3

[a]A significant ANOVA main effect for groups was obtained at Baseline.
[b]Higher scores are favorable; for all others, lower scores are favorable.

Effects on Parent–Adolescent Relationships

BFST was selected as the experimental intervention for this study based on the conviction that reduction of parent–adolescent conflict and improvement in family communication would result in improved diabetes management and diabetic control. Immediate and long-term effects of the three conditions on selected measures of these processes are presented in Table 16.3. These data are presented and discussed in greater detail in Wysocki et al. (1997) and Wysocki et al. (1999, 2000).

Table 16.3 shows that BFST had durable effects on change in family composite scores on the PARQ Overt Conflict and Skill Deficits scale and the PARQ Extreme Beliefs scale, with greater improvement on each scale for the BFST group. Each ANCOVA yielded a significant main effect for groups and post hoc analyses confirmed that BFST yielded more improvement than did either of the other groups at all three follow-up evaluations. No comparable effects were seen on the PARQ Family Structure scale. Table 16.3 shows similar benefits for BFST in terms of its effects on family composite scores on the Diabetes Responsibility and Conflict scale—a measure of diabetes-related conflict between parents and adolescents. In this case, a significant main effect for groups was found on the ANCOVA, and post hoc analyses show that BFST yielded more improvement than either ES or CT at posttreatment and 6-month follow-up; there were no between-group differences at the 12-month follow-up.

Table 16.3 also shows the effects of the three conditions on direct observation measures of family communication scored using the Interaction Behavior Code, as reported in greater detail by Wysocki et al. (in press-b). The negative communication behaviors of mothers and adolescents, but not fathers, decreased significantly more for BFST families than did those in the other two groups. No similar effects were obtained for positive communication. BFST families demonstrated significantly more improvement in negative reciprocity and problem resolution than did families in the other groups. There were no significant between-group effects on positive reciprocity or problem-solving process.

Finally, Wysocki et al. (1997) presented a comparison of family scores on the Treatment Evaluation Questionnaire, on which parents in the BFST and ES rated the social validity of their respective interventions as treatments for parent–adolescent relationship problems. These data indicate that significantly higher scores on this scale were obtained from BFST parents at all three measurement points. Certain other self-report measures of family relations (e.g., 24-Hour Recall Interview Conflict measures, issues checklist) did not reveal comparable treatment effects. In most of these cases, there was excessive variability in family scores.

Although the lack of between-group equivalence before treatment complicated the data analyses, the data presented earlier reveal fairly consistently that BFST did result in consistent and durable improvements in many of the key family interactions that were targeted for treatment. Whether examining self-report questionnaires (PARQ, DRC), directly observed family discussions (IBC), or social validity ratings (TEQ), BFST

TABLE 16.3

Change in Mean Scores Relative to Baseline at Posttreatment and at 6-Month and 12-Month Follow-Ups. Measures Are Those for Which a Significant ANCOVA Between-Group Effect Was Found Favoring the BFST Group

Measure	Posttreatment			6-Month			12-Month		
	CT	ES	BFST	CT	ES	BFST	CT	ES	BFST
Parent–Adolescent Relationship Questionnaire									
Overt conflict and skill deficits	-.02	-1.60	-2.81	-.80	-1.41	-2.33	-.48	-1.10	-2.59
Extreme beliefs	-.03	-1.22	-4.06	-1.21	-.80	-3.87	-.62	-.59	-3.08
Interaction Behavior Code									
Adolescent negative communication	.49	-.56	-.92	.84	-.46	-1.08	.61	-.09	-1.02
Mother negative communication	.38	-.06	-1.21	1.03	-.09	-1.05	.82	-.19	-.93
Negative reciprocity	-.02	.07	-.22	.21	.10	-.11	.18	.11	-.14
Problem resolution	.13	.08	-.20	.10	.11	-.18	.09	.09	-.13
Diabetes Responsibility and Conflict Scale	-2.87	-3.12	-6.79	-2.64	-4.57	-7.03	-3.84	-4.86	-6.01

families consistently showed more improvement than did the other two groups. In no case did either the CT or ES group prove superior to BFST.

Effects on Treatment Adherence and Adjustment to Diabetes

There were no significant between-group effects at the three follow-up evaluations on the five adherence factor scores derived from the Johnson et al. (1986) 24-Hour Recall Interview procedure. For some other measures of behavioral and affective adjustment to diabetes, significant group by sex and group by age interaction effects were found, although these were transient. For example, Fig. 16.2 shows that, on the Self-Care Inventory, more improvement in treatment adherence was found for younger children in the BFST group at posttreatment. This effect dissipated by the 6-month follow-up. Similarly, Fig. 16.3 shows that, in response to BFST, scores on the Teen Adjustment to Diabetes Scale improved for boys and deteriorated for girls. Precisely the opposite effect was found for families in the ES group. Again, this interaction effect had disappeared by the two follow-up evaluations. Therefore, despite the obtained improvements in parent–adolescent relationships, BFST did not yield comparably robust or durable improvements in diabetes treatment adherence.

Effects on Diabetic Control and Health Care Utilization

Not surprisingly, given the absence of between-group effects on treatment adherence, BFST conferred no overall advantage over the other two groups in terms of GHb levels, hospitalization rates, or emergency room use at any

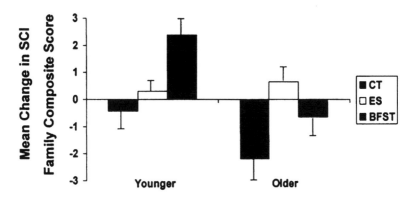

FIG. 16.2. Mean change in family composite scores for younger (< 14.3 years) and older (> 14.3 years) adolescents on the Self-Care Inventory for each group at the posttreatment evaluation.

of the three follow-up measurement points. Further exploration of the data, as shown in Fig. 16.4, reveals that BFST sustained moderate improvement in GHb for boys (0.6% decrease) and younger girls (0.9% decrease) at post-treatment, but not for older girls (2.3% increase). This interaction effect, like that on the Self-Care Inventory, disappeared by the 6-month follow-up. By the 12-month follow-up, all three groups demonstrated statistically signifi-cant deterioration in diabetic control relative to baseline.

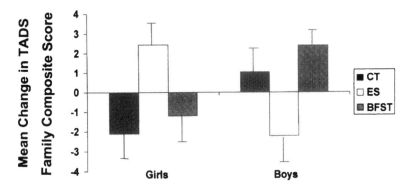

FIG. 16.3.   Mean change in family composite scores for boys and girls on the Teen Adjustment to Diabetes Scale for each group at the posttreatment evaluation.

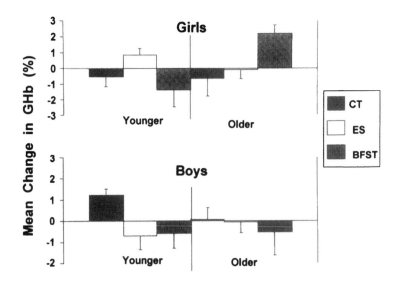

FIG. 16.4.   Mean change in GHb (% ± 1 S.E.M.) for younger and older boys and girls in each group at the posttreatment evaluation.

CONCLUSIONS

Several important practical lessons were learned from this study. First, it is feasible to recruit a sufficiently large sample of clinically appropriate families to participate in such a trial and maintain their participation for over 1 year. Second, careful randomization is not always effective in yielding equivalent groups. This study would have been greatly improved had we stratified our sample based on one or more clinically important outcome measures, thus greatly enhancing the likelihood of pretreatment equivalence of the groups. Finally, we learned that the degree of improvement produced by BFST in parent–adolescent relationships, although valued by families, was not sufficient to yield substantial benefits in diabetes outcomes such as treatment adherence or metabolic control.

This randomized, controlled trial of BFST was conducted in an effort to demonstrate that reduction of parent–adolescent conflict and improvement in family communication could have demonstrable effects on important diabetes outcomes such as treatment adherence and diabetic control. Although not every measure of family interactions was affected equally, there was a consistent pattern of greater improvement in the targeted family processes for BFST families than for those in the CT and ES groups. In most cases, these effects were durable over follow-ups as long as 12 months posttreatment. In no case was ES a more effective treatment than BFST for any measure of parent–adolescent relationships.

Unfortunately, and equally consistently, BFST exerted little or no beneficial effect on diabetes treatment adherence, diabetic control, or health care utilization. What few effects were found on these variables were short-lived and dependent on the adolescent's age or gender. There would appear to be several plausible explanations for this paradox:

⟨ Although several cross-sectional and longitudinal studies point to family conflict as a determinant of treatment adherence and diabetic control, the obtained associations may be so weak as to lack clinical significance. Although parent–adolescent conflict may be a significant impediment to effective management of diabetes by many families experiencing excessive conflict, the presence of family conflict does not guarantee that this is the only barrier to successful adaptation to diabetes. In fact, within our sample, pretreatment correlations between measures of treatment adherence and family conflict were generally nonsignificant. However, this may reflect a restriction of range problem because families recruited for this study had unfavorable status on both dimensions of functioning before treatment. There are, of course, many other factors that could obstruct family adaptation to diabetes that may function independently of family communication and problem solving.

⟨ The magnitude of change in parent–adolescent relationships may have been too small to yield broadly generalized benefits in terms of diabetes outcomes. Positive influence on outcomes as diverse and complex as diabetic control and treatment adherence may require profound changes in family communication and problem solving. The treatment effects reported here may fall short of that criterion.

⟨ BFST may be more appropriate as a preventive intervention for younger adolescents than as a remedial intervention for older adolescents. For example, Delamater et al. (1990) reported more durable and beneficial effects of a diabetes self-management training program for younger, newly diagnosed patients.

⟨ For BFST to affect treatment adherence and diabetic control more convincingly, it may be necessary to identify and target for treatment more explicitly each adolescent's specific barriers to better diabetes outcomes. For example, resolving family conflict over whether an adolescent records blood glucose test results reliably may have less impact on diabetic control than would efforts to promote the adolescent's use of those test results effectively to correct unwanted blood glucose fluctuations. Diary procedures such as those described by Quittner and Opipari (1994) may be one method to identify valid treatment targets.

It remains for future research to determine which, if any, of these conjectures is accurate.

ACKNOWLEDGMENT

Preparation of this chapter was supported in part by grant #RO1-DK43802 from the National Institutes of Health (National Institutes of Diabetes, Digestive, and Kidney Disease) of the U.S. Public Health Service. Additional support was provided by the Pediatric and General Clinical Research Centers (Grants #RR06021 and RR00036) of Washington University in St. Louis. We wish to thank Drs. Diana Guthrie and Arthur L. Robin for their assistance as consultants to this project.

REFERENCES

American Diabetes Association. (1990). *Diabetes support groups for young adults: A facilitator's manual*. Alexandria, VA: Author.

Bobrow, E. S., AvRuskin, T. W., & Siller, J. (1985). Mother–daughter interactions and adherence to IDDM regimens. *Diabetes Care, 8*, 146–151.

Delamater, A. M., Bubb, J., Davis, S. G., Smith, J. A., Schmidt, L., & White, N. H. (1990). Randomized, prospective study of self management training with newly diagnosed diabetic children. *Diabetes Care, 13*, 492–498.

Greco, P., La Greca, A. M., Auslander, W. F., Spetter, D., Skyler, J. S., Fisher, E., & Santiago, J. V. (1990). Assessing adherence in IDDM: A comparison of two methods. *Diabetes, Suppl. #2*, 108A (Abstract).

Johnson, S. B. (1995). Managing insulin-dependent diabetes mellitus in adolescence: A developmental perspective. In J. L. Wallander & L. J. Siegel (Eds.), *Advances in pediatric psychology: Adolescent health problems. Behavioral perspectives* (pp. 265–288). New York: Guilford.

Johnson, S. B., Silverstein, J., Rosenbloom, A., Carter, R., & Cunningham, W. (1986). Assessing daily management in childhood diabetes. *Health Psychology, 5*, 545–564.

Johnson, S. B., Tomer, A., Cunningham, W. R., & Henretta, J. C. (1990). Adherence in childhood diabetes: Results of a confirmatory factor analysis. *Health Psychology, 9*, 493–501.

Lorenz, R. A., & Wysocki, T. (1991). The family and childhood diabetes. *Diabetes Spectrum, 4*, 261–292.

Miller-Johnson, S., Emery, R. E., Marvin, R. S., Clarke, W. L., Lovinger, R., & Martin, M. (1994). Parent–child relationships and the management of insulin-dependent diabetes mellitus. *Journal of Consulting and Clinical Psychology, 62*, 603–610.

Montemayor, R., & Hanson, E. (1985). A naturalistic view of conflict between adolescents and their parents and siblings. *Journal of Early Adolescence, 5*, 23–30.

Prinz, R. J. (1977). *The assessment of parent–adolescent relations: Discriminating distressed and non-distressed dyads*. Unpublished doctoral dissertation, State University of New York at Stony Brook.

Quittner, A. M., & Opipari, L. C. (1994). Differential treatment of siblings: Interview and diary analyses comparing two family contexts. *Child Development, 65*, 800–814.

Robin, A. L., & Foster, S. L. (1989). *Negotiating parent–adolescent conflict: A behavioral-family systems approach*. New York: Guilford.

Robin, A. L., Koepke, T., & Moye, A. (1990). Multidimensional assessment of parent–adolescent relations. *Psychological Assessment, 10*, 451–459.

Rubin, R. R., Peyrot, M., & Young-Hyman, D. L. (1989). Parent–child conflict and responsibility for diabetes management. *Diabetes, 38*, 7A (Abstract).

Wysocki, T. (1993). Associations among teen–parent relationships, metabolic control and adjustment to diabetes in adolescents. *Journal of Pediatric Psychology, 18*, 443–454.

Wysocki, T., & Greco, P. (1997). Self-management of childhood diabetes in family context. In D. S. Gochman (Ed.), *Handbook of health behavior research: Volume II. Practitioner determinants* (pp. 169–187). New York: Plenum.

Wysocki, T., Greco, P., Harris, M. A., Harvey, L. M., McDonell, K., Elder-Danda, C. L., Bubb, J., & White, N. H. (1997). Social validity of support group and behavior therapy interventions for families of adolescents with insulin-dependent diabetes mellitus. *Journal of Pediatric Psychology, 22*(4), 443–457.

Wysocki, T., Harris, M. A., Greco, P., Bubb, J., Elder-Danda, C. E., Harvey, L. M., McDonell, K., Taylor, A., & White, N. H. (2000). Randomized, controlled trial of behavior therapy for families of adolescents with insulin-dependent diabetes mellitus. *Journal of Pediatric Psychology, 25*(1), 23–33.

Wysocki, T., Hough, B. S., Ward, K. M., & Green, L. B. (1992). Diabetes mellitus in the transition to adulthood: Adjustment, self-care and health status. *Journal of Developmental and Behavioral Pediatrics, 13*(3), 194–201.

Wysocki, T., Miller, K. M., Greco, P., Harris, M. A., Harvey, L. M., Elder-Danda, C. E., Taylor, A., McDonell, K., & White, N. H. (1999). Behavior therapy for families of adolescents with diabetes: Effects on directly observed family interactions. *Behavior Therapy, 30*, 507–525.

Wysocki, T., White, N. H., Bubb, J., Harris, M. A., & Greco, P. (1995). Family adaptation to diabetes: A model for intervention research. In J. L. Wallander & L. J. Siegel (Eds.), *Advances in pediatric psychology* (Vol. 2, pp. 262–304). New York: Guilford.

CHAPTER SEVENTEEN

Adherence to Medical Treatments in Adolescents With Cystic Fibrosis: The Development and Evaluation of Family-Based Interventions

Alexandra L. Quittner
University of Florida, Gainesville, FL

Dennis Drotar
Carolyn Ievers-Landis
Nancy Slocum
Rainbow Babies and Children's Hospital, Cleveland, OH

Dawn Seidner
Indiana University, Bloomington, IN

Jessica Jacobsen
Riley Hospital for Children, Indianapolis, IN

Cystic fibrosis (CF) is the most common, terminal genetic disease of White populations, and affects approximately 1 in 2,500 live births (Fitzsimmons, 1993). The genetic defect, discovered in 1989 (Riordan et al., 1989), leads to the production of thick, sticky mucus in several organs—most notably the lungs and the pancreas. The buildup of mucus in the lungs can cause infection and damage, and blockage of the pancreas leads to problems with digestion and absorption of food. Major advances in the diagnosis and treatment of the disease have been made over the past two decades, significantly increasing life expectancy to a median age of 32. However, reduction in the mortality of CF patients has been based on arduous, time-consuming treatment regimens prescribed two to four times a day depending on illness severity. Treatments typically involve aerosolized medications and chest physical therapy (CPT) or some other form of airway clearance, increased calorie intake, and replacement enzymes with each meal and snack (Stark, Jelalian, & Miller, 1995). Thus, CF imposes extensive treatment demands on patients and their families (Drotar & Ievers, 1994; Quittner, Tolbert, Regoli, Orenstein, Hollingsworth, & Eigen, 1996) that can affect every aspect of daily life, including recreation time, family interactions, and peer relationships (Quittner & DiGirolamo, 1998).

EXTENT OF ADHERENCE PROBLEMS

Although adherence problems are widely recognized as a significant problem for patients, families, and members of the health care team, they have received surprisingly little empirical attention (Stark et al., 1995). Earlier, anecdotal research suggested that children with CF were more likely to adhere to their treatments than children with other chronic conditions. However, more recent studies indicate that compliance rates for this population are similar to those reported for other populations and vary with the complexity of the demands. Adherence to medications tends to be highest (Gudas, Koocher, & Wypji, 1991; Passero, Remor, & Solomon, 1981), whereas adherence to those aspects of the treatment regimen regarded as most critical to health (CPT, diet) are lowest (DiGirolamo, Quittner, Ackerman, & Stevens, 1997; Stark et al., 1995), especially among adolescents (Gudas et al., 1991; Schultz & Moser, 1992). For example, Czajkowski and Koocher (1986) studied adherence behaviors in a controlled hospital setting and found that 35% of the hospitalized teens were noncompliant with CPT. The extent of noncompliance is likely to be much higher in ambulatory patients, who are at home and must fit the treatment regimen into their daily activities.

In a recent study of 45 adolescents with CF at two major CF Centers (Indianapolis and Pittsburgh), adherence to aerosol treatment was significantly higher than adherence to CPT (DiGirolamo et al., 1997). According to parent reports, the majority of adolescents (42%) were doing their aerosol treatments twice a day. When frequency of aerosol treatment was compared to what the physician had prescribed, 71% of teens were categorized as *adherent* and 39% were *nonadherent* (see Fig. 17.1). For CPT, 34% of adolescents were doing CPT twice a day; when this was compared to physician recommendation, fewer than 50% of adolescents were categorized as *adherent* (see Fig. 17.2).

Increasing adherence to CF treatment is important for several reasons. First, there is evidence that aerosol treatments and airway clearance techniques are effective in delaying the progression of lung damage, which is the primary contributor to mortality (Desmond, Schwenk, Thomas, Beaudry, & Coates, 1983; Patterson, Budd, Goetz, & Warwick, 1993; Warwick & Hansen, 1991). Second, although initial human trials of gene therapy have begun and may hold significant promise for halting the progression of lung disease in patients with CF, lung damage cannot be reversed

A

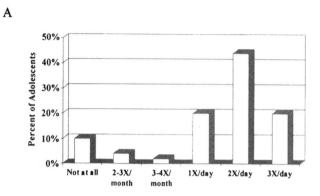

B

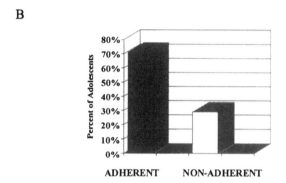

FIG. 17.1. (A) Frequency of aerosol treatment; (B) parent-reported aerosol adherence.

once it has occurred. Thus, effective management of the disease is critical for those who may eventually benefit from gene therapy. Third, adherence problems are a major source of conflict for families of patients with CF, particularly adolescents, and reducing this source of stress would be beneficial (DiGirolamo et al., 1997; Patterson et al., 1993).

The authors of this chapter recently received funding from the National Institutes of Health to develop and evaluate a randomized, controlled trial of two family-based interventions designed to increase adherence to treatment in adolescents with CF. The major objectives of this chapter are to review the methodological, assessment, and treatment issues that have shaped our current intervention trial. We describe the design of the treatment trial, the challenges we have encountered in developing and implementing these intervention programs, and the clinical and scientific implications of this work for the broader field of treatment adherence.

A

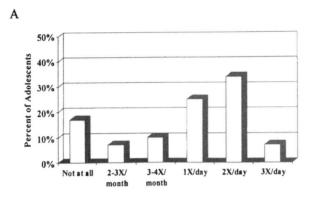

B

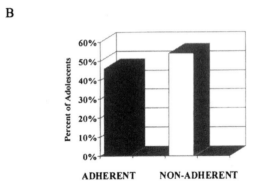

FIG. 17.2.   (A) Frequency of chest physical therapy treatment; (B) parent-reported chest physical therapy adherence.

FACTORS THAT INFLUENCE ADHERENCE

As in other chronic health conditions, the variables that influence adherence to treatment for adolescents with CF are multidimensional, including developmental, educational, and familial factors (Karoly, 1993; La Greca & Schuman, 1995). In terms of developmental factors, there is consistent evidence that age is strongly associated with adherence behaviors. A recent study of 50 children and teens with CF (ages 9–17 years) indicated that age was inversely related to adherence (Ricker, Delamater, & Hsu, 1998), with older children less likely to adhere to treatment regimens than younger ones. In a hierarchical regression analysis, age accounted for a greater proportion of the variance than family functioning and perceived competence. In a series of studies comparing the problematic situations encountered by school-age children and adolescents with CF, adherence problems increased around age 10 and plateaued at age 16 (DiGirolamo et al., 1997; Quittner et al., 1996). This is consistent with data indicating that adolescents' desire for greater independence may conflict with the demands of their medical condition (Czajkowski & Koocher, 1986; Johnson, Freund, Silverstein, Hansen, & Malone, 1990). One factor that may be critical to maintaining good adherence during this developmental period is involvement and monitoring by parents (Drotar & Ievers, 1994).

The relationship between knowledge of CF and adherence may be less straightforward. General or global knowledge about CF (e.g., etiology, effects on organ systems) does not appear to be strongly related to better management of the disease (Nolan, Desmond, & Herlich, 1986; Parcel et al., 1994). However, information that is directly related to the prescribed regimen or corrects misconceptions about the reasons for the regimen or how it should be performed have been associated with better adherence (Henley & Hill, 1990; Ievers et al., in press). Ievers and colleagues (1999) recently found strong relationships between an accurate understanding of a physician's recommendations for treatment and rates of adherence in a sample of school-age children with CF. Between 12% and 33% of mothers in this study did not have correct information about the types of treatment that had been prescribed (see Ievers-Landis & Drotar, chap. 11, this volume).

Finally, family variables such as communication, conflict, and levels of stress have also been found to be associated with adherence patterns (Patterson et al., 1993; Quittner et al., 1996). Patterson, McCubbin, and Warwick (1990) found some of the strongest evidence in a series of prospective studies in which they assessed the predictive relationship among family stress (including conflict), parental availability, positive family coping, and two health outcomes—pulmonary functioning and nutritional status. At the 3- and 15-month follow-ups, lower family stress, parental availability, and integrative family coping were linked to positive changes in pulmonary functioning and weight gain. Patterson et al. (1993) extended these findings to document interrelationships between family functioning and pulmonary measures over a 10-year period. Their findings indicate that balanced family coping (use of several positive strategies) and decreased family stress are related to 10-year trends in pulmonary functioning. Although these studies have documented that family processes affect health, the specific mechanisms through which dimensions of family interactions affect adolescents with CF has not been clearly established. The Patterson et al. data (1993) suggest that compliance with CF treatment was a likely mediator of these effects, but significant limitations in their assessment of compliance made it difficult to establish a causal link. In the current randomized intervention trial, we can more rigorously test the pathways among family functioning, adherence, and long-term health outcomes.

INTERVENTION STUDIES

Given the scope of adherence problems in adolescents with CF and their critical relationship to the maintenance of health, it is surprising that so few intervention studies aimed at improving adherence have been developed and evaluated. A search of literature indicates that fewer than a handful of published studies exist (Bauman, Drotar, Leventhal, Perrin, & Pless, 1997; Bauman et al., in press; Stark, Miller, Plienis, & Drabman, 1987). Several reasons for this lack of intervention research may be cited. First, over the past two decades, the majority of studies in the CF area have been descriptive in nature, focusing on comparing general indexes of adjustment in CF and non-CF samples (Quittner & DiGirolamo, 1998). Although these studies have demonstrated that chronic illness is a major risk factor for child and family adjustment, the global level at which these constructs have been measured (e.g., self-esteem, depression) have provided little information about the specific tasks and demands that families face (Quittner, 1999). This information is critical for the development of effective family-based interventions. Recent efforts to identify the key problematic situations encountered by adolescents and their parents have proved useful in targeting the specific barriers to adherence in our intervention study (DiGirolamo et al., 1997; Quittner et al., 1996).

A second reason for the lack of intervention research with this population is the relative paucity of data suggesting that adherence behaviors can be increased and that better adherence leads to improvements in health outcomes. Although some data demonstrate that daily aerosol treatments, airway clearance, and improved calorie intake are associated with improved physical functioning (Patterson et al., 1993; Stark et al., 1998; Warwick & Hansen, 1991), there is currently no large-scale randomized trial similar to the DCCT trial for diabetes in the CF population (Diabetes Complications and Control Trial Research Group, 1993). A longitudinal study comparing three forms of airway clearance in a national sample is about to begin, but the data will not be available for several years. In addition, less attention has been focused on the daily management of CF because the long-term outlook for children with this disease, up to now, has been fairly bleak. It has only been in the last decade that the median survival age has exceeded 30. This shift—from a primarily pediatric disease to one that extends into adulthood—has heightened awareness of the role that treatment adherence plays in preserving physical functioning and quality of life. Thus, interventions targeting adherence behaviors may be greeted with greater enthusiasm now by the health care team and by patients and family members.

Finally, a major stumbling block in developing a methodologically sound adherence trial is the problem of objectively measuring adherence behaviors. To determine whether an intervention has had the desired effect, it is critical to establish that the dependent variable is measured reliably. There is an extensive literature detailing the multitude of problems associated with the measurement of adherence behaviors, which include, but are not limited to, problems with the validity of patient and physician reports (Johnson, 1993; La Greca & Schuman, 1995). However, new technologies hold considerable promise for providing objective indicators of compliance with several aspects of the treatment regimen (e.g., metered-dose inhalers, aerosol machines), which can be combined with different methods of eliciting self-report. Given the central importance of adherence behaviors in maintaining adolescent health and positive family functioning, we developed a controlled trial comparing two family-based interventions for increasing adherence in adolescents with CF.

FAMILY INTERVENTIONS TO INCREASE ADHERENCE TO MEDICAL TREATMENT

Goals of the Study

This study is the first controlled evaluation of interventions aimed at increasing adherence to treatment in adolescents with CF. The major goal of the study is to improve adherence to the multiple components of the CF treatment regimen and thereby improve long-term health outcomes and quality of life. The specific objectives of the study are as follows:

1. To conduct a randomized, controlled trial comparing the effects of standard medical care (SC) to two structured interventions: Family Learning Program (FLP) and Behavioral Family Systems Therapy (BFST);

2. To compare the effects of these three conditions on four major outcomes: (a) adherence behaviors (enzyme use, inhaled medications, and airway clearance); (b) family conflict, communication, and coping skills; (c) long-term health outcomes (health status, morbidity, and health-related quality of life); and (d) cost-effectiveness (cost of the interventions in relation to cost savings for medical care);

3. To evaluate mechanisms that may mediate the effectiveness of the two family interventions, such as therapeutic alliance, increased knowledge, and treatment satisfaction; and

4. To examine maintenance of treatment effects over an 18-month period.

Design and Recruitment

The design of the study is a multisite, randomized controlled trial with repeated measurements over a 2-year period. Both of the structured interventions are equivalent in terms of contact time with the therapist. Families are currently being enrolled at two major CF Centers—Riley Hospital for Children in Indianapolis and Rainbow Babies and Children's Hospital in Cleveland. Because the PI recently moved to the University of Florida, additional families will be recruited from the CF Center there (see Fig. 17.3).

Issues in Ensuing Equivalence of Treatment Groups.   Our plan is to enroll 120 families of adolescents with CF who meet the following criteria: (a) ages 10.5 to 16.5 years; (b) diagnosed a minimum of 1 year; (c) illness severity, as measured by FEV_1, greater than 35% predicted; (d) no other chronic disease (other than CF-related diabetes); and (e) no history of psychiatric treatment within the past year. Younger adolescents were targeted for this intervention trial because of prior data that indicate that problems with adherence emerge around age 10 and plateau at about age 16. Family conflict related to adherence follows a similar developmental pattern based on the reports of both parents and teens (DiGirolamo et al., 1997; Quittner & DiGirolamo, 1998).

One of the most important methodological issues to consider when designing a controlled trial is how to ensure equivalence of the treatment groups. If the groups differ on some important demographic variable, such as socioeconomic status (SES) or family composition, or on one of the primary outcomes, it becomes difficult to establish that it was the treatment condition alone that was responsible for the observed effect (Hsu, 1998; Stout, Wirtz, Carbonari, & Del Boca, 1994). Although random assignment to conditions is one way to prevent a systematic bias from appearing in one of the treatment arms, this strategy is most effective when the sample size is fairly large. In many behavioral interventions, we rarely have more than 100 to 200 participants, thus randomization may not be enough to ensure equivalence of the groups (Wysocki et al., 2000). It may be critical to identify, a priori, key demographic and dependent variables that are likely to have an impact on the hypothesized outcomes and to stratify the sample on these variables prior to random assignment to conditions. Given prior findings suggesting that family demographic characteristics (e.g., single vs. two-parent families, teen's age), extent of family conflict, and severity of illness may influence adherence behaviors (Geiss, Hobbs, Hammersley-Maercklein, & Kramer, 1992; La Greca & Schuman, 1995; Ricker et al., 1998), we screened and stratified our families on these variables prior to randomization.

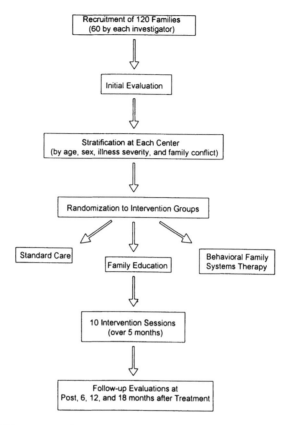

FIG. 17.3.   Design of the multisite adherence trial for adolescents with CF.

Measurement of Outcome Variables

After random assignment to one of the three arms of the clinical trial (SC, FLP, or BFST), families complete a comprehensive evaluation. The most important outcome for this intervention trial is improved treatment adherence. Given the plethora of problems associated with measuring adherence behaviors, such as the difficulty of obtaining accurate reports from parents and teens and the technical limitations of monitoring devices, we have used a multiple measures approach, gathering data on adherence behaviors using several sources and methods. In addition, because several studies have established a strong relationship between adherence and family functioning, we have also measured family variables such as conflict, communication, and coping skills using several different methods. Finally, we are evaluating the impact of these interventions on several long-term health outcomes, including pulmonary functioning, days admitted to hospital, days absent from school, and perceived quality of life. These are the traditional health indicators used in CF research and are not described in detail here. However, a disease-specific measure of quality of life for patients with CF has just been developed and information on this new measure is provided later.

Measures of Treatment Adherence

Electronic Monitors. One challenge we faced in designing this study was to identify measures of adherence that would be more objective than self-report. New microchip technologies have the potential to provide objective data on the performance of certain treatment behaviors, such as the use of nebulized medications and the rhythmic movements of CPT. Our goals are to demonstrate that teens can increase their adherence to daily medical regimens, and identify which family intervention is more effective in modifying these behaviors. Given the complex nature of the CF treatment regimen, which includes inhaled medication (e.g., bronchodilators, antibiotics, recombinant DNA), several methods of clearing mucus (e.g., CPT, flutter device, mechanical oscillation of the chest wall), and enzyme medications with meals and snacks, it was difficult to identify monitoring devices for all of these aspects of the treatment regimen. However, a number of new commercially available products can be used for this purpose; in other cases, we have made creative applications.

To assess adherence to inhaled medications, we provide teens with the Doser-CT (Medalogic Corporation), which attaches to a metered-dose inhaler (MDI) and records the date and frequency of use of the MDI over a 24-hour period. This information is stored in the device for up to 45 days and can then be read manually and entered into a data entry file (see Fig. 17.4). For nebulized medications (e.g., rhDNase, inhaled Tobramycin), we developed a partnership with American Biosystems (which manufactures the ThAIRapy vest) to develop a monitor that can be plugged into the nebulizer machine to record time, date, and duration of the electrical current generated when the nebulizer machine is turned on (see Fig. 17.5).

Measuring adherence to some form of airway clearance was difficult because adolescents now have several options for clearing mucus from their lungs: (a) traditional manual CPT, which requires assistance from parents; (b) a flutter device into which the teen blows for 12 to 15 minutes; or (c) the ThAIRapy vest, which is worn by the teen and vigorously oscillates the chest wall. For adolescents using manual percussion, we provided parents with digital wrist actigraphs, which are the size of small watches and generate an internal signal each time they are moved above a preset thresh-

Teen's Use of Inhaler

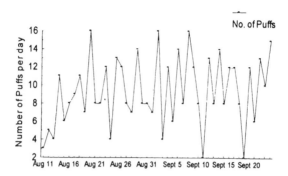

FIG. 17.4.   Daily use of metered-dose inhaler.

Teen's Aerosolized Medication Use

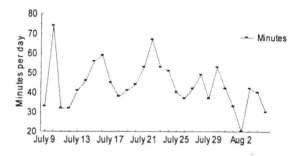

FIG. 17.5.   Duration (in minutes) of aerosolized medications.

old. Parents wear the wrist actigraphs while they perform CPT and the device records wrist movements in .5-second intervals. These data are then downloaded into a computer file for analysis. We were not able to find any device that measures compliance with the flutter valve and could not interest medical technology companies in developing one. The ThAIRapy vest currently comes with an updated monitoring device that records the date, time, and duration of its activation. Engineers have redesigned this monitoring device so that it is activated only when the vest is exerting pressure on a vibrating chest wall and not when it is sitting on a chair in the corner turned on. Data can be stored on this microchip for over 1 year.

Although regular use of enzyme medication is a critical part of CF care, and there is substantial evidence to suggest that compliance is a major problem (Henley & Hill, 1990; Quittner et al., 1996), we could not find any appropriate monitoring devices. Medication caps, which are commonly used to measure compliance in drug trials, are not useful for enzyme medications because the size of the prescription bottle is quite large and teens often transfer their daily meal and snack doses into smaller containers.

Self-Report. In addition to the monitoring data, we also collect self-report data on adherence from the adolescent and both parents. The Treatment Adherence Questionnaire (TAQ–CF; Quittner et al., 1996) is a 10-item self-report measure that focuses on three components of CF treatment: aerosolized medications, CPT, and enzyme use. For each component of the treatment regimen, teens and parents report the frequency and duration of that aspect of treatment and report their physician's most recent treatment recommendation. In a prior study, agreement between parents and teens on the TAQ–CF was moderate to high (r = .55 for aerosol medications, r = .78 for CPT), and test–retest reliabilities over 1 year ranged from .62 to .73 for adolescent reports and .76 to .88 for parent reports (DiGirolamo et al., 1997; Quittner et al., 1996). More recently, Ievers and colleagues (1999) administered the TAQ–CF to school-age children and their mothers and found somewhat higher levels of agreement (r = .69 for aerosol frequency, r = .88 for airway clearance). For this study, we have substantially revised the TAQ–CF. First, because the treatment regimen for CF has been expanded to include new drugs and methods of airway clearance, we added new items to measure compliance with these treatments. Second, we have added items that assess compliance with oral antibiotics and vitamins and efforts to boost calories. The revised TAQ–CF now contains 57 items.

One of the major challenges we have faced in this study is determining precisely what treatments have been prescribed for an individual teen. Given the variability in treatment recommendations both between CF centers and among physicians within the same center, it has been difficult to establish what the adolescent is supposed to be adhering to. As noted earlier, often the parents and patients are not clear about the specifics of the daily regimen (Ievers et al., in press). Because it is essential to know what the prescribed treatment regimen is to measure the degree of adherence to it, we developed a brief form for physicians to complete during an adolescent's clinic visit that documents what treatment recommendations have been made. The Prescribed Treatment Form (PTF) is a six-item checklist that includes the most commonly prescribed medications and components of treatment, along with typical dosages. The physician or nurse can simply circle what is currently recommended.

Daily Phone Diary. We are also using the Daily Phone Diary (DPD; Quittner & Espelage, 1999; Quittner & Opipari, 1994) to assess adherence to medical treatments. The DPD is a cued recall procedure that tracks activities and interactions over the previous 24 hours. For all activities lasting 5 minutes or longer, respondents report the type of activity, its duration, who was present, and a rating of their mood. This measure has been used in a variety of studies to assess activity patterns, compliance with medical regimens, and role strain among caregivers (Quittner & Opipari, 1994; Quittner et al., 1998). The DPD has yielded reliable stability coefficients over a 3-week period with CF populations (rs = .61–.71, $p <$ .01) and high levels of interrater agreement (over 90%) for two independent coders (Quittner & DiGirolamo, 1998).

One major advantage of the DPD procedure is the unobtrusive nature of the assessment process. In tracking adolescents and parents through their activities and interactions during the day, from awakening in the morning until going to bed at night, the behaviors that are being targeted in the evaluation are less obvious. We are able to assess both what they did in terms of their treatment regimen and how much time they spent doing it. Figure 17.6 shows the daily activity patterns of two randomly selected teens in our study—one who is spending a large percentage of time on treatment activities (i.e., 13%) and one who is not (i.e., 2%). An examination of the Treatment Adherence Questionnaire completed by both of these teens and their parents revealed that Adolescent 1 is complying with his prescribed regimen (i.e., airway clearance three times a day for 15 minutes, inhaled medications three times a day for 10 minutes, and inhaled Tobramycin three times a day for 15 minutes = 120 minutes of treatment per day), but that Adolescent 2 is not (i.e., airway clearance two times a day for 20 minutes a day and inhaled medications two times a day for 15 minutes = 70 minutes of treatment per day).

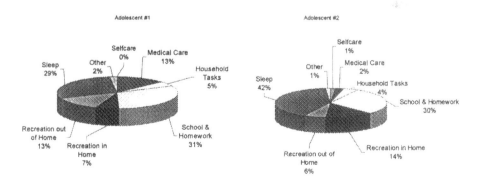

FIG. 17.6. Time spent doing medical treatment as assessed by the Daily Phone Diary.

Measures of Family Conflict, Communication, and Coping Skills

Self-Report. Two measures of family conflict and communication are completed by adolescents and parents. The Conflict Behavior Questionnaire (Robin & Foster, 1989) is used to screen families for extent of conflict prior to random assignment. It is a 20-item scale to which respondents rate each statement as *true* or *false* in terms of conflictual behaviors that have occurred over the past 2 weeks. The Parent–Adolescent Relationship Questionnaire (PARQ; Robin, Koepke, & Moye, 1990) is also completed by the teen and his or her parents. This measure consists of 250 to 300 true–false items that cluster into 16 scales. For the purposes of this study, we have included items from the Communication, Problem-Solving, Beliefs, and School Conflict scales. We have also developed a CF-specific scale that measures conflict related to adherence.

Audiotaped Role-Play Vignettes. To assess the frequency and difficulty of common problematic situations encountered by adolescents with CF and their parents, and the competence of coping strategies used in those situations, we have families complete the Role-Play Inventory of Situations and Coping Strategies (RISCS; DiGirolamo et al., 1997; Quittner et al., 1996; Quittner & DiGirolamo, 1998). Based on a sequential series of steps aimed at identifying the most salient problems for a specific population, two versions of the RISCS measure have been developed: one for adolescents with CF ages 12 to 18 and one for parents of adolescents with CF. The adolescent version consists of 25 vignettes that assess the frequency and difficulty of problems in seven domains, including treatment adherence, parent–teen conflicts, and school issues. Teens listen to each audiotaped situation, produce a coping strategy they would use to deal with that situation, and then rate their perception of the frequency and difficulty of this problem. A rater's manual has been developed using expert judges to score the effectiveness of the coping strategies that are recorded. The parent version consists of 28 vignettes and follows a similar set of procedures.

Videotaped Family Discussions. Level of family conflict and problems with communication are assessed in two 10-minute family discussions that are videotaped and coded using a modified version of the Interaction Behavior Code (IBC; Robin & Foster, 1989). Topics for the family discussion are chosen from a list of issues that often cause conflict between parents and teens, with the content representing both CF (doing aerosol treatment on time) and non-CF (following a curfew) problems. These videotaped family discussions are coded by independent raters in terms of 36 categories of positive and negative interactions (e.g., yelling, making positive suggestions) that yield summary scores for each family member's positive and negative communication behaviors, positive and negative reciprocity, and problem-solving process and resolution. Several investigations using the IBC have reported consistently high interrater agreement ranging from .82 to .97 (Foster et al., 1983; Wysocki et al., 1999). We are in the process of expanding the coding system to make it more sensitive and comprehensive.

Measures of Health-Related Quality of Life

The Cystic Fibrosis Questionnaire (CFQ; Henry, Aussage, Grosskopf, & Launois, 1996; Henry et al., 1998; Quittner, Sweeny, Watrous, Munzenberger, & Henry, 1998; Quittner et al., 1999). Over the past two decades, considerable progress has been made in defining and measuring health-related quality of life (Drotar, 1998; Schipper, Clinch, & Olweny, 1996). In addition, there is growing recognition that for chronic health conditions, in particular, measures of quality of life (QOL) provide unique information about the impact of an illness and the effectiveness of various treatments (both pharmacological and behavioral). Until recently, researchers in the CF area have relied on generic measures of QOL, which ask general questions about symptoms and daily functioning that can be completed by patients with a variety of chronic conditions (Orenstein, Nixon, Ross, & Kaplan, 1989). The major disadvantage of these generic measures is their lack of sensitivity to the specific challenges posed by CF (Czyzewski & Bartholomew, 1998; Czyzewski, Mariotto, Bartholomew, LeCompte, & Sockrider, 1994), which make it more difficult to quantify changes in QOL that result from new treatments or as part of the natural progression of the disease (Quittner, 1998). In addition, few measures of health-related QOL have been designed specifically for children and adolescents, which has limited their validity and clinical utility. The need for a disease-specific measure of QOL was recognized more than a decade ago (Eigen, Clark, & Wolley, 1987), but one has become available only recently.

The Cystic Fibrosis Questionnaire (CFQ; Henry et al., 1996; Quittner et al., 1999) is a disease-specific QOL measure for CF. Originally developed in France, there are three versions of the measure—one for children with CF ages 6 to 13, one for parents of children with CF ages 6 to 13, and one for adolescents and young adults with CF ages 14 and older. Psychometric studies of the CFQ in France have indicated that it has strong internal consistency, good test–retest reliability over a 10-day period and converges significantly with the Nottingham Health Profile. As part of the linguistic validation of the instrument in the United States, we have completed a forward and backward translation of the measure and two phases of cognitive testing with 60 participants to determine whether the items are clear, comprehensible, and relevant to the target populations (Quittner et al., 1999). We are now beginning a national psychometric evaluation of the measure at 20 CF Centers in the United States.

Intervention Programs

After completing the comprehensive evaluation outlined earlier, adolescents and their parents are randomly assigned to one of three groups: (a) Standard Care, (b) Family Learning Program (FLP), or (c) Behavioral Family Systems Therapy (BFST). Those assigned to SC attend their regular clinic visits in addition to monitoring their pulmonary functioning on a daily basis using the AirWatch monitor. Families assigned to either the FLP or BFST program complete a 10-session manualized intervention that occurs over 5 months. The first half of the intervention program is conducted with the family on a weekly basis. At Session 5, sessions are scheduled every 2 to 3 weeks to give the family extra time to practice new skills and complete the homework assignments. A booster session is scheduled 3 months after completion of the tenth session. Families in both intervention programs are seen as a unit (mother, father, teen) for 60 to 90 minutes and have the same amount of contact time with the therapist.

Family Learning Program (FLP).   This is a psychoeducational program that was initially based on the booklets developed by Bartholomew and colleagues for the Family Education Program (Bartholomew et al., 1997). A nurse with some knowledge of CF as well as teaching experience was chosen at each site to conduct the sessions. Each of the 10 sessions is structured to: (a) provide specific information about CF that is likely to promote adherence to treatment, (b) include an activity that engages the teen and parents in the learning experience, and (c) end with a homework assignment that reinforces the content of the current session or focuses the teen on a behavior that is relevant for the next session. For example, several sessions are devoted to how CF affects the lungs and why clearing the lungs of mucus is so important. Activities include experimenting with different thicknesses of mucus (e.g., corn syrup, water), reading and interpreting a pulmonary function test, and completing a brief exercise tolerance test. Homework assignments focus on having the teen monitor what he or she currently does for airway clearance and how often (keeping a treatment log) and asking parents to complete a simulated regimen for 3 days to increase their empathy and understanding (see Table 17.1 for a list of the sessions). We have tried to make the sessions fun, engaging, and interactive as opposed to didactic and, from a teen's perspective, boring.

Behavioral Family Systems Therapy (BFST).   Originally developed by Robin and Foster (1989), BFST integrates principles from both behavioral and family systems theory. Based on this model and consultation from Dr. Rubin, we tailored the intervention to specific challenges faced by families in managing their CF. A psychologist who has experience with teens and families was hired at each site to conduct the family therapy sessions.

TABLE 17.1
Family Learning Program (FLP)

Session Number	Topic
1	Introductions/getting the most from your food!
2	Keep on boosting!
3	Lungs: Keeping them healthy!
4	Airway clearance: Mucus on the move!
5	Lungs: Bugs and other stuff!
6	Lungs and keeping fit!
7	"What's up Doc?"/Communicating with the health care team!
8	More communication fun!
9	New ways to handle stress!
10	How's it working?
Booster	Checking in and moving on!

The 10-session intervention has been manualized and structured to include goals and interactive exercises for each session; homework for parents and teen is also assigned at the end of each session. Four major components of change are targeted: problem solving, communication skills, cognitive restructuring, and functional/structural family issues (see Table 17.2 for a list of the sessions). Problem-solving and communication training are standard components of many interventions, but for this program we have made a concerted effort to keep the focus on adherence-related problems rather than generic parent–teen conflicts. For example, in the sessions on cognitive restructuring, the common problem of developing negative, even catastrophic belief systems for families of children with chronic illnesses (e.g., if you do not do treatment for 1 day, your health will decline) are addressed. In consultation with Dr. Robin, we have also adapted the program to increase the intervention period from its usual 10 to 20 weeks (with the same number of sessions), and we utilize information from the initial assessment measures (CBQ, RISCS) to focus in on the specific barriers to compliance that are reported. For example, results on the RISCS measure may indicate that procrastination in doing airway clearance treatments is a major source of parent–teen conflict. Adherence behaviors are monitored throughout the intervention; as data from the various monitors become available, they are presented to the families to show them their progress.

Difficult Methodological and Clinical Issues

Developing and evaluating clinical interventions within the context of a research project poses some unique methodological challenges. We raise them here to stimulate discussion and potentially assist others who are in the midst of this process. First, although both interventions were developed out of existing frameworks (BFST has been applied to children with atten-

TABLE 17.2
Behavioral Family Systems Therapy (BFST) Sessions

Session Number	Topic
1	Assessment and engagement
2	Parenting styles/beliefs and expectations
3	Problem solving
4	More problem solving
5	Communication skills training
6	Advanced communication skills training
7	Social disclosure issues
8	Filling in the gaps
9	Moving toward closure
10	Disengagement/closure
Booster	Problem solving ~ adherence issues

tion deficit hyperactivity disorder [ADHD] and teens with diabetes; the FLP program was drawn, in part, from Bartholomew's FEP), we have made substantial modifications in adapting them to the specific context of CF and the developmental period of early adolescence. In addition, after our manuals were written, we made changes and refinements to the sessions and activities in response to the therapists' and families' comments. This seemed particularly important in our case because there are no other CF adherence intervention studies to draw on, and this clinical trial is the first and largest of its kind. Although we believe that this iterative process has led to significant improvements in our intervention programs, it raises some questions about evaluating the effects of the intervention. When is an intervention fully developed and ready for an effectiveness study? How much liberty can interventionists take in modifying or refining a manualized intervention? How can program evaluators account for the inevitable improvements over time in the therapist's skill in administering the intervention and in working with the target population? Clearly this is a grey area with few clear-cut answers.

A related issue concerns the development and use of manualized interventions. To be most effective, clinical interventions should be tailored to the individual needs of each family, as well as the therapist and family's style of interacting. One limitation of manualized treatments is their potential to be applied in a dry, automated fashion. Therapists may feel that their autonomy and freedom to use clinical judgment has been restricted by the need to adhere to a manual, and so may resist structured interventions. Given the importance of the therapeutic relationship in effecting behavioral change, it may be critical to include process-oriented comments in the manual and explicit directions for solving difficult therapeutic dilemmas that arise in the course of treatment (Kendall, 1998). In developing both our family therapy and psychoeducational interventions, we have addressed this issue by asking the therapists to track and record the process issues that arise for each session. This information has been used to develop the manual for the interventions. A set of overarching issues designed to maximize the effectiveness of the interventions are included in the manual, as well as specific issues that are frequently encountered in each session.

A third issue that plagues most interventions aimed at increasing adherence to medical treatment is the problem of clearly establishing what the medical regimen is. If the research or clinical team cannot determine precisely what the teen is supposed to be doing each day to manage his or her medical condition, it becomes difficult, if not impossible, to promote success and establish empirically whether positive changes have occurred. For researchers, this means not knowing what the dependent variable is. There are several reasons for this ambiguity.

One reason may be problems in the communication process among the physician, patient, and family members (Ievers et al., 1999). Physicians may not clearly state (or write in the chart) what the daily medical regimen should be in terms of specific medications, dosages, and other aspects of the treatment regimen (e.g., how long to do CPT), or they may not review what has been prescribed at each clinic visit (see Ievers-Landis & Drotar, chap. 11, this volume). In addition, adolescents and family members may not listen carefully or fully comprehend what is being said. They may be reluctant to ask follow-up questions or take the physician's time to clarify these details.

We have also found that CF treatment information is often not updated or adjusted for increased developmental maturity. For example, many school-age children are still taking their enzyme medications halfway through the meal, which was recommended when they were infants and toddlers with erratic eating habits, but is not as effective as taking them just before a meal (Orenstein, Nixon, Ross, & Kaplan, 1989).

Another problem is that the treatment regimen for CF is increasing in its complexity as new medications and delivery systems are developed. For example, one commonly used antibiotic is now available in an inhaled form and may be added to the list of regular inhaled medications. Antiinflammatory drugs and medications designed to thin mucus are also being added to an already time-consuming and complex daily routine. Given the dizzying array of medications and treatment techniques that are now available for CF, it is critical that health care providers emphasize what the patient is supposed to do, when, and for how long.

Unlike other chronic pediatric conditions, such as asthma and diabetes, there are no national guidelines for treating a patient with CF. This leads to a final and far more subtle problem. There is tremendous variability from center to center, and among pulmonologists within the same center, in the treatment regimen that is prescribed. This makes it difficult to establish consistency across health care team members (physician, nurse) in what patients are told. It also makes it more difficult to develop interventions to increase adherence across centers because there are such diverse expectations about what patients are supposed to do. In addition, there is little agreement about the long-term health benefits that can be expected for those who regularly comply with even the most standard treatments, such as daily aerosolized bronchodilators and airway clearance. This may lead to treatment recommendations that are made with less certainty, less urgency, and in a tone that is more skeptical than assertive. If physicians do not believe that adherence to prescribed treatments will make an important clinical difference, why should patients and their family members?

SUMMARY AND FUTURE DIRECTIONS

In summary, we are at an exciting crossroads in the treatment of patients with CF. New medical treatments are being developed that are likely to increase life span and quality of life, and the medical community is beginning to recognize that adherence is as important to the process of disease management as the development of new medications and surgical techniques. We have now identified some of the key problems that adolescents and parents face in complying with daily treatments, and this has enabled us to tailor our intervention programs to the issues that are most relevant for these families and most likely to promote behavior change.

From our review of the adherence literature and our experience over the last several years in designing and implementing an adherence intervention trial, we have identified several key principles that have guided our research and may be useful in directing future efforts. First, the assessment and intervention process must be matched to the specific context in which the intervention occurs. The context in its entirety is complex, including the developmental age of the child and family, the medical regimens and challenges of the particular chronic condition, and the structure and dynamics of the family system (Quittner et al., 1996; Quittner & DiGirolamo, 1998). For example, an adherence intervention program for preschool-age children and their parents should have a very different focus than one designed for adolescents. Similarly, although there are some commonalities in treatment regimens prescribed for different chronic conditions (e.g., dietary alterations for CF and diabetes), the underlying rationales and routines vary dramatically (e.g., boosting calories vs. managing blood sugars). A wealth of evidence also indicates that family-centered interventions, which include components of negotiation of responsibility and improved communication between adolescent and parent, are likely to have the greatest impact and most long-lasting effects (Robin,

1998; Wysocki et al., 1999). Although a contextual approach substantially increases the complexity of program development and evaluation, a variety of data indicate that this is the one we should pursue (Glueckauf, in press; Lavigne & Faier-Routman, 1992; Quittner & DiGirolamo, 1998).

A second key principle in developing adherence interventions concerns the role that monitoring, feedback, and reinforcement can play in *building for success*. By asking adolescents and parents to attend an intervention program aimed at improving adherence to treatment, we are increasing the demands on their time and energy. It is important to acknowledge that we are adding to what they already do, potentially making their daily lives more hectic and stressful. We are also asking them to work hard to change long-standing, difficult behavior patterns (e.g., mothers preparing daily aerosol medications). This is a lot to ask of families, and we have found that it is critical to engage them early on in this process and help them achieve some measurable success. Specifically, we recommend that the intervention include several components that may facilitate this process: (a) assist them in monitoring the behaviors that are targeted for change (e.g., diary logs recording each use of the flutter), (b) provide regular and frequent feedback on their progress in treatment (e.g., graphs of daily airway clearance), and (c) give them frequent and tangible reinforcement for the improvements they are making (e.g., video coupons for teens who have increased their daily aerosol treatments, communication games in session with prizes given to the winners). Psychologists have been on the forefront in developing and using these tools in behavioral interventions, and we have found that they can be applied to adherence interventions in fun and creative ways.

Finally, we think there are several pragmatic issues that need to be addressed in developing adherence interventions for pediatric chronic conditions. First, there is the enormous problem of access to these interventions for families that live at a distance from a major children's hospital where they are likely to be offered. In our intervention trial, some families that were interested in participating in the adherence program were not able to travel the several hundred miles that were required, which was exacerbated by our requirement that fathers participate in the intervention. Other families did make the commitment to travel several hours each way, but this clearly places a significant burden on families who are already *stretched* to the limit. We have considered several solutions for this problem, including the development of a structure for disseminating established, manualized interventions to smaller hospitals and clinics and the use of new technologies to deliver interventions remotely into families' homes (Glueckauf et al., 1999; Hufford, Glueckauf, & Webb, 1999).

A related problem concerns the low prevalence of many pediatric chronic conditions and the need, therefore, to conduct adherence intervention trials at multiple sites. This raises a new set of pragmatic challenges, including differences in patients' prescribed treatment regimens at different centers, standardization of the intervention sessions across sites, and difficulties in organizing and maintaining uniform data collection and entry procedures. We have tried to address these problems in several ways, including scheduling regular videoconferences between sites, detailing process-oriented suggestions for the therapists for each session, and utilizing double data entry and verification procedures. The use of new telehealth technologies may also prove useful in maintaining consistency in the delivery of interventions at geographically distant sites.

A final issue concerns the duration of adherence-based interventions for chronic conditions. Given the life-long nature of chronic illnesses such as CF and the difficulty of maintaining good adherence to the various components of treatment over time, we may need to consider how intervention programs can be extended and reinforced to preserve their effectiveness. Intervention programs may need to include regular developmental updates (e.g., changes in the treatment regimen after puberty), booster sessions that include the family and significant others (e.g., close friends, boyfriends), and the possibility of establishing ongoing contact and support with a member of the CF team. At this point, the ideal duration and intensity of interventions with this or other chronic illness populations is not known, and future research needs to address this issue. Behavioral scientists have made substantial progress in developing and evaluating family-based interventions that hold promise for improving adherence behaviors and family functioning.

ACKNOWLEDGMENT

This research was supported in part by grants from the National Institutes of Health to the first and second authors (Research Career Development Award K04 # HL02892 and R01 # HL47064) and a Clinical Research Grant from the Cystic Fibrosis Foundation.

REFERENCES

Bartholomew, L. K., Czyzewski, D. I., Parcel, G. S., Swank, P. R., Sockrider, M. M., Mariotto, M. J., Schidlow, D. V., Fink, R. J., & Seilheimer, D. K. (1997). Self-management of cystic fibrosis: Short-term outcomes of the CF Family Education Program. *Health Education Quarterly, 24*(5), 652–666.

Bauman, L. J., Drotar, D., Leventhal, J. M., Perrin, E. C., & Pless, B. I. (1997). A review of psychosocial interventions for children with chronic health conditions. *Pediatrics*.

Czajkowski, D. R., & Koocher, G. P. (1986). Predicting medical compliance among adolescents with cystic fibrosis. *Health Psychology, 5*, 297–305.

Czyzewski, D., & Bartholomew, L. (1998). Quality of life outcomes in children and adolescents with CF. In D. Drotar (Ed.), *Measuring health-related quality of life in children and adolescents* (pp. 203–218). Mahwah, NJ: Lawrence Erlbaum Associates.

Czyzewski, D., Mariotto, M., Bartholomew, K., LeCompte, S., & Sockrider, M. M. (1994). Measurement of quality of well-being in a child and adolescent cystic fibrosis population. *Medical Care, 23*, 965–972.

Desmond, K. J., Schwenk, W. K., Thomas, E., Beaudry, P. H., & Coates, A. L. (1983). Immediate and long-term effects of chest physiotherapy in patients with cystic fibrosis. *Journal of Pediatrics, 103*, 538–542.

Diabetes Control and Complications Trial Research Group. (1993). The effect of intensive treatment of the development and progression of long-term complications in insulin-dependent diabetes mellitus. *The New England Journal of Medicine, 329*, 977–986.

DiGirolamo, A. M., Quittner, A. L., Ackerman, V., & Stevens, J. (1997). Identification and assessment of ongoing stressors in adolescents with a chronic illness: An application of the Behavior Analytic Model. *Journal of Clinical Child Psychology, 26*, 53–66.

Drotar, D. (1998). *Measuring health-related quality of life in children and adolescents: Implications for research and practice.* Mahwah, NJ: Lawrence Erlbaum Associates.

Drotar, D., & Ievers, C. (1994). Preliminary report: Age differences in parent and child responsibilities for management of cystic fibrosis and insulin-dependent diabetes mellitus. *Journal of Developmental and Behavioral Pediatrics, 15*, 367–374.

Eigen, H., Clark, N., & Wolley, J. (1987). NHLBI Workshop summary: Clinical behavioral aspects of cystic fibrosis. Directions for future work. *American Review Respiratory Disease, 136*, 1509–1513.

Fitzsimmons, S. (1993). The changing epidemiology of cystic fibrosis. *Journal of Pediatrics, 122*, 1–8.

Foster, S. L., Prinz, R. J., & O'Leary, K. D. (1983). Impact of problem-solving communication training and generalization procedures on family conflict. *Child and Family Behavior Therapy, 5*, 1–23.

Geiss, S., Hobbs, S., Hammersley-Maercklein, G., & Kramer, J. (1992). Psychosocial factors related to perceived compliance with cystic fibrosis treatment. *Journal of Clinical Psychology, 48*(1), 99–103.

Glueckauf, R. L. (in press). The family and disability assessment system. In J. Touliatos & B. F. Perlmutter (Eds.), *Handbook of family measurement techniques* (Vol. 2). Newbury Park, CA: Sage.

Glueckauf, R. L., Hufford, B., Whiton, J., Baxter, J., Schneider, P., Kain, J., & Vogelgesang, S. (1999). Telehealth: Emerging technology in rehabilitation and health care. In M. G. Eisenberg, R. L. Glueckauf, & H. H. Zaretsky (Eds.), *Medical aspects of disability: A handbook for the rehabilitation professional* (2nd ed., pp. 625–639). New York: Springer Publishing Company.

Gudas, L. J., Koocher, G. P., & Wypji, D. (1991). Perceptions of medical compliance in children and adolescents with cystic fibrosis. *Journal of Developmental and Behavioral Pediatrics, 12*, 236–242.

Henley, L. D., & Hill, I. D. (1990). Global and specific disease-related information needs of cystic fibrosis patients and their families. *Pediatrics, 85*(6), 1015–1021.

Henry, B., Aussage, P., Grosskopf, C., & Goehrs, J.-M. (1998). Evaluating quality of life (QOL) in children with cystic fibrosis (CF): Should we believe the child or the parent? *Pediatric Pulmonology, 26*(Suppl.), Abstract.

Henry, B., Aussage, P., Grosskopf, C., & Launois, R. (1996). Constructing a disease-specific quality of life questionnaire for children and adults with cystic fibrosis. *Isreali Journal of Medical Science, 32*(Suppl.), S181.

Hsu, L. M. (1998). Random sampling, randomization, and equivalence of contrasted groups in psychotherapy outcome research. In A. E. Kazdin (Ed.), *Methodological issues &*

strategies in clinical research (2nd ed., pp. 119–133). Washington, DC: American Psychological Association.

Hufford, B. J., Glueckauf, R. L., & Webb, P. M. (1999). Home-based videoconferencing for adolescents with epilepsy and their families. *Rehabilitation Psychology, 44,* 176–193.

Ievers, C. E., Brown, R. T., Drotar, D., Caplan, D., Pishevar, B., & Lambert, R. G. (1999). Knowledge of physician prescriptions and adherence to treatment among children with cystic fibrosis and their mothers. *Journal of Developmental and Behavioral Pediatrics, 20,* 335–343.

Johnson, S. B. (1993). Chronic diseases of childhood: Assessing compliance with complex medical regimens. In N. A. Krasnegor, L. Epstein, S. B. Johnson, & S. J. Yaffe (Eds.), *Developmental aspects of health compliance behavior* (pp. 157–184). Mahwah, NJ: Lawrence Erlbaum Associates.

Johnson, S. B., Freund, A., Silverstein, J., Hansen, C. A., & Malone, J. (1990). Adherence/health status relationships in childhood diabetes. *Health Psychology, 9*(5), 606–631.

Karoly, P. (1993). Enlarging the scope of the compliance construct: Toward developmental and motivational relevance. In N. A. Kransnegor, L. Epstein, S. B. Johnson, & S. J. Yaffee (Eds.), *Developmental aspects of health compliance behavior* (pp. 11–27). Hillsdale, NJ: Lawrence Erlbaum Associates.

Kendall, P. C., Chu, B., Gifford, A., Hayes, C., & Nauta, M. (1998). Breathing life into a manual. *Cognitive and Behavioral Practice, 5*(2), 177–198.

La Greca, A. M., & Schuman, W. B. (1995). Adherence to prescribed medical regimens. In M. C. Roberts (Ed.), *Handbook of pediatric psychology* (pp. 55–83). New York: Guilford.

Lavigne, J. V, & Faier-Routman, J. (1992). Psychological adjustment to pediatric physical disorders: A meta-analytic review. *Journal of Pediatric Psychology, 17,* 133–157.

Nolan, T., Desmond, K., & Herlich, R. (1986). Knowledge of cystic fibrosis in patients and their parents. *Pediatrics, 77*(2), 229–235.

Orenstein, D., Nixon, P., Ross, E., & Kaplan, R. (1989). The quality of well-being in cystic fibrosis. *Chest, 95,* 344–347.

Parcel, G., Swank, P. R., Mariotto, M., & Bartholomew, L. (1994). Self-management of cystic fibrosis: A structural model for educational and behavioral variables. *Social Science & Medicine, 38*(9), 1307–1315.

Passero, M. A., Remor, B., & Solomon, J. (1981). Patient-reported compliance with cystic fibrosis therapy. *Clinical Pediatrics, 20,* 264–268.

Patterson, J. M., Budd, J., Goetz, D., & Warwick, W. J. (1993). Family correlates of a 10 year pulmonary health trend in cystic fibrosis. *Pediatrics, 91*(2), 383–389.

Patterson, J. M., McCubbin, H. I., & Warwick, W. J. (1990). The impact of family functioning on health changes in children with cystic fibrosis. *Social Science Medicine, 31,* 291–301.

Quittner, A. L. (1998). Measurement of quality of life in cystic fibrosis. *Current Opinion in Pulmonary Medicine, 4,* 326–331.

Quittner, A. L. (1999). Improving assessment in child clinical and pediatric psychology: Establishing links to process and functional outcomes. In D. Drotar (Ed.), *Handbook of research methods in pediatric and child clinical psychology* (pp. 119–143). New York: Plenum.

Quittner, A. L., & DiGirolamo, A. M. (1998). Family adaptation to childhood disability and illness. In R. T. Ammerman & J. V. Campo (Eds.), *Handbook of pediatric psychology and psychiatry* (Vol. 2, pp. 70–102). Boston: Allyn & Bacon.

Quittner, A. L., & Espelage, D. (1999). Reliability and validity of a daily phone diary measure to assess daily activities and family interactions. *Psychological Assessment.*

Quittner, A. L., & Opipari, L. C. (1994). Differential treatment of siblings: Interview and diary analyses comparing two family contexts. *Child Development, 65,* 800–814.

Quittner, A. L., Sweeny, S., Watrous, M., Munzenberger, P., & Henry, B. (1998). Initial US validation of a disease-specific quality of life (QOL) measure for cystic fibrosis: The Cystic Fibrosis Questionnaire. *Pediatric Pulmonology, 27*(Suppl. 17).

Quittner, A. L., Tolbert, V. E., Regoli, M. J., Orenstein, D., Hollingsworth, J. L., & Eigen, H. (1996). Development of the Role-Play Inventory of Situations and Coping Strategies (RISCS) for parents of children with cystic fibrosis. *Journal of Pediatric Psychology, 21*, 209–235.

Quittner, A. L., Watrous, M., Sweeny, S., Munzenberger, P., Bearss, K., Gibson-Nitza, A., Fisher, L. A., & Henry, B. (in press). Development of a disease-specific quality of life measure for cystic fibrosis: Linguistic validation of the French CFQ. *Journal of Pediatric Psychology.*

Ricker, J. H., Delamater, A. M., & Hsu, J. (1998). Correlates of regimen adherence in cystic fibrosis. *Journal of Clinical Psychology in Medical Settings, 5*(2), 159–172.

Riordan, J. R., Rommens, J. M., Kerem, B., Alon, N., Rozmahel, R., Grzelczak, Z., Zielenski, J., Lok, S., Plavsic, N., & Chou, J. L. (1989). Identification of the cystic fibrosis gene: Cloning and characterization of complementary DNA. *Science, 245*, 1066–1073.

Robin, A. L. (1998). Training families with ADHD adolescents. In R. A. Barkley (Ed.), *Attention deficit hyperactivity disorder: A handbook for diagnosis and treatment* (2nd ed.). New York: Guilford.

Robin, A. L., & Foster, S. L. (1989). *Negotiating parent adolescent conflict: A behavioral-family systems approach.* New York: Guilford.

Robin, A. L., Koepke, T., & Moye, A. (1990). Multidimensional assessment of parent–adolescent relations. *Psychological Assessment: A Journal of Consulting and Clinical Psychology, 2*, 451–469.

Schipper, H., Clinch, J., & Olweny, C. (1996). Quality of life studies: Definitions and conceptual issues. In B. Spiker (Ed.), *Quality of life and pharmacoeconomics in clinical trials* (2nd ed., pp. 11–23). Philadelphia: Lippincott-Raven.

Schultz, J. R., & Moser, A. (1992). Barriers to treatment adherence in cystic fibrosis. *Pediatric Pulmonology, 11*, 321.

Stark, L. J., Quittner, A. L., Opipari, L., Jelalian, E., Jones, E., Poweres, W., Higgins, L., Maguiness, K., Seidner, D., Hoover, J., Eigan, H., Duggan, C., & Stallings, V. (1998, October). The contribution of behavior therapy to enhancing adherence in school age children with CF: The example of diet. In J. Glazner (Chair), *Innovative approaches to CF education.* Symposium conducted at the Twelfth annual North American Cystic Fibrosis Conference.

Stark, L. J., Jelalian, E., & Miller, D. L. (1995). Cystic fibrosis. In M. C. Roberts (Ed.), *Handbook of pediatric psychology* (pp. 241–262). New York: Guilford.

Stark, L. J., Miller, S. T., Plienis, A. J., & Drabman, R. S. (1987). Behavioral contracting to increase chest physiotherapy. *Behavior Modification, 11*, 75–86.

Stout, R. L., Wirtz, P., Carbonari, J. P., & Del Boca, F. K. (1994). Ensuring balanced distribution of prognostic factors in treatment outcome research. *Journal of Studies on Alcohol, 12*, 70–75.

Warwick, W. J., & Hansen, L. G. (1991). The long-term effect of high-frequency chest compression therapy on pulmonary complications in cystic fibrosis. *Pediatric Pulmonology, 11*, 265–271.

Wysocki, T., Harris, M. A., Greco, P., Bubb, J., Danda, C. E., Harvey, L. M., McDonell, K., Taylor, A., & White, N. H. (2000). Randomized, controlled trial of behavioral therapy for families of adolescents with insulin-dependent diabetes mellitus. *Journal of Pediatric Psychology, 25*(1), 23–33.

Wysocki, T., Miller, K. M., Harvey, L. M., Taylor, A., Danda, C. E., McDonell, K., Greco, P., Harris, M. A., & White, N. H. (1999). Behavior therapy for families of adolescents with diabetes: Effects on directly observed family interactions. *Behavior Therapy, 30*, 507–525.

CHAPTER EIGHTEEN

Adherence to Diet in Chronic Conditions: The Example of Cystic Fibrosis

Lori J. Stark
Children's Hospital Medical Center, Cincinnati, OH

Nutritional recommendations are part of the management of many chronic illnesses of childhood, such that children are instructed to eat more foods, avoid foods, eat at prescribed times, and/or eat different foods. For example, children with Type 1 diabetes are instructed to avoid foods high in sugar and to eat at regular times corresponding to insulin injections. Children with phenylketonuria (PKU) are instructed to avoid foods containing phenylalanine. Children with cystic fibrosis (CF) are instructed to consume increased energy of 120% to 150% of the recommended daily allowance (RDA) for healthy children. Children with juvenile rheumatoid arthritis (JRA) need a high-protein diet. There is also research indicating that a special ketogenic diet may be an important treatment for children with intractable seizure disorders (Kinsman, Vining, Quaskey, Mellits, & Freeman, 1992).

In addition to the modification of diet for the treatment of chronic conditions, childhood is also seen as the optimal time to intervene on diet to prevent chronic health conditions in adulthood. For example, the American Heart Association advocates a diet low in concentrated fat and high in fiber at all ages to prevent the risk of heart disease in adulthood. Research has found that some precursors to heart disease—such as elevated blood cholesterol, high blood pressure, and obesity—are evident in childhood (Center for Disease Control, 1994; Gortmaker, Dietz, Sobol, & Wehler, 1987), and children with these risk factors are likely to carry them into adulthood (Ernst & Obarzanek, 1994). More recently, investigators have

begun to examine the effects of calcium intake during childhood and adolescence in the prevention of osteoporosis in adulthood. Calcium intake
during childhood and adolescence appears critical because it is during this
stage of development that 40% of the skeletal structure is built and
enlarged, making it a critical time for bone mass optimization (Christiansen, Rodbro, & Throgen, 1975).

Despite our growing knowledge about the importance of diet in the
management and prevention of these diseases, there is little information
on children or their family's ability to adhere to these recommendations
or the toll such adherence takes on the family (Linscheid, Budd, & Rasnake, 1995). Although diet is an important component of many chronic
conditions, the current chapter examines the issue of dietary adherence in
the context of cystic fibrosis (CF). CF is a genetically inherited disease primarily affecting Whites, in which nutritional status is strongly correlated
with physical outcome on a short-term (Gurwitz, Corey, Francis, Crozier,
& Levison, 1979; Kraemer, Rudeberg, Hadorn, & Rossi, 1978) and long-
term (Corey, McLaughlin, Williams, & Levison, 1988; Shepherd et al.,
1986) basis. For example, patients with better nutritional status, as indicated by higher weight percentiles, have been found to have longer survival (Corey et al., 1988; Kraemer et al., 1978) as well as better pulmonary
function (Gurwitz et al., 1979) and faster recovery from respiratory infections (Gurwitz et al., 1979; Kraemer et al., 1978). This chapter provides an
in-depth review of what is known about dietary adherence in CF and a
working model of the contribution of behavioral intervention to improve
adherence to diet in this population. As such the chapter provides an
overview of the disease, the importance of diet in the treatment of CF, a
review of adherence to diet in this population, models of adherence and
data supporting these models, and a behavioral model for improving
adherence to diet.

CYSTIC FIBROSIS AND WHY DIET IS IMPORTANT

CF is a complex, autosomal recessive disease. It primarily affects Whites
and has an incidence rate of approximately 1 in 2,500 live births. The
exocrine glands of several major organ systems are affected such that the
epithelia of the exocrine glands in the respiratory, digestive, pancreas, kidney, liver, and reproductive systems produce an abnormal mucus that is
thick, viscous, and sticky. The most serious manifestations of the disease
are in the respiratory and pancreatic systems. The major cause of death is
cardiovascular failure (Cystic Fibrosis Foundation, 1998). Accumulation
of the viscous mucus in the bronchi and bronchioles of the lungs leads to
obstruction and infection. Over time the cycle of obstruction and infec-

tion damages the lungs and leads to respiratory insufficiency and death (Holsclaw, 1980). In terms of pancreatic functioning, 85% of patients with CF suffer from pancreatic insufficiency. The enzymes responsible for the breakdown of proteins and fats are either missing or blocked by the thick mucus (Kopelman, 1991). Therefore, patients must take pancreatic enzyme supplements to aid in the absorption of proteins, fats, and fat-soluble vitamins.

Thus, nutritional status in patients with CF is compromised in several ways. Energy needs are increased secondary to pulmonary disease (Ramsey, Farrell, & Pencharz, 1992) and an increased metabolic rate via the genetic defect (O'Rawe et al., 1992). Malabsorption of fats and proteins continues to occur, to some degree, even with enzyme replacement therapy (Ramsey et al., 1992). To offset these increased energy needs, patients with CF are recommended to follow a high-energy, high-fat diet. Specifically, they are recommended to consume 120% to 150% of the recommended daily allowance (RDA) of energy for healthy individuals (Ramsey et al., 1992) with 35% to 40% coming from fat (MacDonald, Holden, & Harris, 1991). Optimal nutritional status is increasingly being recognized as important in the management of the disease (Foster & Farrell, 1996; Ramsey et al., 1992) because of the strong correlation between nutritional status and survival (Corey et al., 1988; Shepherd et al., 1986) and recovery from acute pulmonary infections (Gurwitz et al., 1979; Kraemer et al., 1978). When the recommended energy intake of 20% to 50% above the RDA for healthy individuals is supplied to patients by enteral (directly into the gut by gastrostomy or nasogastrostomy tube; Levy, Durie, Pencharz, & Corey, 1985; Shepherd et al., 1986) or parenteral (via vein; Lester, Rothberg, Dawson, Lopez, & Corpuz, 1986; Mansell et al., 1984) supplementation, improved weight gain and pulmonary functioning has been reported. Thus, improved energy intake has been associated with improved nutritional and pulmonary status.

Although optimizing nutritional status in patients with CF is gaining recognition (Ramsey et al., 1992), it continues to be somewhat controversial in the actual implementation. That is, prevention of low weight status and early intervention to optimize weight status is not universally accepted. The impetus for the recommendation to optimize nutritional status early in the treatment of the disease comes from correlational studies. Perhaps the most compelling of these studies was a comparison of two large CF Centers in North America (Corey et al., 1988). In this study, one center had a mean survival age of 30 years, whereas the mean survival age in the second center was 9 years less at 21 years. In the center with the greater survival curve, patients also had better heights and weights and were on normal to high-fat diets. Other researchers have also reported significant correlations between relative underweight and survival (Kraemer et al.,

1978) and between malnutrition and decline in pulmonary functioning (Gurwitz et al., 1979).

Although the relationship between survival and nutritional status and pulmonary function and nutritional status has been strong, it is only correlational. Thus, it is also possible that poor weight is secondary to lung disease and that improving weight will not affect survival. As stated earlier, a handful of studies have reported improved pulmonary functioning following nutritional rehabilitation in severely malnourished CF patients. However, these studies are compromised by the small sample size and lack of a prospective control group. Thus, although improving nutritional status is advocated, data have not yet been collected demonstrating a clear cause and effect between weight status and disease status. Until such studies are conducted, there will probably continue to be a discrepancy between recommendations for the provision of dietary treatment and actual clinical implementation and inconsistency in the implementation of treatment across CF Centers.

ADHERENCE TO DIETARY RECOMMENDATIONS

Dietary recommendations prior to 1980 were for a high-energy, low-fat diet. Early studies of patients with CF found that when fat was restricted, patients could not even achieve the RDA for energy of healthy individuals. Most studies reported an intake of approximately 80% of the RDA for energy (Chase, Long, & Lavin, 1979; Hodges et al., 1984; Hubbard & Mangrum, 1982; Parson, Beaudry, Dumas, & Pencharz, 1983) during that time. However, in 1980, the dietary recommendations were revised to advocate a normal to high-fat diet of 35% to 40% fat. It was assumed that liberalization of fat intake would improve the energy intake of patients and allow them to meet the prescribed 20% to 50% increase in the RDA for energy. Subsequent studies of children with CF have consistently demonstrated that liberalization of fat in the CF diet have allowed patients to achieve a normal intake of 100% RDA for energy (Buchdahl, Fullylove, Marchant, Warner, & Brueton, 1989; Daniels, Davidson, & Cooper, 1987; Stark et al., 1995, 1997; Tomezsko, Stallings, & Scanlin, 1992). However, they are not achieving the CF dietary requirements, nor are they achieving a 35% to 40% fat intake (Stark et al., 1995, 1997; Tomezsko et al., 1992). In these studies, children with CF were achieving a similar percent of their intake in fat, only 32% to 33%, to the healthy controls (Stark et al., 1995, 1997; Tomezsko et al., 1992).

Thus, it appears that children with CF are able to achieve oral energy intake similar to healthy peers, but they are unable to achieve the recommended energy intake for CF. Adherence studies in CF have found diet to be one of the least complied with components of treatment (Carter, Kronenberger, & Conradsen, 1993; Gudas, Koocher, & Wypij, 1991). In examining factors that interfere with achieving the CF dietary recommendations, we have adopted the typologies of noncompliance identified by Koocher, McGrath, and Gudas (1990). Specifically, Koocher et al. (1990) proposed three typologies for understanding noncompliance in CF: educated noncompliance, inadequate knowledge, and psychosocial resistance. Although this model has not been validated, it provides a useful framework for conceptualizing potential barriers to adherence. In this model, *educated noncompliance* refers to the patient and/or family making a reasoned analysis of the perceived costs and benefits of complying with treatment and choosing not to follow the treatment recommendations as given. *Inadequate knowledge* refers to instances of noncompliance due to lack of information or inadequate information. Lack of information can result from the patient not receiving the information on treatment or its rationale from the health care provider or not understanding the information that was given. The third typology, *psychosocial resistance*, includes control struggles with parents or authority figures, responding to cultural or peer pressures for conformity, denial of the disease, and a chaotic home environment (Koocher et al., 1990).

In reviewing the literature, little evidence has been found to support educated noncompliance in regard to dietary treatment. However, there is evidence that parents of children with CF do not have adequate knowledge to meet the dietary requirements of the disease. Gudas et al. (1991) found that parents and patients often did not understand that diet was a formal treatment recommendation. Henley and Hill (1990) reported that in a survey of patients and their parents, many were unaware of the importance of fat in the CF diet. In addition, anecdotal data from parents participating in behavioral treatment studies targeting dietary adherence indicate that they are confused by the public health messages to lower overall fat consumption in the U.S. population. Many families of children with CF voice concern about their child's cardiovascular health and hence are hesitant to serve a high-fat diet.

The third typology for conceptualizing noncompliance to dietary adherence in CF is *psychosocial resistance*. There are numerous studies that provide data supporting the potential influence of psychosocial factors. A survey study of treatment (Quittner, DiGirolamo, & Winslow, 1991) reported that 94% of families of young children with CF reported mealtimes to be a problematic aspect of treatment (Quittner et al., 1991). In fact, mealtimes were one of the most frequently endorsed problems by these families. In another study, parents of young children with CF, ages 1 to 7 years, were compared to parents of healthy children (Crist et al., 1994). In this study, parents of the children with CF reported a higher number of problematic mealtime behaviors, including long meals, delay of eating by talking, and spitting out food. Crist et al. (1994) also reported that higher rates of problem behaviors were found to be significantly correlated with lower caloric intake in the children with CF. Parents of children with CF also reported that they engaged in higher rates of ineffective parenting strategies, such as coaxing and making a second meal, than the parents of the control children. The types of behavioral factors described by parents, such as long meals, delay of eating by talking, and spitting out food, are similar to behaviors reported for children with feeding disorders (Sanders, Patel, LeGrice, & Shepherd, 1993). Children exhibiting such behaviors in response to food and eating are often difficult to treat (Linscheid et al., 1995). It has been hypothesized that, once established, these child behaviors are maintained by maladaptive parental response (Palmer & Horn, 1978; Sanders et al., 1993) that provide increased parental attention (e.g., coaxing) to behaviors incompatible with eating. Thus, a wide range of behavioral factors appear to contribute to the problems of poor dietary adherence in children with CF and may present challenges to adherence that go beyond psychosocial resistance.

UNDERSTANDING BARRIERS TO NONADHERENCE: BEYOND SELF-REPORT

In our own research, we have attempted to more specifically identify barriers to achieving dietary adherence in CF and to understand them in the context of family functioning. In this regard, we have recently completed an observational study of the mealtime behaviors of 32 children with CF, ages 2 to 5 years, and 29 nonchronically ill children matched on age, gender, socioeconomic status (SES), number of siblings, and number of parents present at dinner (Stark et al., in press). In this study, we hypothesized that, given the literature on the self-report of problems experienced by parents of children with CF, parents and children with CF would demonstrate more maladaptive behaviors during the mealtime compared with families of healthy controls. To examine this question, three videotaped meals per subject were examined for 17 parent and child mealtime behaviors. These data were analyzed for the meal overall and by the meal phase, first half verses second half.

In this population, the children with CF were previously found to have a meal length that was significantly longer by an average of 6 minutes than the healthy controls (Stark et al., 1995). When time was held constant, children with CF did not differ from their peers in the proportion of behaviors that occurred across the meal. Similarly, when time was held constant, parents of children with CF did not differ in the proportion of behaviors exhibited from parents of controls. In general, when parent and child eating behaviors were examined across the two phases of the meal, first half and second half, similar patterns emerged for the families of children with CF and controls. Across the meal, children in both groups demonstrated a decrease in the number of bites taken in the second half of the meal as compared with the first and an increase in behaviors incompatible with eating. Specifically, children were away from the table more frequently, refused food more often, and were more noncompliant with commands to eat. Thus, it appeared that, across the meal, children demonstrated less interest in food and more behaviors incompatible with eating. During the same time the children were showing less interest in food, parents demonstrated an increase in their attempts to get their children to eat regardless of group (CF or control). Specifically, parents issued more direct and indirect commands to the child to eat and engaged in more coaxing, physical prompts, and feeding of the child during the second half of the meal compared with the first half of the meal.

Because certain child behaviors and parent responses were hypothesized to be stressful in the meal situation, we felt that controlling for time may not fully capture the mealtime setting. Thus, we felt it would be important to look at absolute frequency of these behaviors. When frequency was examined, children with CF were found to engage in more behaviors incompatible with eating than their healthy peers. For example, children with CF were away from the table, refused food, and were more noncompliant with commands to eat than control children. Of note, children with CF did not differ from their peers on the frequency of their request for food. Parents of children with CF also differed from the parents of the control children in the absolute frequency of direct and indirect commands issued, the frequency of feeding the child, and provision of physical prompts and coaxing. The parents of children with CF engaged in these behaviors more frequently. There was no difference in the frequency of reinforcement parents gave the children, which was low in both groups.

From these data, we concluded that children with CF and their parents did not differ from nonchronically ill children and their parents in the types of behaviors they exhibited. That is, the children with CF and their parents did not exhibit maladaptive or pathological interactions during mealtime. Instead it appears from these data that the main strategy parents of children with CF used to increase their child's caloric intake was to keep the children at the meal longer than parents of control children. In this sample, longer mealtimes led to an increase in typical parenting strategies and typical child mealtime responses.

The data on the oral intake of children with CF indicate that these children are eating a similar amount of food to healthy children as indicated by their caloric intake and percent RDA of energy. However, the dietary recommendations for CF require that children with CF exceed this typical intake by 20% to 50%. Such an increase may present special challenges because the children may need to go beyond their satiety point to accommodate these energy needs (Bowen & Stark, 1991). In addition, there may be some aspects of the disease that make food less appealing and therefore make it more difficult to increase food consumption. For example, hunger may be suppressed secondary to subclinical glucose intolerance (present in 30%–50% of children with CF; Handwerger et al., 1969; Park & Grand, 1981). In the face of such challenges, it appears from our observational study that parents of children with CF keep their children at the meal longer and use typical parenting strategies at an increased rate. The results of these efforts are twofold: Mealtimes are perceived as *stressful* and families are unsuccessful in meeting the CF dietary requirements.

INTERVENTIONS TO IMPROVE DIETARY ADHERENCE

Over the past 10 years, our research team has been developing treatment protocols to address the challenges of meeting the dietary treatment recommendations in CF. Beginning in 1990 (Stark, Bowen, Tyc, Evans, & Passero, 1990), we published the first of four intervention studies exploring the efficacy of behavior therapy to increase the caloric intake of preschool and school-age children with CF. This protocol and its subsequent refinements (Stark et al., 1993, 1996; Stark, Powers, Jelalian, Rape, & Miller, 1994) have focused on the premise that nutritional education is necessary, but not sufficient, to change dietary intake, and that behavior therapy skills such as child management strategies and shaping would enhance dietary adherence. Borrowing from successful protocols on other diet behaviors with this age group, such as obesity (Epstein, Wing, Steranchak, Dickson, & Michelson, 1980), the intervention was designed to be conducted in a group format. Parents and children were seen simultaneously, but in separate parent–child groups. The groups have been conducted over six (Stark et al., 1990) to seven (Stark et al., 1993, 1996) sessions of 60 to 90 minutes each.

In all studies, the initial session served as a baseline during which anthropometric measures (weight, height, skinfolds) were taken on the children, and parents and children were instructed on dietary monitoring procedures. Baseline data on calorie intake was kept via weighed 7-day food diaries. Active intervention occurred during Sessions 2 to 7. During these sessions, one meal/snack was targeted for increased calorie consumption. Treatment typically began with targeting snacks and proceeded across sessions to include breakfast, lunch, and dinner. Using a shaping paradigm, snack was the initial target meal because it was hypothesized to be the easiest meal in which to effect change. Snacks were typically underutilized by parents to maximize energy intake, and parents were not as invested in the child's food consumption at snacktime as they were at other meals. That is, parents did not report increased anxiety if their child did not consume a snack. Children's calorie goals were set at a 250-calorie per day increase at the targeted meal and maintenance of their intake at nontargeted meals. Intervention gradually progressed across meals and, because it was assumed that dinner was the most difficult meal, it was targeted last. Dinner was assumed to be difficult because it was a time the family was together and was possibly perceived by parents as their last opportunity to get their child to eat.

In the parent group, parents received nutritional education regarding the targeted meal and were instructed in child behavior management focusing on motivating their child to eat presented foods. Nutritional education focused on alternate cooking methods, which emphasized increasing caloric density instead of volume; frying instead of baking; adding calorie boosters such as extra butter, cream, and syrups; and choosing higher calorie foods than those typically served. Parents received calorie comparison guides and individualized calorie boosters based on their child's baseline oral intake. The parents were also taught child behavior management strategies. The sequence of the strategies followed the general principles of parent training recommended by Forehand and McMahon (1981). During the initial sessions, parents were taught to use differential attention (praising and ignoring). During subsequent sessions, parents were taught the use of contingent privileges (i.e., awarding a privilege contingent on meeting a mealtime calorie goal). Emphasis was placed on providing social rewards for achieving calorie goals, such as special time with a parent.

The children's treatment group focused on providing nutritional education at a developmentally appropriate level through fun and educational activities. For example, children learned the importance of food to provide energy for growth, development, and play through the use of body drawings. Information about specific foods at the targeted meals were taught through activities such as collages and games (i.e., high-energy bingo). In addition, children were provided with star charts to track their progress on meeting their energy goals at home. Parents were initially instructed to accompany the giving of stickers with verbal praise. As treatment progressed, the stickers were redeemable for home-based privileges. Throughout treatment, trophies were awarded in the treatment sessions for children meeting their energy goals on 5 out of 7 days per week. Children were also provided an opportunity to practice meeting their calorie goals via consumption of a high-calorie meal and behavioral reward program in the treatment group. The child group leaders also used behavioral management strategies, such as praising and describing to promote appropriate behavior in the group setting and manage in session meals. In the latter studies (Stark et al., 1993, 1996), a relaxation protocol was implemented at Session 4. Relaxation provided the children with a coping mechanism for dealing with feelings of fullness and also provided a break in the sequence of increasing caloric intake.

The three published studies using this intervention showed similar gains in calorie and weight across the intervention. Specifically, in the first two studies, the treatment children served as their own controls and increased their daily calorie intake by approximately 900 to 1,000 calories per day representing a 25% to 43% (Stark et al., 1990) and 32% to 60% (Stark et al., 1993) increase above their baseline intake. In these studies, the children achieved or surpassed the recommended 120% RDA for energy. The children also demonstrated significant increases in weight pre- to posttreatment of 1.48 kg (Stark et al., 1990) and 0.66 kg (Stark et al., 1993). In both studies, the treatment gains were maintained at 9 months (Stark et al., 1990) and 24 months (Stark et al., 1993) posttreatment.

In the third study (Stark et al., 1996), five children with CF receiving the behavioral intervention were compared to four children with CF on a wait-list for treatment. The waitlist group control continued to receive standard of care for nutrition via the routine clinical visits. In this study, the behavioral intervention group increased their caloric intake pre- to posttreatment significantly more than the controls—an averaged increase of 1,032 cal/day for the treatment group versus 244 cal/day for the controls. Children receiving the behavioral intervention also gained significantly more weight (average 1.7 kg) than the controls (average 0.0 kg) pre- to posttreatment. Although this treatment study was one of the few to employ a control group, the limited sample size prevented matching on disease severity or weight percentile prior to the intervention.

IMPLICATIONS OF OUR PREVIOUS STUDIES

The results of the prior studies have been promising. The data indicate that adherence to dietary treatment in children with CF may be enhanced by providing parents and children with behavioral skills to meet the challenge imposed by the demand to eat more and differently (high-fat food) than others. A recent meta-analysis compared the effect of the behavioral treatment on caloric intake and weight gain in patients with CF to medical interventions that supply sufficient energy via enteral and parenteral feeds (Jelalian, Stark, Reynolds, & Seifer, 1998). In this comparison, the calorie increases produced in the behavioral studies were comparable to those found with enteral and parenteral nutrition. Furthermore, the increased caloric intake of the subjects in the behavioral studies were associated with significant weight gain. A meta-analysis of behavioral, enteral, and parenteral studies for effect size with respect to weight gain in patients with CF demonstrated that the behavioral studies have an effect size comparable to enteral nutrition (1.58 vs. 1.69 standard deviation units, respectively; Jelalian et al., 1998). Although the effect size of the behavioral intervention was less than the effect size of 2.19 standard deviation units for parenteral supplementation, the three interventions (behavioral, enteral, and parenteral) did not statistically differ from each other with respect to weight gain.

Although the behavioral intervention has shown effects for caloric intake and weight, the design of the studies has precluded evaluation of the intervention on physical outcome such as pulmonary functioning or respiratory infections. For example, effects of improved nutritional status on pulmonary functioning has been difficult to assess because of ceiling effects. Most participants in the behavioral intervention studies have had optimal to good pulmonary functioning with little room for improvement. The studies also lacked a control group and long-term follow-up to compare pulmonary function, which is expected to decline over time in CF. In all studies, pulmonary functioning was stable across the intervention and follow-up, and parents anecdotally reported the children had improved activity levels. Because the behavioral treatment protocol is conceptualized as an early intervention, long-term follow-up with prospectively identified controls is necessary to evaluate the effect on measures of physical health.

EVALUATING THE ROLE OF BEHAVIOR THERAPY TO ENHANCE ADHERENCE TO DIETARY TREATMENT

The previous studies of behavior therapy to enhance adherence to dietary treatment have been promising. Participants have demonstrated an increase in caloric intake and corresponding increase in weight. However, the limited sample size and absence of a comparison group that controls for professional contact and nutrition information limit our understanding of the contribution of the behavioral component of the intervention. To address this question, we are currently conducting a multisite clinical trial in which behavioral intervention plus nutrition education is compared to nutrition education alone (Stark & Quittner, 1996). This study seeks to understand the additive effect of behavioral treatment to nutrition education. Children with CF and their families are randomly assigned to a Behavior Intervention (BI) or Nutrition Education (NE) group. The BI group receives the standard training as described earlier. The NE group is structured similarly to the BI in terms of the number of sessions (one baseline and six active treatment sessions), length of session (90 minutes), and nutritional content. Similar to the BI group, parents and children in the NE group are provided calorie goals that increase by 250 calories per meal, one meal per session. The parents are given the same intensive nutrition education materials, but no instructions on how to manage their child at meals. The children are not provided star charts, nor do they earn trophies for meeting calorie goals. In the NE group, children are given trophies noncontingently for attendance at group sessions. The children in the NE group are provided a sample meal in sessions like the children in the BI group. However, unlike the children in the BI condition, children in the NI condition are not required to eat the foods to receive in-session rewards. The NE condition is an active treatment condition that is far more intense and focused than the current standard of care for nutrition in CF.

Preliminary analysis of the first 33 participants was presented at the 12th Annual North American CF Conference (Stark et al., 1998). The results of this analysis are interesting in that an effect was found for both BI and NE conditions. Contrary to previous studies of nutrition education in which no changes in dietary behavior were found (Bell, Durie, & Forstner, 1984), the present protocol is demonstrating a calorie increase of approximately 475 cal/day pre- to posttreatment for nutrition education. However, the BI condition is demonstrating an increase in calories that is nearly double that found for the NE condition—788 cal/day. The associated weight change for children in these conditions also supports the differential calorie changes. The children in the BI condition gained twice the weight (average 1.47 kg) of the children in the NE condition (average 0.78 kg) pre- to posttreatment. This supports that the change in calories is not due to self-report bias that may be inherent in caloric monitoring.

The change found for the NE condition is worthy of comment. This condition was designed to control for contact time and nutritional content. As such, it necessarily incorporated some behavioral aspects of treatment delivery such as shaping and feedback. The structure of the NE sessions mirrored that of the BI condition. Only one meal was targeted at a time and calories were systematically increased across weeks. Similarly, parents in both groups received graphs displaying their child's progress on a weekly basis. Thus, the structure, intensity, feedback, and nutrition content differ from the manner in which most nutrition education is delivered. In typical CF care, families are given global recommendations across meals in one to two sessions that may be months apart. Although such intervention may be useful in raising awareness and/or knowledge, it has little effect on behavior. Our preliminary results would suggest that changing the structure of how dietary information is delivered may increase the efficacy of this approach on actual eating behavior.

Although the results of the NE condition demonstrate the promise of this approach, it also points out the limitations. The children in the NE group were only half as successful as the children in the BE group. From our experience, the behavioral program has probably been more successful for several reasons. First, the child management skills taught to the parents were derived from our assessment study and specifically targeted the child behaviors that parents have found most problematic at meals. Second, the group setting and educational component of the BI condition also contributed to parents' acceptance and implementation of the behavioral child management strategies. For example, parents are informed about the findings of our assessment study. Specifically, they are told that our data indicate that children with CF are not engaging in unusual behaviors, they are just engaging in a higher frequency of typical child behaviors. Similarly, they are informed that parents of children with CF are responding to these behaviors as parents typically would. However, because of the increased awareness of diet and weight in this population, parents tend to extend the mealtime and engage in more of these typical behaviors (such as prompting and coaxing) than parents of healthy children.

Directly educating the parents about the unique challenge CF brings to their meals and providing data showing their child's actual intake set the stage for parents to understand that the typical response parents use to encourage eating in a nonill child is probably not sufficient for a child with CF. The BI condition provides the parents with strategies (e.g., contingent privileges) to manage their child when the child is resistant to dietary changes. This education component sets the stage for parents to try the novel approach provided by the behavioral intervention. This education about child behavior and meals is important because many of the behavior management techniques are counterintuitive, such as ignoring dawdling or complaining at meals. However, the parents in the NE group were not taught new strategies to manage child resistance and thus were most likely limited on what they could achieve in modifying their child's diet.

A third factor that is hypothesized to be critical to the success of the program is the intervention group for the children. In the BI condition, the children are directly accountable for their progress. The use of sticker charts and ingroup rewards for meeting calorie goals are hypothesized to increase the child's motivation to cooperate with the parents during meals as the parents are acquiring new management skills. Children in both the BI and NE conditions receive the same nutritional information and are given the same instructions to increase their energy intake. However, only the children in the BI condition earn stickers on a daily basis at home and must have 75% of their stickers to earn the trophy at the next treatment session. Parents in the BI condition often anecdotally report that their child was immediately more cooperative with meals and tried to eat more and different foods after beginning treatment. Parents, in turn, report feeling successful using the behavioral skills of differential attention and can clearly see the effects of contingency management. Thus, implementation of the behavioral techniques by the parents appear to be enhanced by direct intervention with the children in which contingency management is utilized in the treatment group.

CONCLUSIONS

Eating is a common everyday occurrence. Because everyone has experience with eating, the ability to change dietary patterns such as types of foods eaten or timing of meals may appear to be easy or something anyone could do with appropriate education. However, research would show that, in fact, diet is a lifestyle behavior that is resistant to modification (Martin & Dubbert, 1984). Education programs to modify diet have demonstrated changes in knowledge but little effect on behavior in healthy or chronically ill populations (Bell et al., 1984; Contento, Manning, & Shannon, 1992). In children with a chronic illness, diet modification may be further compromised by normal development of feeding and eating (Linscheid et al., 1995). As reviewed by Linschied et al. (1995), feeding typically proceeds from a parent-controlled situation to a shared parent–child-controlled situation. Children are expected to exhibit strong food preferences and demonstrate increased noncompliance between ages 1 to 2 years. It has been hypothesized that the way in which parents respond to these typical child behaviors influences whether such behaviors become problematic or are successfully negotiated between parent and child.

Dietary treatment recommendations such as mandated timing and type of food in diabetes, or increased volume in CF, may place the parent of a child with a chronic illness at a disadvantage in negotiating these common stages of feeding and child development. That is, the parent may feel so much pressure to meet the dietary recommendations or begin to define their job as a parent based on their child's food intake that they become overly reliant on less effective strategies such as substituting foods, coaxing (Crist et al., 1994), and/or feeding (Linscheid et al., 1995). Because meals occur several times daily, these patterns of interaction become overlearned and difficult to change. As reviewed here, we have found that children with CF exhibit similar types of behaviors in the mealtime situation as nonill children. However, parents of children with CF appear to differ from parents of nonill children in that they respond to these behaviors by extending the mealtime (Stark et al., 1995). This extended mealtime provides the setting for an increase in the frequency of both typical child and typical parent behaviors. Unfortunately, the extended mealtime and increase in typical parent behaviors does not appear effective in meeting the dietary recommendations. In fact, we hypothesize that the increased frequency of parent behaviors may inadvertently be maintaining the very child behaviors the parent is trying to change (i.e., food refusal, noncompliance with eating) by increasing the attention the parent gives to these behaviors.

Based on this hypothesis, we have developed an intervention designed to modify dietary patterns in children with CF that provides parents with training in specific skills to assist them in managing their child's resistance to dietary change and support them in the implementation of new skills as they are being acquired. As reviewed here, our pilot studies have shown intensive nutrition plus behavioral intervention to have a positive impact on caloric intake and weight. In our current multisite clinical trial comparing nutrition education plus behavioral child management to nutrition education alone (Stark et al., 1998), the addition of behavior therapy to nutrition education appears to maximize the effect of treatment. If these trends on caloric intake and weight gain continue, as additional data are collected, the importance of behavioral skill training in dietary treatment with children with CF will be better understood.

FUTURE RESEARCH DIRECTIONS

Although the current chapter focused on dietary adherence in CF, it is important to note that diet is part of almost all chronic illness regimens. It is unknown how generalizable the problems noted in dietary adherence in CF are to other illness populations. Assessment of dietary adherence in other pediatric illnesses has been limited by several factors. First, dietary behavior has typically been assessed as only one part of adherence to a multicomponent treatment regimen. Thus, specific problems and barriers to diet are rarely identified. As the current chapter illustrates, there may be specific difficulties associated with diet that warrant specific assessment of adherence and barriers to adherence to diet separate from assessment of adherence to medication. If knowledge about the role of diet in the treatment of chronic conditions and the prevention of disease is to advance, we need to understand the specific challenges that dietary recommendations bring forward for families of children.

Second, unlike adherence to some aspects of medical treatment for pediatric chronic illness, the impact of diet behaviors is often not evident for months or years even with excellent adherence. Thus, it is often difficult to measure the impact of dietary adherence on a short-term basis. Consequently, interventions to improve adherence to diet with long-term follow-up would advance our knowledge about the importance of diet to health in chronic illness. In addition, research needs to develop and evaluate the most efficacious method for delivering dietary treatment. For most diseases, dietary treatment is in the form of brief education sessions embedded in the context of a medical visit. Our current research on CF would indicate that such teaching is not optimal for modifying eating behaviors. The development and implementation of more intensive interventions that include parent training on behavioral child management skills should be evaluated in other illness populations. Finally, we need to go beyond treating problem adherence and investigate prevention. We are currently evaluating an early intervention program with young children with CF ages 6 months to 3 years that provides early behavioral intervention shortly after diagnosis (Powers et al., 1999). This intervention provides parents with education on the child's developmental level in regard to expected eating behaviors and behavioral management techniques to effectively intervene to meet dietary treatment recommendation before problem behaviors occur. Evaluation of early intervention and prevention of problematic mealtime behaviors through the behavioral skills teaching to parents may be useful in improving adherence to dietary treatment with other chronic illness populations as well and is an important area of future research.

REFERENCES

Bell, L., Durie, P., & Forstner, G. G. (1984). What do children with cystic fibrosis eat? *Journal of Pediatric Gastroenterology and Nutrition, 3*, S137–S146.
Bowen, A. M., & Stark, L. J. (1991). Malnutrition in cystic fibrosis: A behavioral conceptualization of cause and treatment. *Clinical Psychology Review, 11*, 315–331.
Buchdahl, R. M., Fullylove, C., Marchant, J. L., Warner, J. O., & Brueton, J. J. (1989). Energy and nutrient intakes in cystic fibrosis. *Archives of Diseases of Childhood, 64*, 373–378.
Carter, B. D., Kronenberger, W. G., & Conradsen, E. (1993, April). *Marital quality, parenting stress and compliance in families of children with cystic fibrosis.* Paper presented at the Florida conference on Child Health Psychology, Gainesville, FL.
Center for Disease Control. (1994). Prevalence of overweight among adolescents—United States. *Morbidity and Mortality Weekly Report, 43*, 818–821.
Chase, H. P., Long, M. A., & Lavin, M. H. (1979). Cystic fibrosis and malnutrition. *Journal of Pediatrics, 95*, 337–347.
Christiansen, C., Rodbro, P., & Throgen. (1975). Bone mineral content and estimated total body calcium in normal children and adolescents. *Scandinavian Journal of Laboratory and Clinical Investigation, 35*, 507–510.
Contento, I. R., Manning, A. D., & Shannon, B. (1992). Research perspective on school-based nutrition education. *Journal of Nutrition Education, 24*, 247–260.

Corey, M., McLaughlin, F. J., Williams, M., & Levison, H. (1988). A comparison of survival, growth, and pulmonary function in patients with cystic fibrosis in Boston and Toronto. *Journal of Clinical Epidemiology, 41*, 583–591.

Crist, W., McDonnell, P., Beck, M., Gillespie, C. T., Barrett, P., & Mathews, J. (1994). Behavior at mealtimes and nutritional intake in the young child with cystic fibrosis. *Developmental and Behavioral Pediatrics, 15*, 157–161.

Cystic Fibrosis Foundation. (1998, August). *Patient registry: 1997 annual data report.* Bethesda, MD: Author.

Daniels, L., Davidson, G. P., & Cooper, P. M. (1987). Assessment of nutrient intake of patients with cystic fibrosis compared with healthy children. *Human Nutrition: Applied Nutrition, 41A*, 151–159.

Epstein, L. H., Wing, R. R., Steranchak, L., Dickson, B., & Michelson, J. (1980). Comparison of family-based behavior modification and nutrition education for childhood obesity. *Journal of Pediatric Psychology, 5*, 25–35.

Ernst, N. D., & Obarzanek, E. (1994). Child health and nutrition: Obesity and high blood cholesterol. *Preventive Medicine, 23*, 427–436.

Forehand, R. L., & McMahon, R. J. (1981). *Helping the noncompliant child.* New York: Guilford.

Foster, S. W., & Farrell, P. M. (1996). Enhancing nutrition in cystic fibrosis with comprehensive therapies. *Journal of Pediatric Gastroenterology and Nutrition, 22*, 238–239.

Gortmaker, S. L., Dietz, W. H. J., Sobol, A. M., & Wehler, C. A. (1987). Increasing pediatric obesity in the United States. *American Journal of Diseases of Children, 141*, 535–540.

Gudas, L. J., Koocher, G. P., & Wypij, D. (1991). Perceptions of medical compliance in children and adolescents with cystic fibrosis. *Developmental and Behavioral Pediatrics, 12*, 236–242.

Gurwitz, D., Corey, M., Francis, P. S., Crozier, D., & Levison, H. (1979). Perspectives in cystic fibrosis. *Pediatric Clinics of North America, 26*, 603–615.

Handwerger, S., Roth, J., Gorden, P., DiSant'Agnese, P., Carpenter, D., & Peter, G. (1969). Glucose intolerance in cystic fibrosis. *New England Journal of Medicine, 281*, 451–461.

Henley, L. D., & Hill, I. D. (1990). Errors, gaps, and misconceptions in the disease-related knowledge of cystic fibrosis patients and their families. *Pediatrics, 85*, 1008–1014.

Hodges, P., Sauriol, D., Mann, S. F. P., Reichart, A., Grace, R. M., Talbot, T. W., Brown, N., & Thompson, A. B. R. (1984). Nutrient intake of patients with cystic fibrosis. *Journal of American Dietetic Association, 84*, 664–669.

Holsclaw, D. J. (1980). Cystic fibrosis: Overview and pulmonary aspects in young adults. *Clinics in Chest Medicine, 1*, 407–421.

Hubbard, V. S., & Mangrum, T. J. (1982). Energy intake and nutrition counseling in cystic fibrosis. *Journal of the American Dietetic Association, 80*, 127–131.

Jelalian, E., Stark, L. J., Reynolds, L., & Seifer, R. (1998). Nutrition intervention for weight gain in cystic fibrosis: A meta-analysis. *Journal of Pediatrics, 132*, 486–492.

Kinsman, S. L., Vining, E. P., Quaskey, S. A., Mellits, D., & Freeman, J. M. (1992). Efficacy of the ketogenic diet for intractable seizure disorders: Review of 58 cases. *Epilepsia, 33*, 1132–1136.

Koocher, G. P., McGrath, M. L., & Gudas, L. J. (1990). Typologies of nonadherence in cystic fibrosis. *Developmental and Behavioral Pediatrics, 11*, 353–358.

Kopelman, H. (1991). Gastrointestinal and nutritional aspects of cystic fibrosis. *Thorax, 46*, 261–267.

Kraemer, R., Rudeberg, A., Hadorn, B., & Rossi, E. (1978). Relative underweight in cystic fibrosis and its prognostic value. *Acta Paediatrica Scandanavica, 67*, 33–37.

Lester, L. A., Rothberg, R. M., Dawson, G., Lopez, A. L., & Corpuz, Z. (1986). Supplemental parenteral nutrition in cystic fibrosis. *Journal of Parenteral and Enteral Nutrition, 10*, 289–295.

Levy, L. D., Durie, P. R., Pencharz, P. B., & Corey, M. L. (1985). Effects of long term nutritional rehabilitation on body composition and clinical weight status in malnourished children and adolescents with cystic fibrosis. *Journal of Pediatrics, 107,* 225–230.

Linscheid, T. R., Budd, K. S., & Rasnake, L. K. (1995). Pediatric feeding disorders. In M. Roberts (Ed.), *Handbook of pediatric psychology* (2nd ed., pp. 501–515). New York: Guilford.

MacDonald, A., Holden, C., & Harris, G. (1991). Nutritional strategies in cystic fibrosis: Current issues. *Journal of the Royal Society of Medicine, 84*(Suppl. 18), 28–35.

Mansell, A. L., Anderson, J. C., Muttart, C. R., Ores, C. N., Loeff, D. S., Levy, J. S., & Heird, W. C. (1984). Short-term pulmonary effects of total parenteral nutrition in children with cystic fibrosis. *Journal of Pediatrics, 104,* 700–705.

Martin, J., & Dubbert, P. M. (1984). Behavioral management strategies for improving health and fitness. *Journal of Cardiac Rehabilitation, 4,* 200–208.

O'Rawe, A., McIntosh, I., Dodge, J. A., Brock, D. J. H., Redmond, O. B., Ward, R., & MacPherson, A. J. S. (1992). Increased energy expenditure in cystic fibrosis is associated with specific mutation. *Clinical Science, 82,* 71–76.

Palmer, S., & Horn, S. (1978). Feeding problems in children. In S. Palmer & S. Ekvall (Eds.), *Pediatric nutrition in developmental disorders* (pp. 107–129). Springfield, IL: Charles C. Thomas.

Park, R. W., & Grand, R. J. (1981). Gastrointestinal manifestations of cystic fibrosis: A review. *Gastroenterology, 81,* 1143–1161.

Parson, H. G., Beaudry, P., Dumas, A., & Pencharz, P. B. (1983). Energy needs and growth in children with cystic fibrosis. *Journal of Pediatric Gastroenterology and Nutrition, 2,* 44–49.

Powers, S. W., Schindler, T., Schwarber, L., Deeks, C., Byars, K., Zeller, M., Arthur, S., Piazza, C., & Johnson, M. J. (1999, April). *Increasing calorie intake in toddlers with cystic fibrosis.* Paper presented at the 7th annual Florida conference on Child Health Psychology, Gainesville, FL.

Quittner, A. L., DiGirolamo, A. M., & Winslow, E. B. (1991, April). *Problems in parenting a child with cystic fibrosis: A contextual analysis.* Paper presented at the Florida conference on Child Health Care Psychology, Gainesville, FL.

Ramsey, B., Farrell, P., & Pencharz, P. (1992). Nutritional assessment and management in cystic fibrosis: Consensus conference. *American Journal of Clinical Nutrition, 55,* 108–116.

Sanders, M. R., Patel, R. K., LeGrice, B., & Shepherd, R. W. (1993). Children with persistent feeding difficulties: An observational analysis of the feeding interactions of problem and non-problem eaters. *Health Psychology, 12,* 64–73.

Shepherd, R., Holt, P. T., Thomas, B. J., Kaye, L., Isles, A., Francis, P. J., & Ward, L. C. (1986). Nutritional rehabilitation in cystic fibrosis: Controlled studies of effects on nutritional growth retardation, body protein turnover, and course of pulmonary disease. *Journal of Pediatrics, 109,* 788–794.

Stark, L. J., Bowen, A. M., Tyc, V. L., Evans, S., & Passero, M. A. (1990). A behavioral approach to increasing calorie consumption in children with cystic fibrosis. *Journal of Pediatric Psychology, 15*(3), 309–326.

Stark, L. J., Jelalian, E., Mulvihill, M. M., Powers, S. W., Bowen, A. M., Spieth, L. E., Keating, K., Evans, S., Creveling, S., Harwood, I., Passero, M. A., & Hovell, M. F. (1995). Eating in preschool children with cystic fibrosis and healthy peers: A behavioral analysis. *Pediatrics, 95,* 210–215.

Stark, L. J., Jelalian, E., Powers, S. W., Mulvihill, M. M., Opipari, L. C., Bowen, A., Harwood, I., Passero, M. A., Lapey, A., Light, M., & Hovell, M. F. (in press). Parent and child mealtime behaviors in families of children with cystic fibrosis. *Journal of Pediatrics.*

Stark, L. J., Knapp, L., Bowen, A. M., Powers, S. W., Jelalian, E., Evans, S., Passero, M. A., Mulvihill, M. M., & Hovell, M. (1993). Behavioral treatment of calorie consumption in children with cystic fibrosis: Replication with two year follow-up. *Journal of Applied Behavior Analysis, 26,* 435–450.

Stark, L. J., Mulvihill, M. M., Jelalian, E., Bowen, A. M., Powers, S. W., Tao, S., Creveling, S., Passero, M. A., Harwood, I., Light, M., Lapey, A., & Hovell, M. F. (1997). Descriptive analysis of eating behavior in school-age children with cystic fibrosis and healthy control children. *Pediatrics, 99,* 665–671.

Stark, L. J., Mulvihill, M. M., Powers, S. W., Jelalian, E., Keating, K., Creveling, S., Brynes-Collins, B., Miller, D. L., Harwood, I., Passero, M. A., Light, M., & Hovell, M. (1996). Behavioral intervention to improve calorie intake of children with cystic fibrosis: Treatment vs. wait-list controls. *Journal of Pediatric Gastroenterology and Nutrition, 23,* 240–253.

Stark, L. J., Powers, S. W., Jelalian, E., Rape, R., & Miller, D. L. (1994). Modifying problematic mealtime interactions of children with cystic fibrosis and their parents via behavioral parent training. *Journal of Pediatric Psychology, 19,* 751–768.

Stark, L. J., & Quittner, A. L. (1996). Behavioral treatment of weight gain in cystic fibrosis. *NIH Grant #R01 50092.*

Stark, L. J., Quittner, A. L., Opipari, L. C., Jelalian, E., Jones, E., Powers, S. W., Higgins, L., Maguiness, K., Seidner, D., Hoover, J., Eigan, H., Duggan, C. P., & Stallings, V. (1998, October). The contribution of behavior therapy to enhancing adherence in school age children with CF: The example of diet. In J. Glassner (Chair), *Innovative approaches to CF education.* North American Cystic Fibrosis Conference, Toronto, Canada.

Tomezsko, J. L., Stallings, V., & Scanlin, T. F. (1992). Dietary intake of healthy children with cystic fibrosis campared with normal control children. *Pediatrics, 90,* 547–553.

CHAPTER NINETEEN

Promoting Adherence to Growth Hormone Therapy Among Children With Growth Failure

David E. Sandberg
Tom A. Mazur
Rebecca A. Hazen
Dana E. Alliger
John Buchlis
Margaret H. MacGillivray
Children's Hospital of Buffalo, Buffalo, NY

There are numerous causes of short stature (Lifshitz & Cervantes, 1996). A breakdown by diagnosis of children referred to pediatric endocrinologists for a growth evaluation suggests that approximately half exhibit normal variants of short stature (i.e., height that falls below the conventional cutoff of −2.0 height standard deviations [*SD*s]), but show normal growth increments that parallel growth channels for the general population (Lifshitz & Cervantes, 1996; Sandberg, Brook, & Campos, 1994). In the category of pathological causes of short stature, growth hormone deficiency (GHD) stands out as a key endocrinologically based cause of poor growth.

A major objective of growth hormone (GH) therapy is to accelerate growth velocity during childhood and adolescence to achieve an adult height commensurate with estimated genetic potential. Because the sole source of GH prior to 1985 was cadaveric pituitaries, there was never a sufficient supply available to adequately meet the needs of children with GHD. The treatment was therefore restricted to children with the most severe and unequivocal GHD. The diagnosis of GHD was based then, as it is today, on the level of GH released from the pituitary in response to pharmacological stimulation. With the introduction of biosynthetic GH and its unlimited supplies, the GH cutoff for making the diagnosis has crept higher from <3–5 ng/dl to today's conventionally accepted level of <10ng/dl (Allen, Johanson, & Blizzard, 1996). Although the threshold for initiating treatment has been lowered, current practice remains consistent with the long-standing tradition in endocrinology of providing hormone replacement when endogenous production is deficient.

GH availability ensures that children who are deficient in this hormone will have adequate access to replacement therapy. It has also created the opportunity to treat various patient groups with growth failure and short stature who test GH-sufficient. As time passes, some of these newer, nontraditional applications are gradually becoming the standard of care in the United States (Lippe & Nakamoto, 1993).

The treatment of short, GH-sufficient youths is predicated on the widespread belief that GH-induced increases in height will improve the child's psychological adjustment (Sandberg, 1996b). Moreover, it is thought that increased growth will reduce or eliminate the at-risk status of these individuals for the development of future problems. Children's complaints of stature-related psychosocial stresses, and the prevalent societal belief about the disadvantages of short stature, have all contributed to the broadening use of this relatively intensive, chronic, and costly hormonal intervention (Cuttler et al., 1996).

At present in the United States, the use of GH in GH-sufficient youths exceeds the number of GHD-treated patients (Allen et al., 1996). This aspect of clinical practice remains controversial, however (Allen et al., 1996; Guyda, 1998). There are a number of assumptions implicit in the psychological rationale for GH therapy in nontraditional applications. First, it is believed that short stature exerts a strong negative influence on children's psychosocial and psychoeducational adaptation (Sandberg, 1996b). The research evidence in support of this assumption is equivocal, however. Most recent studies of clinic-referred (Skuse, Gilmour, Tian, & Hindmarsh, 1994; Sandberg et al., 1994; Sandberg & Michael, 1998; Zimet et al., 1995) and community samples of youths with short stature (Downie, Mulligan, Stratford, Betts, & Voss, 1997; Vance, Ingersoll, & Golden, 1994; Wilson et al., 1986) have failed to detect significant deficits in adaptation, although there continue to be sporadic reports to the contrary (e.g., Stabler et al., 1994, 1998).

A second assumption implied by the practice of providing GH therapy to poorly growing, GH-sufficient children is that hormone-induced increases in growth velocity will result in improved psychological adaptation. Here, too, the clinical research literature provides contradictory findings. For example, in a well-controlled study of the psychological response to GH treatment of 15 children with GH-sufficient short stature, investigators did not detect statistically significant effects on IQ, educational performance, behavior problems, or self-concept at baseline, after 3 years, or after 5 years of treatment. This is compared with either untreated short children or a group of average stature control subjects (10th to 90th percentiles) who were all drawn from the same school-based sample as the treated group (Downie et al., 1996). This absence of group differences was observed despite substantial improvements in growth and height in the GH-treated group (from −2.44 to −1.21 heights SDs) over 5 years of treatment.

In a much larger study (N = 131) of the psychological benefits of GH therapy in GHD and GH-sufficient youths with short stature, Stabler and colleagues (1998) detected statistically significant decreases in parent-reported behavior problems of both groups early in the 3-year course of treatment. In contrast, academic achievement test scores and rates of school problems did not change significantly. Interestingly, the decline in behavior problems was not correlated with change in height SDs over the 3 years of treatment (from −2.59/−2.84 to −1.28/−1.39 for the GHD and GH-sufficient short youths, respectively). Clouding interpretation of these findings was the absence of an adequate control group and sole reliance on parents as informants of the child's behavioral adaptation.

Although the rationale behind GH therapy is essential in clinical deliberations regarding the costs/risks versus benefits of treatment, the medical and psychological underpinnings for this treatment are not the focus here. Instead, the work described herein is concerned with adherence to the GH treatment regimen across patient groups with a range of diagnoses. Despite the controversy over the clinical indications for GH therapy and its high cost, relatively little clinical research has been directed toward the question of treatment adherence. This is surprising considering the first-hand experience that most pediatric endocrinologists have with problems of adherence in the clinical management of insulin-dependent diabetes mellitus (IDDM; Johnson, 1995). This chapter is concerned with a summary of what is known about GH treatment adherence, how it might be improved, and whether there are ways to enhance satisfaction with treatment that, in turn, would improve adherence.

FEATURES OF GH THERAPY

Although taller adult height in poorly growing children is predicted by initiation of treatment at a younger age, most children with isolated GHD begin therapy around 10 to 11 years of age when the condition is first diagnosed. Once started on therapy, the mean duration of treatment is 5 to 6 years, and the treatment involves daily or near daily subcutaneous injections (Blethen et al., 1997). In addition to the injections, children typically undergo a pretreatment MRI of the head and annual bone-age X-ray to assess skeletal maturation. Once treatment has started, patients typically return to clinic at 3-month intervals to assess growth velocity and modify the dose of hormone injected based on changes in body weight.

Blood tests are intermittently ordered. One feature of GH therapy that has drawn considerable attention, and that has fueled the treat-or-not-to treat debate is its high cost. The annual cost of treatment is approximately $28,000 for a child weighing 40 kg (Abramowicz, 1994).

STUDIES OF ADHERENCE TO THE GH THERAPY REGIMEN

There are reports that adherence to the GH therapy treatment regimen is far from perfect. In one of the first and most notable studies on this topic, British investigators reported that slightly over half of the patients were showing either intermittent or poor adherence as indicated by the number of self-reported missed injections. Confusion about dosage was a major limiting factor. Only 40% of the individuals responsible for giving the GH injection had an adequate understanding of the treatment (Smith, Hindmarsh, & Brook, 1993). These investigators identified family knowledge regarding GH treatment as a robust predictor of treatment adherence. Thus, families who were most knowledgeable about the treatment (focusing on the individual in the home responsible for administering injections) showed the highest degree of adherence.

The importance of adequate knowledge regarding details of the treatment regimen was underscored by Stanhope and colleagues (Stanhope, Moyle, & McSwiney, 1993) in a separate study also conducted in the United Kingdom. In their review of 107 consecutive children receiving GH therapy, understanding of the regimen exceeded 90%. Even so, as many as 10% admitted missing three or more injections per month. This apparent relative success over that reported by Smith and colleagues (1993) was attributed to providing the families with an unrestricted choice of GH injection devices as well as the availability of a dedicated growth research nurse to teach families about the regimen and assist in maintaining adherence over the long term.

Similar (low) rates of missed injections (3.4% of the sample missed between 5% and 10% of their injections since their last clinic visit and 2.5% missed greater that 10% of injections) were recently reported in a study conducted in Spain of 473 patients (Oyarzabal et al., 1998). Close to 60% of patients and/or relatives, however, stated that they would like to receive more information on GH treatment.

In a different Spanish study of 88 patients receiving GH therapy, investigators reported that patients' (8 years and older) knowledge of regimen details was poorer than their compliance with the treatment (López Siguero, Martinez Aedo, López Moreno, & Martínez Valverde, 1995). Approximately 40% of the children were incorrect in their knowledge of the prescribed volume they were supposed to inject, and close to 6%

reported having missed more than five injections since their last clinic visit. The vast majority were inaccurate in their knowledge of the volume of water needed to be added to the GH powder in preparation for injection. These statistics are worrisome in view of the fact that 43% of the children and adolescents reported *I do it myself*—referring to the injection of GH. Finally, the investigators reported that both the knowledge of therapy and adherence to the regimen were significantly higher among those patients who had attended a workshop on growth problems and specifically on GH treatment.

Considering factors other than knowledge of the treatment regimen, Gács and Hosszu (1991) in a chart review study examined the role of family and individual characteristics prior to initiating therapy as predictors of adherence to the GH treatment regimen. These investigators reported in a sample of 78 patients with GHD that higher paternal educational background predicted younger age at referral for evaluation and treatment of growth failure and better adherence to GH therapy recommendations. There also tended to be a higher proportion of girls in the poorly adherent group. (Insufficient information in the medical chart precluded investigating the influence of maternal education.)

Although not specifically designed to assess adherence in GH therapy, studies examining the comparative acceptability to patients and families of different GH delivery systems (e.g., conventional syringe and needle, pen injector, or Auto Injector) have shown that levels of convenience and pain vary across delivery systems (Gluckman & Cutfield, 1991; Stanhope, Albanese, Moyle, & Hamill, 1992). The authors quite appropriately imply a relationship among convenience and comfort and adherence to treatment recommendations, although these studies did not examine the question directly.

Authorities in the area of treatment adherence would not find it surprising that a high level of treatment adherence is predicated on a solid knowledge base. It is also clear that knowledge alone is generally insufficient to ensure strong adherence (Meichenbaum & Turk, 1987). Adherence is a complex phenomenon, and the perceived and anticipated psychosocial liabilities associated with short stature, along with beliefs and expectations regarding the benefits of treatment, are likely to influence adherence and satisfaction with treatment. These additional constructs have not been linked in empirical investigations of GH treatment adherence.

None of the studies described herein, nor any other published reports that we are aware of, assess adherence behaviors more directly. For instance, all data concerning the number of missed injections is based on parents' self-reports. An alternative strategy that heretofore has not been utilized would be to count empty vials at follow-up visits and compare this number against that calculated assuming full adherence to the injection regimen. Although an improvement over self-report alone, such counting of permanent products is not foolproof (La Greca & Schuman, 1995). An additional factor further complicating interpretation of adherence data in GH therapy stems from the practice of having clinical staff directly involved in the child's treatment either interview or administer questionnaires to patients (or their parents). This arrangement may unduly bias results in the direction of higher reported adherence. Only one study (Oyarzabal et al., 1998) had nurses observe patients' injection technique to assess competency. Even here, accuracy in dosing was not ascertained. Clearly more systematic and detailed studies of adherence to specific aspects of the GH treatment regimen, including attempts at validating patient/parent reports, are needed.

An important means of assessing adherence is in terms of clinical outcome. In other words, if the GH-treated youth exhibits clinical benefit by an observed narrowing of his or her height deficit, it might be assumed that the patient/family was adherent (Meichenbaum & Turk, 1987). Although relationships among dose of GH, frequency of injections, growth velocity, and adult height have been shown (Allen et al., 1996), there are many factors (e.g., timing of onset, tempo of puberty) that could invalidate these relationships in the individual case.

ADHERENCE IN GH THERAPY: SHOULD
WE ANTICIPATE PROBLEMS?

There are potentially several factors, in addition to limited knowledge of the child's medical condition and details of the treatment regimen, that may serve to reduce adherence to GH therapy. Youths prescribed GH in this new era of treatment (and their families) face daily burdens associated with therapy. First, there are the challenges associated with daily (or almost daily) injections of the hormone. This treatment recommendation represents a significant increase in treatment intensity over the previous three injections per week commonly adopted in the pituitary derived era of hormone replacement therapy (Allen et al., 1996). In addition to the increased time commitment involved, fear of needles and injections is common in a pediatric population (McGrath, 1990), which could serve as a barrier to adherence in a characteristically nonlife-threatening medical condition. Furthermore, the negative influence of this factor can become amplified among those individuals in which the parent, who is often responsible for administering GH, personally shares such fears (Gittelman, 1986; McGrath, 1990).

An additional factor that should be considered in the context of adherence to the GH therapy treatment regimen is patient and parental expectations regarding the anticipated benefits of therapy. Even with the current advantages of unlimited supplies of GH and improved dosing and injection regimens, the adult height of treated GHD patients falls below the mean for the general population (−1.6 to −0.7 height SDs; Blethen et al., 1997). The same is true for GH-sufficient clinical groups (e.g., Turner syndrome; Rosenfeld et al., 1998; idiopathic growth failure; Cowell, 1997; Hintz, Attie, Baptista, & Roche, 1999; Kawai et al., 1997). It has been reported that both patient and family expectations for improvements in relative height with GH therapy are typically unrealistically high (Grew, Stabler, Randall, Williams, & Underwood, 1983; Kusalic & Fortin, 1975). This tendency could result in a sense of disappointment and frustration when expectations for growth have not been fully realized, further complicating adherence to this long-term treatment.

Although not a common reason for nonadherence with GH therapy, our clinical experience has shown us that some patients interpret the recommendation for treatment as an expression of parental dissatisfaction with the child's physical appearance (e.g., "My mother doesn't want me to be short"). There are other children, in special circumstances, who express the belief that increased height will jeopardize their excellence in a particular sport (e.g., gymnastics) or otherwise threaten the social niche they have created for themselves, in which short stature offers certain social benefits. This latter state has been referred to as the *readjustment syndrome* (Money & Pollitt, 1966).

More generically, individual differences in patient behavioral and emotional functioning may facilitate or interfere with GH treatment (e.g., Kusalic & Fortin, 1975) as they do in adherence to any extended regimen. In studies of children with medical disorders not specifically involving growth failure, children with more positive self-esteem and fewer behavioral or emotional problems exhibit better adherence (Hanson et al., 1989; Korsch, Fine, & Negrete, 1978). The patient's level of understanding of the need to closely follow the prescribed treatment regimen is an additional factor that significantly determines adherence, in particular for adolescents (La Greca & Schuman, 1995).

Parental emotional distress and family functioning undoubtedly play an important role in the child's medical management. The medical treatment, including follow-up visits to the hospital, may require significant changes in family routine and thereby serve as a stressor. Several studies have demonstrated that families experiencing conflict do not typically support positive treatment adherence (Hauser et al., 1990). Parents' level of understanding of the child's medical condition and knowledge regarding the treatment regimen are additional family factors that predict the degree of adherence to the medical regimen, particularly for younger children (La Greca, Follansbee, & Skyler, 1990).

The costs of GH therapy nonadherence on the child and family, health care provider, and health care system (in particular third-party payers) are

complex. For the patient, chronic nonadherence, or potentially even intermittent nonadherence during particularly crucial phases of growth, can
result in an attenuation of adult height with associated disappointment
and emotional distress related to the limited outcome of the therapy.
Among those individuals for whom GH therapy is only one aspect of a
more comprehensive regimen of hormone replacement (as in the case of
pan-hypopituitarism), dissatisfaction with the final results of therapy could
jeopardize adherence to other lifelong and life-preserving aspects of
patient health care. In those families in which treatment nonadherence is
conceptualized as one consequence of poorly adaptive family functioning,
failure in following the recommended treatment guidelines could serve to
reinforce already negative perceptions held by family members regarding
their ability to constructively problem solve.

From the clinician's perspective, concealed nonadherence (with associated poor treatment response) can result in confusion regarding the accuracy of the child's medical diagnosis and suitability of the recommendation of GH therapy. In the contrasting situation in which nonadherence is
either openly disclosed or can be inferred by such physical evidence such
as unused prescriptions, physicians may develop a sense of frustration
with patients and families who are perceived as consciously jeopardizing
the effectiveness of an elective but extremely costly therapy during a period in which *cost-containment* is the watchword of the health care industry. The associated mistrust on the part of the medical staff can subsequently threaten the integrity of the collaborative relationship that must
be maintained to ensure optimal health care within that subgroup of
patients requiring lifelong care.

Because nonadherence to GH therapy is only atypically associated with
medical sequelae requiring additional medical services such as emergency
room or inpatient hospitalization, insurers of medical services will not
encounter additional financial costs. On the contrary, poor adherence—in
the extreme case resulting in premature termination of treatment—would
result in cost savings. This situation is markedly different from other
endocrine disorders such as diabetes mellitus or hypo/hyperthyroidism in
which nonadherence would potentially result in increased health care
costs both in the short and long term.

APPLICATIONS OF THE HEALTH BELIEF MODEL
TO GH THERAPY ADHERENCE

Estimates of treatment nonadherence for a variety of ailments (both acute
and chronic) in pediatric populations is considered to be quite high (Eney
& Goldstein, 1976). To take into account the multiplicity of factors pro-

ducing variability in treatment adherence, several health behavior models have been generated. Possibly the best known among these is the Health Belief Model (Becker et al., 1978). An interpretation of the Health Belief Model as applied to the instance of GH therapy predicts that treatment adherence is dependent on: (a) the individual's (and/or parents') belief that the child's present height deficit will persist and/or intensify over time without medical intervention; (b) the perceived seriousness for the patient (and/or family) of short stature at present and/or in the future; and (c) the patient and parental belief that GH therapy, if adhered to as recommended, will yield significant increases in growth velocity and relative height. Factors that interfere with treatment adherence are conceptualized as barriers and, in the case of GH therapy, may include fear of needles, unfulfilled expectations regarding treatment effects, behavioral and emotional problems of the child, family discord, and parental psychopathological symptoms. Overall, enhanced adherence to the GH treatment regimen would be predicted in cases in which the anticipated benefits of therapy exceed the burdens.

Intervention approaches that have yielded improved treatment adherence in a range of pediatric conditions include: education of the patient and family regarding the justification and importance of treatment along with the development of new behavioral skills for successful treatment implementation, interventions emphasizing monitoring and supervision, and the use of rewards to the patient for cooperation with treatment adherence (La Greca & Schuman, 1995).

With the limited research base concerning adherence in GH therapy, in conjunction with the controversy that surrounds treatment of particular patient subgroups (i.e., medical indications and costs), we wanted to learn how closely patients and parents follow specific treatment recommendations—most notably, the regularity of injections and accuracy in dosing. An additional objective of our work was to identify predictors of enhanced adherence. Finally, we set as a goal the development of a psychoeducational intervention designed to improve adherence and increase satisfaction with treatment results. To the best of our knowledge, there are as yet no published studies of a clinical intervention designed to optimize adherence to GH therapy.

STUDY DESIGN AND DESCRIPTION OF INTERVENTION

On obtaining written informed consent, the (ongoing) study commences with a pretreatment assessment of the child's psychosocial adaptation and aspects of family functioning using both the patient and parent as informants (Table 19.1). Questionnaires are administered and their completion

TABLE 19.1
Study Design and Methods

Pretreatment Assessment		Intervention	3-Month Assessment	6-Month Follow-Up Assessment
Patient Report	*Parent Report*			
	Experiences Related to Height and GH Therapy Questionnaire (patient and parent versions)	Psychoeducational Intervention *plus* Standard of Care		Readministration of pretreatment assessment
Youth Self-Report	Child Behavior Checklist		Empty vial count and nursing evaluation	Empty vial count and nursing evaluation
Self-Perception Profile		Standard of Care		
	Family Assessment Device			
	Brief Symptom Inventory			

supervised by a research staff person not involved in the child's clinical care to minimize one source of potential response bias. This is followed by a stratified randomization of 40 patients each to either the three-session Psychoeducational Intervention plus Standard of Care group or a group that only receives the Standard of Care preparation for therapy. GH treatment begins immediately thereafter.

Adherence is monitored at the routine 3-month follow-up visit through an empty vial count and nursing evaluation. At 6 months, the patient and parent are reassessed using the pretreatment protocol, with only minor changes, including a patient and parent report of adherence during the preceding 3-month interval since their last endocrine clinic visit. An empty vial count is repeated as is the nursing evaluation to assess adherence to various aspects of the regimen. Families are provided two $25 participation payments—one at the time of the pretreatment assessment and again after completing the 6-month follow-up.

Table 19.2 summarizes the topics that a pediatric psychologist covers with patients and their parents over the three sessions of the psychoedu-

TABLE 19.2
Psychoeducational Intervention to Enhance Adherence to GH Therapy

Session Number	Overview of Content

1. Growth disorders and their treatment	Correct name and implications of child's diagnosis
	Causes of growth disorder
	Biological control of growth (handouts provided)
	Patient/parent expectations for . . .
	    short-term (3 months) growth and adult height
	    changes in social/emotional function
	    educational improvements
	Importance of active involvement and good adherence in successful treatment outcome
	Introduction to relaxation techniques (handouts with homework assigned)

2. Preparation for GH injections	Review topics/answer questions from Session 1 Assess patients' competency with relaxation exercises In vivo rehearsal of injection procedure (using saline) Discussion of side effects of GH Discussion of strategies to reduce GH treatment burden
3. Monitoring of adherence and contingency management	Review topics/answer questions from Session 2 Reassess competency with relaxation techniques Introduction of GH therapy contract (instruction guide provided) Instructions to contact nurse/psychologist immediately in event of problems/concerns (*Coping with Negative Experiences* form provided) Educational pamphlet regarding GH therapy provided

cational intervention. The Health Belief Model, as applied to GH therapy, was used to guide the development and goals of the intervention sessions with the specific content drawn from our own clinical experience and that of others (for review, see Meyer-Bahlburg, 1990).

Each session lasts approximately 1 hour. During Session 1, parent(s) and the child are familiarized with the correct name and implications of the diagnosis; they are informed of the cause of the growth disorder and, in general, the factors that control physical growth. The family's expectations for short-term (3 months) and long-term growth (i.e., adult height) and the possible influences that this therapeutic effect will have on their child's psychosocial and educational adjustment are reviewed; the importance of strong adherence to the details of the regimen are underscored, and the session ends with a brief demonstration (following manual; Cautela & Groden, 1978) of relaxation techniques that the child immediately rehearses during the session. The parent is instructed to supervise the child's practice of the relaxation exercises (following excerpts from the manual) in the interval between Sessions 1 and 2. These same relaxation techniques are to be applied prior to receiving the daily GH injection once treatment begins.

The material covered in the first session is reviewed at the outset of Session 2, and the competency of the parent–child team in performing the relaxation exercises is assessed. With the child in a physically relaxed state, in vivo practice is provided in receiving as well as giving a saline injection. An endocrinologist or pediatric endocrine fellow supervises this aspect of the procedure. The parent is also given the opportunity to practice their injection technique and to receive a saline injection administered by the child. (It should be noted that the children particularly enjoy the opportunity to inject their parent prior to receiving one themselves.) With the endocrinologist present, the topic of potential side effects from the treatment is covered. Finally, a discussion follows in which strategies designed to reduce the burden associated with the GH treatment regimen are reviewed. For example, families are encouraged to incorporate the child's GH injection to their bedtime ritual or, in general, to give the injection at the same time each day to reduce the likelihood that an avoidance strategy develops.

Session 3 begins with a review of earlier material, and the child's competency with the relaxation techniques is reassessed. A key component of this final session is the introduction of the GH therapy contract, which is designed along the lines of a home token economy (Alvord, 1973). Target behaviors include assisting the parent in preparing the GH for injection, accepting the injection, and completing the injection procedure within 3 minutes. Tokens or points are earned for each behavior and points are lost when the child tries to postpone or resist receiving the injection. The points earned are used for mutually agreed on privileges. Parents are encouraged to incorporate behaviors unrelated to the GH treatment into the contract to reduce the salience of the therapy. Behavior management strategies similar to these have been effectively used in other chronic pediatric conditions (e.g., da Costa, Rapoff, Lemanek, & Goldstein, 1997).

At the end of the third training session, the family is strongly encouraged to contact the health care team immediately in the event that they encounter problems. We have found that families can tolerate obstacles to treatment for quite a long time before contacting medical staff. To facilitate the early detection of problems, families are provided with a *GH Injections: Coping with Negative Experiences* form to document difficulties encountered and indicate what steps they took in their attempt to remedy these. Finally, families are provided with the brochure *Growth Hormone Treatment: What to Expect* (Parker & Rieser, 1996), which serves the dual purpose of providing anticipatory guidance as well as an introduction to a national support organization for individuals with growth disorders and their families.

After completing the psychoeducational intervention, all patients (i.e., those who had received the intervention and those who had not) spend between 1 and 2 hours with an endocrine nurse specialist to review the guidelines for drawing up and injecting GH, as well as to discuss expected effects and potential side effects of treatment. A video demonstration of proper injection techniques is included. The first GH injection is given at this time. This session represents the standard of care in our clinic for many years.

Table 19.1 lists the methods employed in the study. The pretreatment assessment includes the *Experiences Related to Height & GH Therapy Questionnaire* (Sandberg, 1996a), which was designed to collect information useful in making predictions concerning adherence based on the Health Belief Model. The Experiences questionnaire is completed by patients 8 years and older (occasionally with the assistance of research staff) and, in all cases, by a parent. Topics covered include: the degree to which the child's short stature is experienced as a problem; the extent to which the parent or child anticipate that GH will remedy problems of psychosocial adaptation; and potential barriers to the treatment procedures such as fear of needles and injections (Table 19.3). The follow-up version of the questionnaire includes a section for both patients and parents concerned with specifics of the GH therapy regimen. Development of certain sections of the *Experiences* questionnaire drew heavily on items from another instrument designed to assess the psychosocial adaptation of youths with short stature (Haverkamp & Noeker, 1998; Noeker & Haverkamp, 1994).

The Youth Self-Report (YSR; Achenbach, 1991a) and Child Behavior Checklist (CBCL; Achenbach, 1991b) provide self- and parent-report infor-

TABLE 19.3

Experiences Related to Height and GH Therapy Questionnaire

Samples of Content[a]

Domains	Patient Version	Parent Version
School	Not assessed in patient version	Has your child experienced any school adjustment problems since kindergarten that you believe are due to his/her height? Did your child have to repeat a grade? How does the school performance of this child compare to that of his/her brothers/sisters?
Experiences related to short stature	Are you currently having any problems that you think are connected to your height? Which worries are more of a concern to you when you think about your height? Present ones? Future ones? I am quickly overlooked by my friends I am embarrassed whenever my height is discussed I have a strong desire to be taller If I do not succeed in something, I often think it's because of my height Does anyone tease you these days because you are shorter than most children your age? Do you think that people treat you as if you are younger than your age?	In addition to asking the same questions from the parents' perspective, this section includes: Is your child *currently* being seen at a child guidance clinic or other mental health agency? For evaluation by a psychologist or psychiatrist? If yes, were the reasons related to your child's height? Has your child ever been seen by a mental health professional?
Medical aspects of growth problem	How do you feel when you go to the doctor and get physical examinations? What is/are the specific name(s) of your growth disorder? What is/are the cause(s) of the growth disorder?	Generally the same questions but from the parents' perspective

What height do you think you will likely reach as an adult without GH therapy? With GH therapy?

In your opinion, what are the chances that you would grow to an acceptable adult height even without GH therapy?

Who will be responsible for giving the GH shots?

Which of the following worries/concerns do you have regarding GH therapy (e.g., blood tests, the shots, side effects, uncertainty of success/failure of the therapy, cost of the treatment)?

How disappointed would the individual members of your family be if the result of GH therapy were unsatisfactory (you're not happy with your growth)? Father, mother, brothers/sisters? Myself?

The following are situations that some people say makes them scared or nervous. Circle those that best describe how scared or nervous you are of them:

    having to go to the hospital

    getting a shot

    the sight of blood

    going to the doctor

Growth hormone therapy regimen

(included in *Follow-Up* version—patient/parent—only)

Which GH do you take?

How many milligrams of GH are in each bottle that you get?

How much diluent (water) is put in each vial of GH? (diagram of syringe provided for participant to shade in response)

How many units of GH are in each shot that you get? (diagram of syringe provided)

How often do you take GH?

Who is usually in charge of remembering that it is time for a GH shot?

Generally the same questions but from the parents' perspective

(Continued)

TABLE 19.3 *(Continued)*

Samples of Content[a]

Domains	Patient Version	Parent Version
	Who is responsible for giving the GH injection?	
	Sometimes people find parts of the GH injections hard to do.	
	How difficult do you find the following parts of the injection to be?	
	mixing	
	drawing up	
	putting needle in	
	pressing down on the plunger	
	other, describe:	
	How long does it take once the syringe is prepared to actually give the treatment?	
	Overall, how willingly do you take the GH injections?	
	How much do you agree with the following statement? *I am in pain when I receive the GH shot.*	
	How many times have you missed an injection since your last endocrine visit?	
	How much of a hassle are the GH injections?	
	Have you told any of your friends that you are receiving GH?	
	If you had a friend who was considering GH treatment, how likely would you be to recommend GH treatment?	

[a]Items are paraphrased. Response options are preformulated and vary from dichotomous to multipoint scales with the opportunity, in specific cases, to clarify through open-ended response.

mation, respectively, concerning the child's social competencies and behavioral/emotional problems. The YSR is administered to patients 11 years or older. The Self-Perception Profile (Harter, 1985, 1988) assesses the child's/adolescent's appraisals of domain-specific competencies and is interpreted as an index of self-concept. The Family Assessment Device (Epstein, Baldwin, & Bishop, 1983) was included to provide information concerning aspects of family functioning such as problem-solving capacity, emotional involvement and responsiveness, and general functioning. Finally, the Brief Symptom Inventory (Derogatis, 1993) was introduced to obtain information concerning emotional distress experienced by the primary caregiver.

PREDICTIONS AND PRELIMINARY FINDINGS

According to elements of the Health Belief Model (Becker et al., 1978), as applied to the GH treatment experience, it is predicted that adherence to the regimen is enhanced if the child's short stature is perceived as a problem. Better adherence is also predicted when the parent and child exhibit a positive psychological adaptation in general and in families showing healthier functioning as a unit. Greater fear of medical procedures (in the child and/or parent) is predicted to exert a negative influence on adherence, as are unrealistic treatment expectations. Feelings of disappointment, frustration, or anger can be triggered by unmet expectations, regardless of whether they are realistic, and they can result in the child giving up. Examples of unrealistic claims regarding the growth-promoting effects of GH can easily be found in newspaper and magazine articles. A front page story published in the *Sun* tabloid claimed, "Growth Hormone Goes Wild. Girl Grows 2 ft. Overnight. We Had to Tilt Photo to Get it on the Page" ("Growth Hormone Goes Wild," 1990, p. 1). A photo of a young girl occupying the full diagonal length of the front page accompanied the headline. Although tabloids such as the *Sun* are not generally considered to be reliable interpreters of medical breakthroughs, they draw a wide readership, including children and adolescents, if only at retail checkout counters. Such obviously inaccurate reports possibly serve to generate or reinforce unrealistic expectations regarding the prospects for growth during therapy. Compare this claim of "2 ft. Overnight" to the actual 7 to 10 centimeters per year that children are likely to achieve while on GH. It would not be surprising to child psychologists to learn that an 8-year-old receiving GROWTH hormone would be thinking in terms of *feet* grown during treatment rather than *centimeters* and would expect whatever changes take place to occur rapidly.

Finally, we make the (unsurprising) prediction that incomplete or inaccurate knowledge about the child's condition or therapy can contribute to poor adherence. Beyond the knowledge required to accurately dilute and inject the GH, false or misleading information about other aspects of the therapy could result in ambivalence toward the treatment, which potentially manifests itself as poorer adherence. For example, as already noted, it is not difficult to find reports about GH in the popular media. Unfortunately, GH's performance-enhancing properties are highlighted and, with it, the potential for negative side effects when illicitly used by adults. *Sports Illustrated* published an article dealing with the abuse of drugs among athletes. The cover page showed a picture of a former (now deceased) football star. The caption read: "I Lied. Former NFL star Lyle Alzado now admits to massive use of steroids and human growth hormone and believes that they caused his inoperable brain cancer" ("I Lied," 1991, p. 1). Regardless of the accuracy of this athlete's attributions regarding his cancer, such stories, of which there are ever-increasing numbers in the media (e.g., rumors have circulated regarding the role of GH and the abuse of anabolic steroids as contributing factors in the recent death of Florence Griffith Joyner, U.S. Olympic track star), may contribute to unwarranted fears and uncertainty about GH therapy.

At the time of this writing, data collection for this study is ongoing and findings pertaining to the outlined hypotheses are not yet available. Nevertheless, we have made some informal observations that are of interest. First, approximately 10% of patients could not be randomly assigned to the psychoeducational intervention or standard care groups because of preexisting emotional or behavioral problems or because of fear of medical procedures. An example of such a case would be a child showing chronic behavior management problems secondary to high levels of negative life events within the household in combination with parents exhibiting limited childrearing skills. Because these problems were expected to interfere with adherence to the treatment regimen, psychologists in our program immediately provided a behavioral intervention before initiating GH treatment. We wonder what would happen at other centers around the country where pediatric psychological services are not as readily available for consultation or provide ongoing care to patients treated by endocrinologists. Certainly we would expect that the adherence to treatment among these children would be quite poor without intervention and that the GH treatment would serve as an additional major stressor for the child and household.

From the perspective of the nurses providing the education on how to prepare and inject GH (i.e., Standard of Care), the task of training has been made much simpler and completed more efficiently in those families that had previously received the psychoeducational intervention. The intervention was accepted by medical staff thereby eliminating one potential barrier to its introduction as a routine procedure, should the findings from this study support its continued application. Further, information gathered with the *Experiences* questionnaire at the 6-month follow-up may be useful to medical staff by highlighting gaps in the initial acquisition of knowledge of the GH treatment regimen or decline in memory for some details. The requirement that families make additional hospital visits was found to be logistically feasible for the majority, providing further evidence that a brief psychological intervention prior to initiating treatment, at a minimum, is accepted by patients and families.

It would be misleading to give the impression that implementing the psychoeducational intervention has not at times been challenging. First, the scheduling of patients for three sessions during the occasionally brief window of time between the physician recommending GH therapy and initiating treatment requires that there be close coordination between research staff and endocrinology nurses. In our case, psychologists and other health care staff in the endocrine program experience the advantage of a long-standing collaborative relationship and close physical proximity of offices to facilitate such scheduling. Even so, the task of coordinating schedules has at times been daunting.

Costs of providing the psychoeducational intervention may also serve as a barrier in the future. At this time, these services are provided free of charge as part of families' participation in a clinical research protocol. Moreover, each family is provided with a financial incentive to participate. Without the financial support of a research grant, it would not be possible in our context to provide such services without directly charging the family. Billing of third-party payers under mental health riders is not a serious option because, according to most contracts, preventive services such as these are not traditionally covered.

An important method of validating reports of treatment adherence in this study has been through an empty GH vial count. Families are mailed a letter by research staff approximately 2 weeks in advance of the 3-month and 6-month follow-up visits reminding them to bring their empty vials to the visit. This procedure may enhance adherence because of families' awareness that their performance is being monitored. On closure of this study, reminder letters are no longer sent and it may not be feasible, for reasons of time constraints, to have nursing staff incorporate this additional feature in their follow-up evaluations.

It has become clear to us, through the course of conducting this ongoing study, that most families appreciate the opportunity to learn about their child's health problem and recommended treatment in a graded approach in a setting removed from the busy circumstances characteristic of our typical outpatient endocrinology clinics. The psychoeducational intervention, which extends over three 1-hour sessions, provides children and their parents the opportunity and encouragement to ask questions and clarify misunderstandings about the child's diagnosis and impending GH treatment. Furthermore, the preparation of the child and parents for the demands of daily injections in the context of otherwise typically busy household schedules will hopefully reduce the burden associated with the treatment. Such an investment of professional services in anticipation of a costly and lengthy medical intervention seems only prudent. Although the intervention described here was specifically designed to address the needs of children (and families) about to commence GH therapy, it seems that a similar outline would be justified and could be applied to any other chronic treatment condition not being initiated on an emergent basis.

Findings from the study may provide information about the link between adherence and treatment outcomes that include both physical and psychological criteria. Such information, in turn, is useful in conducting both cost-benefit and cost-effectiveness analyses of the GH treatment regimen (Yates, 1995).

ACKNOWLEDGMENT

This research was supported in part by a grant from the Genentech Foundation for Growth and Development (#96-52). We are particularly grateful to Wanda Grundner, RN, and Barbara Shine, RN, endocrine nurse specialists, for their instrumental support in helping to coordinate the research and clinical aspects of this study, and to Uhlas Nadgir, MD, for assistance in implementing aspects of the intervention protocol. Finally, the work described here would not have been possible without the dedicated support of the Children's Growth Foundation of Buffalo, which has provided support for the endocrine and psychoendocrine health care staff to work collaboratively at the Children's Hospital of Buffalo in the clinical management of youth with the full range of endocrine disorders.

REFERENCES

Abramowicz, M. (1994). Recombinant human growth hormone. *Medical Letter on Drugs and Therapeutics, 36,* 77–78.

Achenbach, T. M. (1991a). *Manual for the Child Behavior Checklist/4-18 and 1991 Profile.* Burlington, VT: University of Vermont, Department of Psychiatry.

Achenbach, T. M. (1991b). *Manual for the Youth Self-Report and 1991 Profile.* Burlington, VT: University of Vermont, Department of Psychiatry.

Allen, D. B., Johanson, A. J., & Blizzard, R. M. (1996). Growth hormone treatment. In F. Lifshitz (Ed.), *Pediatric endocrinology* (3rd ed., pp. 61–81). New York: Marcel Dekker.

Alvord, J. R. (1973). *Home token economy: An incentive program for children and their parents.* Champaign, IL: Research Press.

Becker, M. H., Radius, S. M., Rosenstock, I. M., Drachman, R. H., Shuberth, K. C., & Teets, K. C. (1978). Compliance with a medical regimen for asthma: A test of the Health Belief Model. *Public Health Reports, 93,* 268–277.

Blethen, S. L., Baptista, J., Kuntze, J., Foley, T., LaFranchi, S., & Johanson, A. (1997). Adult height in growth hormone (GH)-deficient children treated with biosynthetic GH. The Genentech Growth Study Group. *Journal of Clinical Endocrinology & Metabolism, 82,* 418–420.

Cautela, J. R., & Groden, J. (1978). *Relaxation: A comprehensive manual for adults, children, and children with special needs.* Champaign, IL: Research Press.

Cowell, C. T. (1997). Non-growth hormone (GH) deficient short children—what role for GH? *Journal of Pediatric Endocrinology & Metabolism, 10,* 257–260.

Cuttler, L., Silvers, J. B., Singh, J., Marrero, U., Finkelstein, B., Tannin, G., & Neuhauser, D. (1996). Short stature and growth hormone therapy: A national study of physician recommendation patterns. *Journal of the American Medical Association, 276,* 531–537.

da Costa, I. G., Rapoff, M. A., Lemanek, K., & Goldstein, G. L. (1997). Improving adherence to medication regimens for children with asthma and its effects on clinical outcome. *Journal of Applied Behavioral Analysis, 30,* 687–691.

Derogatis, L. R. (1993). *Brief Symptom Inventory: Administration, scoring, and procedures manual.* Minneapolis, MN: National Computer Systems.

Downie, A. B., Mulligan, J., Stratford, R. J., Betts, P. R., & Voss, L. D. (1996). Psychological response to growth hormone treatment in short normal children. *Archives of Disease in Childhood, 75,* 32–35.

Downie, A. B., Mulligan, J. M., Stratford, R. J., Betts, P. R., & Voss, L. D. (1997). Are short normal children at a disadvantage? *British Medical Journal, 314,* 97–100.

Eney, R. D., & Goldstein, E. O. (1976). Compliance of chronic asthmatics with oral administration of theophylline as measured by serum and salivary levels. *Pediatrics, 57,* 513–517.

Epstein, N. B., Baldwin, L. M., & Bishop, D. (1983). The McMaster Family Assessment Device. *Journal of Marital and Family Therapy, 4,* 171–180.

Gács, G., & Hosszu, E. (1991). The effect of socio-economic conditions on the time of diagnosis and compliance during treatment in growth hormone deficiency. *Acta Paediatrica Hungarica, 31,* 215–221.

Gittelman, R. (1986). Childhood anxiety disorders: Correlates and outcome. In R. Gittelman (Ed.), *Anxiety disorders of childhood* (pp. 101–125). New York: Guilford.

Gluckman, P. D., & Cutfield, W. S. (1991). Evaluation of a pen injector system for growth hormone treatment. *Archives of Disease in Childhood, 66,* 686–688.

Grew, R. S., Stabler, B., Randall, W., Williams, B. S., & Underwood, L. E. (1983). Facilitating patient understanding in the treatment of growth delay. *Clinical Pediatrics, 22,* 685–690.

Growth hormone goes wild. (1990, December 25). *Sun,* p. 1.

Guyda, H. J. (1998). Growth hormone therapy for non-growth hormone-deficient children with short stature. *Current Opinion in Endocrinology and Diabetes, 5,* 27–32.

Hanson, C. L., Cigrang, J. A., Harris, M. A., Carle, D. L., Relyea, G., & Burghen, G. A. (1989). Coping styles in youths with insulin-dependent diabetes mellitus. *Journal of Consulting and Clinical Psychology, 57,* 644–651.

Harter, S. (1985). *Manual for the self-perception profile for children.* Denver, CO: University of Denver Press.

Harter, S. (1988). *Manual for the self-perception profile for adolescents.* Denver, CO: University of Denver Press.

Hauser, S. T., Jacobson, A. M., Lavori, P., Wolfsdorf, J. I., Herskowitz, R. D., Millery, J. E., Bliss, R., Wertlieb, D., & Stein, J. (1990). Adherence among children and adolescents with insulin-dependent diabetes mellitus over a four-year longitudinal follow-up: II. Immediate and long-term linkages with the family milieu. *Journal of Pediatric Psychology, 15,* 527–542.

Haverkamp, F., & Noeker, M. (1998). Short stature in children—a questionnaire for parents: A new intsrument for growth disorder-specific psychosocial adaptation in children. *Quality of Life Research, 7,* 447–455.

Hintz, R. L., Attie, K. M., Baptista, J., & Roche, A. (1999). Effect of growth hormone treatment on adult height of children with idiopathic short stature. *New England Journal of Medicine, 340,* 502–507.

I Lied. (1991, July 8). *Sports Illustrated,* cover page.

Johnson, S. B. (1995). Insulin-dependent diabetes mellitus in childhood. In M. C. Roberts (Ed.), *Handbook of pediatric psychology* (2nd ed., pp. 263–285). New York: Guilford.

Kawai, M., Momoi, T., Yorifuji, T., Yamanaka, C., Sasaki, H., & Furusho, K. (1997). Unfavorable effects of growth hormone therapy on the final height of boys with short stature not caused by growth hormone deficiency. *Journal of Pediatrics, 130,* 205–209.

Korsch, B. M., Fine, R. N., & Negrete, V. F. (1978). Noncompliance in children with renal transplants. *Pediatrics, 61,* 872–876.

Kusalic, M., & Fortin, C. (1975). Growth hormone treatment in hypopituitary dwarfs. *Canadian Psychiatric Association Journal, 20,* 325–331.

La Greca, A. M., Follansbee, D., & Skyler, J. S. (1990). Developmental and behavioral aspects of diabetes management in youngsters. *Children's Health Care, 19,* 132–137.

La Greca, A. M., & Schuman, W. B. (1995). Adherence to prescribed medical regimens. In M. C. Roberts (Ed.), *Handbook of pediatric psychology* (2nd ed., pp. 55–83). New York: Guilford.

Lifshitz, F., & Cervantes, C. D. (1996). Short stature. In F. Lifshitz (Ed.), *Pediatric endocrinology* (3rd ed., pp. 1–18). New York: Marcel Dekker.

Lippe, B. M., & Nakamoto, J. M. (1993). Conventional and nonconventional uses of growth hormone. *Recent Progress in Hormone Research, 48,* 179–235.

López Siguero, J. P., Martinez Aedo, M. J., López Moreno, M. D., & Martínez Valverde, A. (1995). Treatment with growth hormone. What do children know and how do they accept it? *Hormone Research, 44*(Suppl. 3), 18–25.

McGrath, P. A. (1990). *Pain in children: Nature, assessment, and treatment.* New York: Guilford.

Meichenbaum, D., & Turk, D. (1987). *Facilitating treatment adherence. A practitioner's guide.* New York: Plenum.

Meyer-Bahlburg, H. F. L. (1990). Short stature: Psychological issues. In F. Lifshitz (Ed.), *Pediatric endocrinology. A clinical guide* (2nd ed., pp. 173–196). New York: Marcel Dekker.

Money, J., & Pollitt, E. (1966). Studies in the psychology of dwarfism: II. Personality maturation and response to growth hormone treatment in hypopituitary dwarfs. *Journal of Pediatrics, 68,* 381–390.

Noeker, M., & Haverkamp, F. (1994). *Short stature in children—a questionnaire for parents.* Bonn, Germany: Pace GmbH.

Oyarzabal, M., Aliaga, M., Chueca, M., Echarte, G., & Ulied, A. (1998). Multicentre survey on compliance with growth hormone therapy: What can be improved? *Acta Pædiatrica, 87,* 387–391.

Parker, S. H., & Rieser, P. (1996). *Growth hormone treatment: What to expect* [Brochure]. Falls Church, VA: Human Growth Foundation.

Rosenfeld, R. G., Attie, K. M., James, F., Brasel, J., Burstein, S., Cara, J. F., Chernausek, S., Gotlin, R., Kuntze, J., Lippe, B. M., Mahoney, C. P., Moore, W. V., Saenger, P., & Johanson, A. J. (1998). Growth hormone therapy of Turner's syndrome: Beneficial effect on adult height. *Journal of Pediatrics, 132,* 319–324.

Sandberg, D. E. (1996a). *Experiences related to height & GH therapy questionnaire.* Unpublished manuscript.

Sandberg, D. E. (1996b). Short stature: Intellectual and behavioral aspects. In F. Lifshitz (Ed.), *Pediatric endocrinology* (3rd ed., pp. 149–162). New York: Marcel Dekker.

Sandberg, D. E., Brook, A. E., & Campos, S. P. (1994). Short stature: A psychosocial burden requiring growth hormone therapy? *Pediatrics, 94*, 832–840.

Sandberg, D. E., & Michael, P. (1998). Psychosocial stresses related to short stature: Does their presence imply psychiatric dysfunction? In D. Drotar (Ed.), *Assessing pediatric health-related quality of life and functional status: Implications for research, practice, and policy* (pp. 287–312). Mahwah, NJ: Lawrence Erlbaum Associates.

Skuse, D., Gilmour, J., Tian, C. S., & Hindmarsh, P. (1994). Psychosocial assessment of children with short stature: A preliminary report. *Acta Pædiatrica, 406*(Suppl. 1), 11–16.

Smith, S. L., Hindmarsh, P. C., & Brook, C. G. D. (1993). Compliance with growth hormone treatment—are they getting it? *Archives of Disease in Childhood, 68*, 91–93.

Stabler, B., Clopper, R. R., Siegel, P. T., Stoppani, C., Compton, P. G., & Underwood, L. E. (1994). Academic achievement and psychological adjustment in short children. *Journal of Developmental and Behavioral Pediatrics, 15*, 1–6.

Stabler, B., Siegel, P. T., Clopper, R. R., Stoppani, C. E., Compton, P. G., & Underwood, L. E. (1998). Behavior change after growth hormone treatment of children with short stature. *Journal of Pediatrics, 133*, 366–373.

Stanhope, R., Albanese, A., Moyle, L., & Hamill, G. (1992). Optimum method for administration of biosynthetic human growth hormone: A randomized crossover trial of an Auto Injector and a pen injection system. *Archives of Disease in Childhood, 67*, 994–997.

Stanhope, R., Moyle, L., & McSwiney, M. (1993). Patient knowledge and compliance with growth hormone treatment [Letter to the editor]. *Archives of Disease in Childhood, 68*, 525.

Vance, M., Ingersoll, G. M., & Golden, M. P. (1994). Short stature in a nonclinical sample: Not a big problem. In B. Stabler & L. E. Underwood (Eds.), *Growth, stature, and adaptation. An international symposium on the behavioral, social, and cognitive aspects of growth delay* (pp. 35–45). Chapel Hill, NC: University of North Carolina Press.

Wilson, D. M., Hammer, L. D., Duncan, P. M., Dornbusch, S. M., Ritter, P. L., & Hintz, R. L. (1986). Growth and intellectual development. *Pediatrics 78*, 646–650.

Yates, B. T. (1995). Cost-effectiveness analysis, cost-benefit analysis, and beyond: Evolving models for the scientist-manager-practitioner. *Clinical Psychology: Science and Practice 2*, 385–398.

Zimet, G. D., Cutler, M., Litvene, M., Dahms, W., Owens, R., & Cuttler, L. (1995). Psychological adjustment of children evaluated for short stature: A preliminary report. *Journal of Developmental and Behavioral Pediatrics, 16*, 264–270.

PART VIII

SUMMARY OF RECOMMENDATIONS TO ENHANCE PRACTICE, RESEARCH, AND TRAINING CONCERNING TREATMENT ADHERENCE IN CHILDHOOD CHRONIC ILLNESS

Treatment Adherence in Childhood Chronic Illness: Issues and Recommendations to Enhance Practice, Research, and Training

Dennis Drotar
Kristin A. Riekert
Erika Burgess
Rachel Levi
Chantelle Nobile
Astrida Seja Kaugars
Natalie Walders
Case Western Reserve University, Cleveland, OH

Conference participants were asked to engage in a series of small-group discussions that focused on the following major themes of the conference: (a) definitions and conceptual models of treatment adherence in chronic childhood illness, (b) understanding the impact of adherence or noncompliance on children and families, (c) measurement of adherence, and (d) development and evaluation of interventions to promote treatment adherence. The conference participants' discussions involved a great deal of interchange and, at times, debate. The purpose of this chapter is to summarize key points in the discussions that are relevant for recommendations to enhance research, practice, and training concerning treatment adherence in childhood chronic illness. Although inclusive of the various points of view that were raised in the discussions, this summary does not reflect a consensus of the conference participants.

DEFINITIONS AND CONCEPTUAL MODELS OF TREATMENT ADHERENCE

Conference participants considered the implications of the definitions of *compliance* versus *adherence* to treatment in childhood chronic illness. Considerable discussion ensued regarding the various implications of the terms used to describe illness self-management perspectives. For example, the term *compliance* was seen by some as implying a unidirectional model of patient care (e.g., the physician giving the child and family advice), whereas *adherence* was perceived as a more collaborative description. Moreover, some felt that the language used to categorize children and families (e.g., as noncompliant) may affect the quality of the patient–physician relationship and hence affect patients' and families' responses to their physicians. Many of the conference participants felt that both *adherence* and *compliance* have significant limitations because they do not emphasize the role of parents and children as informed participants in treatment (Bauman, chap. 4, this volume; Creer, chap. 5, this volume; Donovan & Blake, 1992). For example, although physicians are knowledgeable about the medical aspects of treatment (i.e., what specific treatments are necessary to manage a given chronic condition), children and family members were seen by many conference participants as experts on their own lives as well as on the context in which treatment is conducted (Deaton, 1985). Nevertheless, some participants felt that the differing perspectives and areas of expertise of physicians, patients, and their families are not reflected in terms such as *adherence* or *compliance*, which have been used to characterize patients' response to the clinical management of childhood chronic illness (see Bauman, chap. 4, this volume; Trostle, chap. 2, this volume).

Adherence and *compliance* are also difficult to operationalize because prescribed treatment regimens are often not clear (Ievers-Landis & Drotar, chap. 11, this volume; La Greca, 1990a). Consequently, some conference participants felt that the definitions of *adherence* and *compliance* should be modified to reflect the perspectives of the consumers of treatment—children and families—and involve more neutral terms (e.g., *self-management*) that emphasize patient and family participation in care (see Bauman, chap. 4, this volume; Creer, chap. 5, this volume).

Developing New Conceptual Models to Guide Research and Practice in Treatment Adherence

Conference participants also recognized the need to develop conceptual models to develop hypotheses for research, guide clinical management of treatment adherence, and predict outcomes of adherence-related interventions. Group discussions noted the limitations of current conceptual models for research and clinical care and appreciated that there is no agreed-on or ideal conceptual model that currently guides research and practice related to treatment adherence. Several suggestions were made for expanding and developing models of adherence to treatment in childhood chronic illness. These included culturally sensitive, peer-group, developmental, and interdisciplinary models.

Culturally Sensitive Models.   Many participants felt that, to facilitate better understanding and management of the factors that can affect the treatment adherence of children and families from different cultural contexts, culturally sensitive models of adherence to treatment need to be developed and implemented in clinical care. Methods of clinical management of chronic illness that have shown to be effective with middle-class families do not necessarily translate into other cultures. Moreover, the specific barriers to chronic illness management may reflect cultural issues that are not well understood. Examples include some families that believe that having animals in their homes can prevent asthma in their children and hence are not willing to comply with physicians' admonitions to remove pets from their homes. Moreover, cultural factors also influence the quality of patient–physician communications and relationships. For example, some families of Asian backgrounds may have difficulty questioning their physicians and engaging them in an open dialogue (see DiMatteo, chap. 10, this volume; Kleinman, 1980).

Peer-Group Models.   The conference group felt that models of treatment adherence that mobilize peer-group influences have potential for designing interventions to promote treatment adherence (Anderson, Wolf, Burkhart, Cornell, & Bacon, 1989; Hanson, Henggeler, & Burghen, 1987; La Greca, 1990b). One such example would be the development of a special Internet network so adolescents can log on and communicate with peers who have the same and other chronic conditions (Greenman, 1998).

Conference participants underscored how the Internet can give patients more information about their illness, but also recognized the disadvantages of such technological options. For example, because it may be difficult for patients to discriminate between accurate and inaccurate medical information, they can easily obtain misinformation on the Internet. One possible way to minimize misinformation would be to develop chat rooms that are monitored and moderated by experts.

Developmental Models.   Participants felt that models of treatment adherence in childhood chronic illness needed to include a developmental perspective. For example, it was recognized that many adolescents, including those with a chronic illness, are motivated by short- rather than long-term incentives. For this reason, incentives that are most important to teenagers and their families and promote independence and initiative in self-care need to be considered in developing models to promote adherence to chronic illness treatment in clinical care. Moreover, developmentally relevant issues such as age-appropriate negotiation and decision making between parents and adolescents concerning responsibilities for managing chronic illness treatment need to be included in intervention models (Anderson, Auslander, Jung, Miller, & Santiago, 1990; Hanson, 1992).

Interdisciplinary Models.   Conference participants were interested in the potential application of interdisciplinary models of adherence promotion to the clinical care of children with chronic illness. Moreover, the issue of the most appropriate or effective interdisciplinary model of illness management and promotion of treatment adherence sparked some debate among the conference participants. The group discussion revealed several important, but as yet unanswered, questions: Which professional disciplines should be involved in adherence promotion? At what point in the management of the child's illness should they be involved? What is the most effective role for professional disciplines other than physicians, such as psychologists, nurses, social workers, and so on, in adherence promotion and management of serious adherence problems?

Conference participants also suggested that there is a good deal of variability from setting to setting in how interdisciplinary models of care are defined and implemented (Creer, Levstek, & Reynolds, 1994). Although some physicians ask for help from other professions to manage problematic adherence, an interdisciplinary approach to adherence promotion in childhood chronic illness is not routine practice, at least in the experience of many of the conference participants. Consequently, there is a continuing need to describe innovative models of interdisciplinary care and document the potential effectiveness of interdisciplinary approaches to adherence promotion.

Conceptual Models of Treatment Adherence and Medical Education

Recommendations concerning the development and use of conceptual models of adherence to treatment are shown in Table 20.1. Some conference participants noted that the conceptual models of illness and treatment currently used to guide the teaching of medical students and residents focus much more on treating acute infections than on managing chronic illness, which requires a different perspective such as the need to consider individual variations in patients' situations and lifestyles. Some conference participants felt that, with regard to communication, some physicians may not appreciate that their patients can benefit from an interactional style that is responsive to their individual needs, skills, or attitudes (Francis, Korsch, & Morris, 1969). Moreover, support and advocacy were seen as potentially important but sometimes neglected components of the patient–physician relationship in the management of pedi-

TABLE 20.1
Recommendations Concerning the Development and Use of Conceptual Models
to Guide Research, Practice, and Training

- Develop models of treatment adherence that incorporate the perspectives of children, families, and physicians in managing chronic illness treatment.
- Use terms such as *self-care* or *self-management*, which reflect patients' initiative in managing their illness, as opposed to *adherence* or *compliance*, which emphasize their response to physicians' directions.
- Develop and evaluate models of illness management that use peer-group influences to promote treatment adherence.
- Develop, implement, and evaluate models of treatment adherence that include developmentally relevant incentives for self-management of chronic illness.
- Develop and evaluate the impact of culturally sensitive models of adherence promotion that recognize and appreciate the role of cultural influences on the management of pediatric chronic illness.
- Document the impact of comprehensive interdisciplinary approaches to chronic illness management and adherence promotion, especially on the prevention of adherence problems.
- Determine the most effective and efficient ways to use the talents of different professions to promote adherence to chronic illness treatment.
- Include models of adherence to chronic illness treatment in medical training that enhance physicians' cultural sensitivities and understanding of developmental influences on chronic illness management.

atric chronic illness. For these reasons, conference participants recognized that the models most appropriate to train physicians in chronic illness management need to place the patient, not the disease, at the center of care (see Creer, chap. 5, this volume; DiMatteo, chap. 10, this volume). Such models should include training in specific models of patient care that can promote long-term adherence to treatment and should focus on cultural sensitivity, recognition, and management of developmental influences.

IDENTIFYING FACTORS THAT INFLUENCE TREATMENT ADHERENCE IN CHILDHOOD CHRONIC ILLNESS

A second major theme of the conference centered around factors that can affect treatment adherence in childhood chronic illness. In their discussion of this issue, conference participants raised a number of potential influences, some of which they felt have been neglected or underemphasized in current research and practice. These include illness-related factors as well as patient, family, and physician influences. Recommendations to enhance research, practice, and training concerning the identification of illness related factors as shown in Table 20.2.

TABLE 20.2
Identifying Factors That Influence Treatment in Childhood Chronic Illness:
Recommendations for Research, Practice, and Training

- Document the impact of key illness-related factors such as the stage and course of chronic illness on treatment adherence.
- Identify cultural factors that are associated with positive versus problematic adherence to chronic illness treatment.
- Study physician influences on adherence to treatment in pediatric chronic illness (e.g., the impact of written treatment plans on treatment adherence and illness management).
- Identify specific family influences (e.g., allocation of treatment-related responsibilities that are associated with positive vs. problematic adherence to chronic illness treatment).
- Develop and evaluate interventions to improve physician management of pediatric chronic illness especially enhancing communication skills, providing written treatment plans, or updating treatment plans.
- Develop and evaluate the impact of treatment plans that respond to changes in the child's development or illness course.
- Develop and evaluate the impact of programs designed to intervene with children and families to improve their communication with their physicians in chronic illness management.
- Use the data from research on the impact of risk or protective factors on adherence to design interventions (e.g., by targeting high-risk individuals and families for interventions).

Impact of Illness-Related Factors

The conference group discussion noted that the stage of a child's chronic illness may have an important but as yet unrecognized impact on treatment adherence (Quittner, DiGirolamo, Michel, & Eigen, 1992). For example, the initial *honeymoon phase* of an illness such as diabetes may mask potential compliance problems because high levels of compliance are not necessarily needed to maintain adequate blood sugar control owing to the child's remaining pancreatic function. Some children and adolescents may develop maladaptive habits concerning self-management during this phase of their illness because they do not experience direct consequences of noncompliance on their blood sugar control. In the more advanced phases of a chronic illness such as cystic fibrosis (CF), however, some children and families may experience clinically significant symptoms and even deterioration in their clinical course despite optimal adherence to recommended treatments.

Another potentially important illness-related factor is the impact of intermittent symptoms such as flare-ups of asthma symptoms or symptoms of inflammatory bowel disease on treatment adherence. Because such flare-ups can occur despite excellent adherence to treatment, they may influence patients' attitudes toward adherence to treatment and their behavior (e.g., by stimulating feelings of discouragement and perceptions that their illness cannot be controlled in any way).

Patient-Related Factors

The specific patient-related factors that facilitate or disrupt treatment adherence and management of a chronic illness, especially over long periods of time, have not been identified for many pediatric chronic conditions. Although a wide range of factors have been identified as potential influences on treatment adherence or noncompliance (Delamater, chap. 8, this volume; La Greca & Schuman, 1995), others have been neglected. For example, the factors that facilitate high levels of adherence to chronic illness treatment in children and families may be different than those that contribute to problematic adherence and are largely unknown. Identifying factors that promote positive adherence to chronic illness treatment could give informed direction to the design of effective adherence promotion strategies.

Individual psychological factors such as self-esteem have been found to be associated with positive treatment adherence among children and adolescents (Friedman et al., 1986), whereas psychological dysfunction predicts problematic adherence (Kovacs, Goldston, Obrosky, & Iyengar, 1992). Nevertheless, the precise causal relationship between such psychological factors and adherence to treatment is not clear. It is possible that self-esteem and correlated factors such as level of self-regulation may facilitate the positive development of treatment adherence for childhood chronic illness (i.e., individuals who are most compliant with treatment may already be engaging in healthy behaviors in a variety of contexts). However, adherence problems that are significant enough to threaten a child's health may also disrupt adjustment and self-esteem.

Family Factors

The conference participants noted that several family factors have been identified as potentially important in promoting treatment adherence as well as limiting adherence (e.g., as a barrier to positive self-management of a chronic illness; DiMatteo, chap. 10, this volume; Quittner et al., chap. 17, this volume). For example, the quality of family functioning has been shown to predict adherence to treatment in adolescents with diabetes (Hauser et al., 1990; Jacobson et al., 1990). However, relatively little is known about the impact of specific family interactions—such as the quality of allocation of treatment-related responsibilities, decision making concerning symptom management, and so on—on adherence to treatment in childhood chronic illness. Moreover, interrelationships between serious family dysfunction and adherence to medical treatment and noncompliance on family functioning need to be understood more completely. Although severe family dysfunction has been linked to problematic adherence in illnesses such as diabetes (Golden, Herold, & Orr, 1985), serious compliance problems can also disrupt child and family adjustment.

Physician Influences

Conference participants recognized the importance of understanding the physician's impact on the management of treatment adherence in childhood chronic illness. Several potentially influential physician behaviors were identified, such as the development of clear treatment plans and clinical management plans that are responsive to changes in the child's clinical status. For example, treatment plans that are given to children and families may not be sufficiently specific or communicated clearly enough to promote adherence (see DiMatteo, chap. 10, this volume; Ievers-Landis & Drotar, chap. 11, this volume). In addition, prescribed treatment regimens and clinical management plans may not be sufficiently responsive to changes in the child's condition and/or emerging developmental needs (Koocher, McGrath, & Dudas, 1990). However, developmentally responsive clinical management of pediatric chronic illness considers how the child's changing developmental needs affect their perceptions of their illness and treatment. For example, it is not uncommon for adolescents to resent the demands of adherence to chronic illness treatment because they interfere with their independence.

Moreover, prescribed treatments for childhood chronic illness may also need to be modified in response to advances in medical treatment and changes (i.e., improvement or deterioration) in the clinical course of the child's illness. Changes in the child's health and/or illness course place additional burdens on physicians to revise their treatment plans and communicate such changes to children and their families.

Several studies have also suggested that it may be difficult for physicians to record their treatment plans accurately and communicate these plans to their patients and families (see Ievers-Landis & Drotar, chap. 11, this volume). Consequently, it may be difficult for patients and families to understand the specific details of their treatment regimen and know precisely what they are supposed to do to manage their illness. Such limitations in documentation of treatments also pose significant problems in conducting research on adherence because it may be difficult for researchers to identify the precise standards for prescribed treatments and hence accurately evaluate patients' departures from such standards (La Greca, 1990a).

Implications for Training Physicians

Conference participants also discussed the potential implications of physician influences on treatment adherence for training physicians in the management of pediatric chronic illness. In the context of the increased time constraints imposed by managed care, it may be difficult for many physicians to respond effectively to the needs of children and families' specific treatment plans, updates of treatment regimens, and specific interventions to promote adherence (see Walders, Nobile, & Drotar, chap. 9, this volume). Moreover, to provide updates of treatment and specific interventions to promote treatment adherence, many physicians need additional training to help them effectively communicate such information with children and their families. For this reason, there is a need to develop and evaluate innovative methods of teaching physicians to manage adherence issues in pediatric chronic illness and/or programs that teach children and family members to communicate more effectively with their physicians (see Kaplan, Greenfield, & Ware, 1989, for an interesting application of this model with adults with diabetes).

Group discussions also noted that health care providers need to be educated concerning strategies of illness management and interactions with families, such as working with diverse populations, strategies of promoting adherence, developing more effective methods of engaging families, understanding home environments (e.g., home visits), and sensitively gathering detailed treatment-related information from parents and children.

IMPACT OF TREATMENT ADHERENCE
ON THE HEALTH AND QUALITY OF LIFE

Conference participants raised several key questions about the realistic benefits versus costs of adherence from the perspectives of children with a chronic illness and their families (Bauman, chap. 4, this volume). These were: What is the evidence that successful adherence results in improvement in the symptoms or course of a chronic illness? What are the burdens that are associated with successful compliance to treatment on children and families? What are the consequences of noncompliance with chronic illness treatment on children and families? Recommendations for research, practice, and training that focus on the impact of adherence to treatment on children, families, and providers are shown in Table 20.3.

The Patient's Dilemma: If I Adhere to Treatment
Will I Get Better?

Conference participants identified a significant gap in scientific knowledge that may affect treatment adherence for children with chronic illnesses and their families—the fact that the efficacy of medical treatments in reducing the morbidity associated with pediatric chronic illness is not well established. One exception is the fact that tight blood sugar control has been shown to reduce the rate of complications due to diabetes (Dia-

TABLE 20.3
Impact of Adherence to Chronic Illness Treatment on Children, Families,
and Providers: Implications for Research, Practice, and Training

- Document the psychological burdens that are associated with successful adherence to treatment in pediatric chronic illness.
- Assess the psychological burdens and stressors associated with long-term adherence to chronic illness treatment on families, including siblings.
- Describe the impact of problematic adherence to chronic illness treatment on children, families, and providers.
- Describe the impact of chronic illness management and treatment on the behavior and adjustment of healthy siblings.
- Design and evaluate interventions to reduce the burden of adherence to chronic illness treatment on families by promoting family support.
- Design and evaluate the impact of interventions designed to reduce conflict and promote positive communication concerning illness management among families of children with adherence problems.
- Develop supports to help the treatment team manage its emotional reactions to serious compliance problems.
- Determine the minimal or threshold levels of compliance with chronic illness treatment that are necessary to improve the clinical course of various chronic conditions.
- Assess the impact of noncompliance with chronic illness treatment on the utilization of services, costs of care, and development of health-related problems.

betes Control and Complications Trial Research Group, 1993). However, for the most part, evidence for the impact of medical treatment for other chronic conditions on children's long-term health status is lacking (see Johnson, 1992). Moreover, many patients with chronic conditions do not necessarily experience positive subjective benefits associated with adherence to treatment even for treatments that have long-term benefits on health. Consequently, children and adolescents may believe that their treatment is not effective and/or that their compliance to treatment is not necessary to improve their health or well-being.

Burdens of Adherence: Is It Compatible With Quality of Life for Children and Families?

The impact of successful versus problematic adherence to chronic illness treatment on the well-being and quality of life of children with chronic illness is not well documented. However, conference participants suggested that the demands of adherence to chronic illness treatment may entail significant psychological costs (e.g., increased burdens on child and family) that have not been well documented or appreciated. Conference participants were concerned that the burdens associated with compliance with treatment for chronic illness (e.g., less time for recreation and time spent together) may be significant for families (Quittner, Opipari, Regoli, Jacobsen, & Eigen, 1992). Such burdens intensify maternal psychological distress and disrupt the quality of family relationships. For example, managing chronic illness treatment may cause conflict in families (e.g., parents insisting on a standard of treatment adherence that an adolescent feels is incompatible with their interests). Other stresses may be raised by side effects of treatments or by a prescribed treatment that does not relieve illness-related symptoms. All of these treatment-related burdens may function as barriers to treatment adherence.

Consequences of Noncompliance With Chronic Illness Treatment on Families

Conference participants were also interested in the potential consequences of noncompliance with chronic illness treatment on family life. Although the impact of nonadherence to treatment on families is not well documented, clinical observations suggest that problematic adherence to treatment may cause family distress and conflict. For example, parents may feel distressed by their children's noncompliance because they feel responsible for this problem and concerned about the potential consequences on their children's future health. In addition, some children feel guilty and discouraged about the burdens that their illness and compliance problems can place on their families and parents. Such personal distress and guilt can disrupt communication between parents and children and limit attempts to improve management. Similarly, parent–child conflict, which is another potential consequence of adherence difficulties, can also lead to increasingly problematic interactions in which parents try harder and harder to get their children to do their treatment. Such children may eventually come to resent such interference and become increasingly resistant to their parents' influence (Anderson & Coyne, 1991).

Some conference participants noted that the impact of chronic illness treatment on physically healthy siblings is not well understood, but is a potentially fruitful area of investigation. Although the roles that healthy siblings can play in treatment adherence are poorly defined, they may be substantial. For example, in some families, older siblings may be responsible for helping their chronically ill sibling develop and maintain treatment adherence. The child or adolescent with a chronic illness may perceive such sibling behavior as helpful or intrusive. Furthermore, in some families, the healthy sibling may become jealous or resentful about the time and attention the parent are giving to the child with a chronic illness, which may lead them to become increasingly disruptive to claim the parent's attention. Such behavior may increase the psychological burdens of care on parents.

Potential Consequences of Noncompliance
on the Patient–Physician Relationship
and Health Care Providers

Conference participants recognized that less than optimal adherence to chronic illness treatment can also have negative consequences on the patient–physician relationship. One potential problem is that blame can be placed on children and families who are noncompliant. In some instances, the label of a *noncompliant* child or family may be applied prematurely or even unfairly (e.g., to explain fluctuations in symptoms or difficulties in managing a chronic illness that are not under anyone's control). The psychological implications of such labels for children and families, and its impact on the relationship with their physicians, are not well understood, but need to be clarified. It is possible that parents, children, and family members may feel discouraged by being labeled as *noncompliant* and may even come to feel that their providers do not believe or trust them. Parents and children may become distressed by their own problems in managing their illness (e.g., "I don't understand what happened, I did everything I was supposed to do; I'm doing all that I can. I can't do any more").

To prevent and ameliorate such problems, conference participants suggested that it may be important for providers to develop effective ways to help children and families save face when problems with compliance are identified and to create a spirit of collaboration when managing such problems (e.g., "Let's see how we can work together to help you and your child manage these very difficult treatments the best way we can"). Moreover, in some circumstances, it may be helpful for practitioners to normalize child and family noncompliance with treatment to provide a supportive atmosphere that promotes discussion and mutual problem solving (e.g., "No one is able to do everything that is prescribed all of the time, but we need to work together to help you do better with your treatments"). In the spirit of problem solving, patients and families can also be encouraged to contribute their own ideas concerning illness management to help improve treatment adherence.

Conference participants also underscored the potential impact of noncompliance with treatment on health care providers. Children and families whose problems with noncompliance are chronic and serious enough to threaten the child's health raise difficult problems for the treatment team. For example, it can be demoralizing, threatening, and stressful for the treatment team to encounter repeated instances of noncompliance in their patients and families, especially when such problems threaten the child's health. Consequently, enhancing the team's support to manage these difficulties may be important.

Impact of Noncompliance on the Evaluation of the Clinical Trials Results

One significant problem that was identified by conference participants concerns the impact of the assumption that patients are complying with recommended treatments on the results of data that are obtained from clinical trials of treatment efficacy. To the extent that patients are not complying with prescribed treatment (which occurs relatively frequently with many conditions), researchers may erroneously assume that such a treatment is not working. Consequently, for all of the prior reasons, there is a need to study adherence to treatment in clinical trials, as well as barriers to adherence, and to develop interventions to limit the frequency of nonadherence to research protocols (see Johnson, chap. 13, this volume).

METHODOLOGICAL ISSUES IN DESIGNING AND EVALUATING STUDIES OF ADHERENCE TO CHRONIC ILLNESS TREATMENT

Critical methodological issues in designing and evaluating studies of adherence to chronic illness treatment were considered by the conference participants, including sampling bias, impact of multiple informants on assessment of adherence, and enhancing generalization of findings concerning adherence assessment. Recommendations for research to improve the design of studies of adherence to treatment are shown in Table 20.4.

Sampling Bias

Conference participants noted that research criteria that exclude families from studies of treatment adherence limit the generalization of findings that are obtained from such research. For example, some studies may exclude nonadherent patients who do not show up for appointments. However, families of the most nonadherent children may exclude themselves from studies (Riekert & Drotar, 1999). Moreover, families whose children have the most problematic adherence may not be enrolled in studies (see Johnson, chap. 13, this volume). If a disproportionate number of children with problematic adherence is not included in research designs, whatever results are obtained may not be generalizable to the overall population of individuals with a chronic condition, let alone the population of most noncompliant patients, which is the group of greatest clinical interest.

Sampling bias can also occur when members of the health care team select the patients who are included in studies of treatment adherence. For

TABLE 20.4
Recommendations for Research to Improve the Design
of Research Concerning Treatment Adherence in Chronic Illness

- Evaluate the impact of patient and family nonadherence with research methods on research findings, including findings generated from clinical trials on the efficacy of medical treatment.
- Describe children and family members' experiences in participating in clinical trials, including studies of adherence to chronic illness treatment.
- Develop and evaluate methods of reducing child and family noncompliance with research protocols including clinical trials of the efficacy of medical treatment.
- Evaluate the impact of selective participation and other sampling biases on the findings of studies of adherence to chronic illness treatment.
- Develop and evaluate methods of enhancing child and family adherence to clinical trials of the efficacy of medical and psychological intervention.
- Develop methods to improve participation of children and families in research or adherence trials.
- Develop methods of assessing adherence to treatment that can be used in different chronic illness groups.

example, they may select patients who are especially compliant because they are thought to be good candidates for research or those with serious compliance problems because they are seen as most in need of help.

Selection bias also occurs when some children and families with chronic illness do not elect to participate in research concerning adherence to treatment because they find such research difficult to manage. Those children and families who are already burdened by the management of chronic illness may experience an additional burden by participating in research. To develop methods to facilitate child and family participation in research, it is important to understand their perceptions of their experiences in participating in clinical trials and in studies of adherence to chronic illness treatment.

The Impact of Multiple Measures and Informants in Assessing Adherence to Chronic Illness Treatment

Conference participants raised many questions about how best to manage data from reports of adherence that are generated by patients, family members, and providers. Although there was some agreement that using multiple measures and assessing different family members' perspectives on adherence to chronic illness treatment can be useful, the optimal way to accomplish this task is not at all clear. In the absence of an agreed-on *gold standard* of approaches to measuring treatment adherence, a number of critical questions remain unanswered. For example, how does one know which set of measures to use to assess adherence to chronic illness treatment? Moreover, assuming that multiple informants and methods are needed, what is the best way to integrate information from multiple sources?

Enhancing Generalizability of Information From Studies of Treatment Adherence

The issue of generalizability of data concerning treatment adherence was considered by conference participants, some of whom questioned whether available measures of treatment adherence could ever be validly used across different chronic illness populations. Others felt strongly that the development of measures of treatment adherence that can be used across different chronic conditions would have significant advantages. For example, such measures could be used to compare rates of adherence problems in children with different chronic conditions and assess adherence to treatment among individuals who have comorbid chronic health conditions that occur relatively frequently (e.g., CF and diabetes). Moreover, such measures would be ideal for use in large-sample, multicenter studies that involve children in multiple chronic illness groups. However, the development of such measures requires careful validation and might not be feasible for conditions with highly unusual and specific treatment regimens.

METHODOLOGICAL AND PRACTICAL ISSUES IN MEASURING ADHERENCE TO CHRONIC ILLNESS TREATMENT

Conference participants spent a great deal of time discussing the issues related to the measurement of adherence to chronic illness treatment, including the need for measures that can be used in clinical care as well as the limitations and trade-offs of alternative approaches to adherence to chronic illness treatment.

Issues in Using Objective Versus Subjective Measures of Adherence

Conference participants generally agreed that multiple measurement strategies that include objective measures of adherence data as well as self-report data are necessary for optimal assessment of treatment adherence. Objective measures of adherence such as computerized devices have significant methodological advantages (Rapoff, 1999). However, conference participants were concerned that the use of monitoring devices in clinical care situations could undermine the relationship between health professionals and patients. For example, when patients are not told about the use of monitors, such methods may engender mistrust among patients, families, and physicians.

A related issue in implementing studies of objective measurement of adherence to chronic illness treatment is what is actually done with the information from these devices and how this information is communicated to children and their families. Concerns were raised that patients are not always carefully instructed in the optimal use of these measures and to appreciate the potential of these devices as a means to enhance self-management of their chronic illness. In some instances, such technology can be help children and families conduct their own personal experiments in evaluating the impact of specific adherence behaviors (i.e., changing diets on their health in a convenient manner).

Trade-Offs in Using Alternative Self-Report Measures of Adherence

Conference participants considered the trade-offs (i.e., the costs vs. benefits) of alternative self-report methods. For example, they recognized the trade-offs in using self-report measures of adherence that are more expensive and time-consuming, but assess fine-grained behaviors and information that is highly relevant to clinically relevant processes related to treatment adherence, such as problem solving concerning illness management. In contrast, more feasible and inexpensive self-report measures do not provide the highly specific information that may be needed to closely monitor adherence. Moreover, such methods have not received extensive validation relative to some of the more comprehensive methods, such as the 24-hour recall methods (Freund, Johnson, Silverstein, & Thomas, 1991). However, a disadvantage of such measures is that, even with a 24-hour window, individuals may not recall what treatments they have completed. Moreover, because these measures are costly and labor-intensive in both administration and scoring, they are not possible to use in routine patient care.

Developing Methods to Measure Adherence to Chronic Illness Treatments by Self-Report

Conference participants recognized that self-report methods have an important place in measuring adherence to treatment in childhood chronic illness (Johnson, Silverstein, Rosenbloom, Carter, & Cunningham, 1986). However, given the feasibility problems associated with some available self-report measures, conference participants identified the need to develop and validate new self-report measures of adherence as well as refine available measures to make them more feasible for physicians, nurses, and patients to use in clinical care. Recommendations to enhance measurement of adherence to treatment in childhood chronic illness are shown in Table 20.5.

Understanding the Factors That Influence the Measurement of Self-Reports of Adherence

Conference participants underscored the need for data to evaluate factors that influence child and parental reports of adherence. For example, children and adolescents may present themselves as adhering to treatment either because they do not recall the events or wish to present themselves in a desirable light. Other factors such as gender differences may also influence the accuracy and validity of children's and adolescent's self-reports of adherence.

TRANSLATING RESEARCH FINDINGS CONCERNING TREATMENT ADHERENCE INTO CLINICAL CARE

Conference participants identified a significant gap between the conceptual models that have been used to guide research concerning adherence to chronic illness treatment versus models of clinical care that are currently being used by practitioners to guide their clinical actions in care of children with chronic illness. In general, research concerning factors that predict adherence to chronic illness treatment as well as interventions that have

TABLE 20.5
Recommendations to Enhance Measurement of Treatment Adherence
in Pediatric Chronic Illness

- Study the influences of factors such as age, gender, and culture that may affect the accuracy and validity of self-report measures of adherence.
- Develop and evaluate methods (i.e., prompting to improve the recall of adherence-related behaviors by children and family members).
- Assess the reliability, validity, and feasibility of promising new methods of adherence such as phone diaries.
- Develop and evaluate situation-specific measures of adherence that assess treatment and illness-specific treatment regimens.
- Develop methods to integrate information from different measures of treatment adherence.
- Document the methodological and practical costs and benefits of alternative measures of adherence, including objective and self-report measures.
- Develop and evaluate measures of barriers and supports including self-efficacy to treatment adherence that can be used in clinical care.

been found to improve adherence have not been implemented or evaluated in clinical care settings. Recommendations to improve adherence management in clinical care and to enhance research on this topic are summarized in Tables 20.6 and 20.7. Implementing adherence promotion interventions in clinical practice settings that are based on research findings was recognized as an important future direction by conference participants. Priorities for such research include: evaluation of community-based interventions to promote treatment adherence, translation of the results of descriptive studies of risk and protective practice into studies of clinical interventions to promote adherence, research concerning the effectiveness of adherence promotion interventions that are delivered in clinical practice and research concerning provider education in adherence promotion (see Table 20.8).

Barriers to Implementing Evidence-Based Models of Adherence in Practice

A number of potential barriers to the implementation of evidenced-based models of treatment adherence in practice were identified by conference participants. These include the lack of physician education concerning the complex nature of adherence to chronic illness treatment and potential strategies of intervention to promote adherence. Many conference participants felt that physicians needed more effective tools to learn how best to assess and manage the impact of families' beliefs and expectations concerning treatment on their adherence to treatment. Disincentives such as lack of reimbursement and time for adherence promoting activities were also identified as barriers to evidenced-based clinical management of adherence to chronic illness treatment.

Another barrier to implementing adherence-related interventions in practice is the limited data concerning the efficacy of such intervention. Researchers need to show that they can change adherence behavior before practitioners will believe that methods developed from research will work in practice. For example, although the Health Belief Model (Becker, Drachman, & Kirscht, 1972) has received empirical support (Bond, Aiken, & Somerville, 1992; Brownlee-Duffeck et al., 1987), it may or may not be applicable to clinical practice. Children and families' beliefs about health and illness may not guide their actions. Consequently, it is important to determine to what extent children and families actually use specific beliefs about health and illness to make decisions about treatment adherence in real-world clinical situations. Conceptual frameworks such as learning-based models (Epstein et al., 1981), which focus on specific behaviors and approaches to help patients and families learn to improve adherence behaviors by practice and reinforcement, may prove to be more powerful than Health Belief Models (Rapoff, 1999).

TABLE 20.6
Recommendations to Improve Adherence Management in Clinical Care

Promoting Adherence to Chronic Illness Treatment

- Develop more effective strategies for rewarding children and families for successful adherence behaviors as opposed to targeting only biological outcomes of a chronic illness. For example, in managing diabetes, children who are compliant with blood testing should be rewarded for their compliance with the blood testing procedures, not for the test results.
- Implement strategies to encourage the development and maintenance of positive adherence behaviors (e.g., reinforcing honesty and behavior change).
- Send the message to children and families that changes, including setbacks in the course of a chronic illness, are expected. Moreover, such setbacks may be independent of patient or family compliance with treatment.
- Normalize less than perfect adherence as an inevitable problem. Help children and families recognize that adherence can be improved using a collaborative, problem-solving approach.
- Use the results of adherence assessments to provide positive feedback to children and families concerning chronic illness management.
- Inform families that treatments for chronic illness do not always work as effectively as anticipated and that they can expect *probabilities* but not *certainties* for improved health outcomes.
- Use technology (e.g., computerized measures of disease management and adherence to treatment) to reinforce children's and families' sense of control and creative management of their treatment regimens.
- Ask patients and families specific questions that focus on identifying factors that promote or disrupt their adherence to treatment (e.g., What helps to manage your treatment? What does not? What is hard or difficult about your treatments? What makes them easier to manage?).
- Develop flexible treatment recommendations and prescriptions that individualize treatment regimens for children of different ages.
- Recognize that *improvement* rather than *perfection* in adherence to treatment-related goals is a primary goal.
- Conduct routine assessments of adherence to treatment and use these data to guide in clinical management.

Enhancing Monitoring of Adherence to Treatment

- Present the need to monitor to patients and family adherence as a routine aspect of care.
- Reframe the monitoring of adherence so that children and families experience this as encouraging their participation in their illness management.
- Do not use information from assessments to catch patients and/or families at being noncompliant with treatment.
- Make a concerted effort to facilitate children's and families' understanding and utilization of measures of adherence to chronic illness treatment.
- Give children and family members the option of whether they want to use assessments, procedures, and devices to monitor their adherence to treatment.
- Obtain feedback from patients and families concerning whether assessments to monitor their treatment adherence were helpful.

TABLE 20.7
Recommendations to Enhance Research Concerning Clinical Management
of Treatment Adherence

- Translate information from descriptive studies of risk factors to design studies of effectiveness of interventions to promote chronic illness management and adherence to treatment in clinical settings.
- Assess the economic costs and benefits of adherence promotion interventions, including behavioral interventions.
- Identify the working models that children and families use to make decisions about adherence to chronic illness treatment.
- Develop and evaluate strategies for intervention that identify and intervene with specific risk factors for noncompliance with chronic illness treatment.
- Evaluate the impact of updates of prescribed treatments in response to developmental changes and changes in the child's health status.
- Evaluate the role of technology (e.g., computerized adherence promotion methods) in helping children and families develop self-management skills to enhance adherence to chronic illness treatment.
- Develop strategies to make adherence a desired or challenging goal for children and adolescents.
- Evaluate the impact of methods to improve the quality and salience of treatment and adherence-related information given to children and parents.

TABLE 20.8
Recommendations for Research Concerning Provider Education
in Adherence Promotion in Childhood Chronic Illness

- Develop and evaluate training programs that help physicians learn how to promote adherence to treatment in childhood chronic illness, identify the signs of problems with adherence, and refer children and families for interventions.
- Develop and evaluate models of patient-centered communication and support that teach physicians to manage chronic illness in children.
- Develop and evaluate educational programs to enhance culturally sensitive communication with children with chronic illness and their families.

Designing Methods to Help Patients Take the Initiative in Monitoring and Managing Their Treatment Adherence

Conference participants identified the need to develop methods to enhance child and parental perceptions of how to monitor and improve their adherence to treatment and health outcomes. Another need that was identified was for patient education interventions to focus on helping children and families use information concerning chronic illness treatment in specific clinical situations. In many settings, patients and their families may not be given sufficient instruction in the specific skills, including the problem-solving skills necessary to facilitate adherence to treatment in a range of situations (Farber, Johnson, & Boekerman, 1998; Live et al., 1997).

Incorporating Behavior in Comprehensive Models of Treatment Adherence

Many conference participants were interested in how behavioral and/or psychological factors can best be integrated into medical care to promote optimal adherence to chronic illness treatment. In this regard, some commented on the fact that biological diagnostic and intervention procedures are generally reimbursed at a higher level than behavioral interventions despite that biological procedures are more expensive but are not necessarily more effective than behavioral interventions. This practice may reflect the larger problem of a *biology bias*, defined as a nonempirically based preference for biological as opposed to behavioral methods in research and clinical care. This bias may limit the financial resources allocated for behavioral as opposed to biological or medical interventions by managed care and by government agencies for research. Some participants felt that this bias should be recognized and countered by scientific data. For example, behavioral interventions that promote adherence have the potential of being cost-effective by preventing additional clinic visits and hospitalizations. Consequently, research should focus on documenting the various costs and benefits of providing behavioral interventions that lead to better treatment compliance with chronic illness. Moreover, future research also needs to document how problematic or inefficient patient–physician communication may result in unnecessary utilization of services and hence unnecessary costs.

Extending the Utility of Assessment of Adherence to Chronic Illness Treatment to Clinical Practice

Conference participants addressed the question of how best to implement routine assessments of adherence to chronic illness treatment in clinical practice situations. The lack of direct correspondence among treatment adherence, clinical symptoms, and health status among children with chronic conditions (Johnson, 1992) suggests that it is important for treatment teams to conduct independent assessments of treatment-related behaviors to identify potential adherence problems and prevent them. In this regard, conference participants also recognized the importance of early identification of adherence problems through sequential assessment of adherence behaviors during different illness phases and developmental stages. They also suggested that detailed assessment of individual patterns of adherence to treatment could be used to profile individual risks and identify potential targets of intervention—and hence may also help promote more effective communication with physicians.

There was also recognition that routine assessment of adherence to chronic illness treatment in clinical practice settings is rarely conducted. In many settings, adherence to chronic illness is assessed in response to a significant problem or crisis. Moreover, such assessments of problematic adherence to chronic illness treatment are difficult to conduct. For example, such assessment can involve superficial and potentially accusatory questions such as, "You are taking your medication, aren't you?" To facilitate the more effective assessment of adherence to treatment in clinical practice, conference participants identified the need to develop valid and clinically relevant measures to assess patients' reasons for not taking medications and barriers to adherence that can be used in practice situations.

Targeting Interventions to Promote Adherence

Conference participants identified the need to develop and evaluate interventions that target selected individuals and/or families for specific interventions concerning adherence promotion, as well as those that identify and target individual and family-specific barriers to treatment adherence. Available data suggest that current patterns of clinical care—the majority of clinical interventions provided by psychologists, social workers, and clinical psychologists—are provided to children and adolescents judged as having compliance problems that are significantly interfering with their medical care (Olson et al., 1989). However, it is not clear whether clinical interventions that are provided in practice are actually successful at reducing serious compliance problems. In addition to developing empirically validated interventions for serious compliance problems, there may be some benefit in targeting children who are at risk for adherence problems (see Rapoff, chap. 14, this volume).

Some conference participants noted that variables such as the quality of family allocation of responsibilities for children's chronic illness treatment, communication, and support (Anderson, Miller, Auslander, & Santiago, 1981; Hauser et al., 1990; Hanson et al., 1987) should be considered in targeting interventions to promote adherence to treatment in chronic illness. For example, premature parental withdrawal of control and monitoring of their child's treatment prematurely (e.g., during early adolescence) may contribute to subsequent adherence problems (Anderson et al., 1990). However, parents who remain so involved in their children's chronic illness treatment that they are seen as intrusive by their children may engender significant levels of family distress and conflict even if the children's adherence to treatment improves (Anderson & Coyne, 1991).

REFERENCES

Anderson, B. J., Auslander, W. F., Jung, K. C., Miller, J. P., & Santiago, J. V. (1990). Assessing family sharing of diabetes responsibilities. *Journal of Pediatric Psychology, 15,* 47–49.

Anderson, B. J., & Coyne, J. C. (1991). "Miscarried helping" in the families of children and adolescents with chronic diseases. In J. H. Johnson & L. S. B. Johnson (Eds.), *Advances in child health psychology* (pp. 167–177). Gainesville, FL: University of Florida Press.

Anderson, B. J., Miller, J. P., Auslander, W. F., & Santiago, J. (1981). Family characteristics of diabetic adolescents: Relationship to metabolic control. *Diabetes Care, 4,* 586–594.

Anderson, B. J., Wolf, F. M., Burkhart, M. T., Cornell, R. G., & Bacon, G. E. (1989). Effects of peer-group intervention on metabolic control of adolescents with IDDM: Randomized outpatient study. *Diabetes Care, 3,* 179–183.

Becker, M. H., Drachman, R. H., & Kirscht, J. P. (1972). Predicting mothers' compliance with pediatric medical regimen. *Journal of Pediatrics, 81,* 843–854.

Bond, G. G., Aiken, L. S., & Somerville, S. C. (1992). The health belief model and adolescents with insulin-dependent diabetes mellitus. *Health Psychology, 11,* 190–198.

Brownlee-Duffeck, M., Peterson, L., Simonds, J. F., Goldstein, D., Kilo, C., & Hoette, S. (1987). The role of health beliefs in the regimen adherence and metabolic control of adolescents and adults with diabetes mellitus. *Journal of Consulting and Clinical Psychology, 55,* 139–144.

Creer, T. L., Levstek, D., & Reynolds, R. V. C. (1994). History and evaluation. In H. Kotses & A. Harver (Eds.), *Self-management of asthma* (pp. 379–405). New York: Marcel Dekker.

Deaton, A. V. (1985). Adaptive noncompliance in pediatric asthma: The parent as expert. *Journal of Pediatric Psychology, 10,* 1–14.

Diabetes Control and Complications Trial Research Group. (1993). The effect of intensive treatment of diabetes on the development and progression of long-term complications in insulin-dependent diabetes mellitus. *New England Journal of Medicine, 329,* 977–986.

Donovan, J. L., & Blake, D. R. (1992). Patient non-compliance. Deviance or reasoned decision making? *Social Science and Medicine, 34,* 507–513.

Epstein, L. H., Beck, S., Figueroa, I., Farkas, G., Kazdin, A. E., Daneman, D., & Becker, D. (1981). The effects of targeting improvements in urine glucose on metabolic control in children with insulin dependent diabetes. *Journal of Applied Behavior Analysis, 14,* 365–375.

Farber, H. J., Johnson, C., & Boekerman, R. C. (1998). Younger inner-city children visited in the emergency room for asthma: Risk practice and chronic care behaviors. *Journal of Asthma, 35,* 547–552.

Francis, V., Korsch, B. M., & Morris, M. J. (1969). Gaps in doctor–patient communication: Patients' response to medical advice. *New England Journal of Medicine, 280,* 535–540.

Freund, A., Johnson, S. B., Silverstein, J., & Thomas, J. (1991. Assessing daily management of childhood diabetes using 24-hour recall interviews: Reliability and stability. *Health Psychology 10,* 200–208.

Friedman, I. M., Litt, I. F., King, D. R., Henson, R., Holtzman, D., Halverson, D., & Kraemer, H. C. (1986). Compliance with anticonvulsant therapy by epileptic youth. *Journal of Adolescent Health Care, 7,* 12–17.

Golden, M. D., Herold, A. J., & Orr, D. P. (1985). An approach to prevent recurrent diabetic ketoacidosis in the pediatric population. *Journal of Pediatrics, 93,* 195–200.

Greenman, C. (1998, May 28). Network helps children cope with serious illness. *New York Times,* pp. D6–D7.

Hanson, C. L. (1992). Developing systematic models of the adaptation of youths with diabetes. In A. M. La Greca, L. J. Siegel, J. L. Wallander, & C. E. Walker (Eds.), *Stress and coping in child health* (pp. 212–241). New York: Guilford.

Hanson, C. L., Henggeler, S. W., & Burghen, G. A. (1987). Social competence and parental support as mediators of the link between stress and metabolic control in adolescents with insulin-dependent diabetes mellitus. *Journal of Consulting and Clinical Psychology*, *55*, 529–533.

Hauser, S. T., Jacobson, A. M., Lavori, P., Wolfsdorf, J. I., Herskowitz, R. D., Milley, J. E., Bliss, R., Wertlieb, D., & Stein, J., (1990). Adherence among children and adolescents with insulin-dependent diabetes mellitus over a four-year longitudinal follow-up: II. Immediate and long-term linkages with the family milieu. *Journal of Pediatric Psychology*, *15*, 527–542.

Jacobson, A. M., Hauser, S. T., Lavori, P., Wolfsdorf, J. I., Herskowitz, R. D., Milley, J. E., Bliss, R., Gelfand, E., Wertlieb, D., & Stein, J. (1990). Adherence among children and adolescents with insulin-dependent diabetes mellitus over a four-year longitudinal follow-up: I. Influence of patient coping and adjustment. *Journal of Pediatric Psychology*, *15*, 511–526.

Johnson, S. B. (1992). Methodological issues in diabetes research: Measuring adherence. *Diabetes Care*, *15*, 1658–1667.

Johnson, S. B., Silverstein, J., Rosenbloom, A., Carter, R., & Cunningham, W. (1986). Assessing daily management of childhood diabetes. *Health Psychology*, *5*, 545–564.

Kaplan, S H., Greenfield, S., & Ware, J. E. (1989). Assessing the effects of physician–patient interactions on the outcomes of chronic disease. *Medical Care*, *27*(Suppl.), 5110–5127.

Kleinman, A. (1980). *Patients and healers in the context of cultures*. Berkeley, CA: University of California Press.

Koocher, G. P., McGrath, M. L., & Dudas, L. J. (1990). Typologies of nonadherence in cystic fibrosis. *Journal of Developmental and Behavioral Pediatrics*, *11*, 353–358.

Kovacs, M., Goldston, D., Obrosky, D. S., & Iyengar, S. (1992). Prevalence and predictors of pervasive noncompliance with medical treatment among youths with insulin-dependent diabetes mellitus. *Journal of the American Academy of Child and Adolescent Psychiatry*, *31*, 1112–1119.

La Greca, A. M. (1990a). Issues in adherence with pediatric regimens. *Journal of Pediatric Psychology*, *15*, 285–308.

La Greca, A. M. (1990b). Social consequences of pediatric conditions: Fertile area for future investigation and intervention? *Journal of Pediatric Psychology*, *15*, 285–308.

La Greca, A. M., & Schuman, W. B. (1995). Adherence to prescribed treatment regimens. In M. C. Roberts (Ed.), *Handbook of pediatric psychology* (2nd ed., pp. 55–83). New York: Guilford.

Live, J. A., Quesenberry, C. P., Capra, A. M., Sorel, M. E., Martin, R. E., & Mendoza, G. R. (1997). Outpatient management practice associated with reduced risk of pediatric asthma hospitalization and emergency department visits. *Pediatrics*, *100*, 334–381.

Olson, R. A., Holden, E. W., Friedman, A., Faust, J., Kenning, M., & Mason, P. J. (1989). Psychological consultation in a children's hospital. An evaluation of services. *Journal of Pediatric Psychology*, *13*, 479–482.

Quittner, A. L., DiGirolamo, A. M., Michel, M., & Eigen, H. (1992). Parental response to CF: A contextual analysis of the diagnosis phase. *Journal of Pediatric Psychology*, *17*, 683–704.

Quittner, A. L., Opipari, L. C., Regoli, M. J., Jacobsen, J., & Eigen, H. (1992). The impact of caregiving and role strain on family life: Comparisons between mothers of children with cystic fibrosis and matched controls. *Rehabilitation Psychology*, *37*, 275–290.

Rapoff, M. A. (1999). *Adherence to pediatric treatment regimens*. New York: Kluwer Academic/Plenum.

Riekert, K. A., & Drotar, D. (1999). Who participates in research on adherence to treatment in insulin-dependent diabetes mellitus? Implications and recommendations for research. *Journal of Pediatric Psychology*, *24*, 253–258.

Author Index

Subject Index

21864931R00307

Printed in Poland
by Amazon Fulfillment
Poland Sp. z o.o., Wrocław